DIAGNOSTIC METHODS
IN
SPEECH PATHOLOGY

DIAGNOSTIC METHODS
in SPEECH PATHOLOGY

WENDELL JOHNSON, ph.D.
Professor of Speech Pathology and Psychology
University of Iowa

FREDERIC L. DARLEY, ph.D.
Consultant in Speech Pathology, Mayo Clinic
Associate Professor of Speech Pathology, Mayo Foundation

D. C. SPRIESTERSBACH, ph.D.
Professor of Speech Pathology
Department of Speech Pathology and Audiology
Department of Otolaryngology and Maxillofacial Surgery
University of Iowa

HARPER & ROW, PUBLISHERS
NEW YORK, EVANSTON, AND LONDON

CONTENTS

FORMS

FOREWORD

This book is designed as a handbook for speech clinicians and for students in courses concerned with the diagnostic aspects of speech pathology. It opens with a consideration of the philosophy of diagnosis and appraisal, and this is followed by a discussion of principles and techniques of case study interviewing. A general case history outline is presented along with supplementary outlines for cases of cerebral palsy, cleft palate, dysphasia (aphasia), laryngectomy, and stuttering. Subsequent chapters include functional descriptions of basic speech, voice, and language examination procedures, test materials and clinical forms, tables of norms, and statements of principles and specific suggestions regarding the reporting of findings of case examinations. Substantial background information, including reviews of research data, provides a basis for the discriminating use of the various procedures and interpretation of examination findings. Attention is given to the speech pathologist's patterns of interprofessional relationships, and to principles of referral for audiological, psychological, and medical evaluation.

A forerunner of this book was the authors' *Diagnostic Manual in Speech Correction* (Harper & Brothers, 1952). The present book, while similar in purpose, differs greatly in reflecting the advances made in clinical speech pathology during the past ten years. Although new procedures or refinements and elaborations of old ones are to be found in all chapters, recent developments are to be noted particularly in Chapter 4, "Testing Articulation," Chapter 7, "Appraisal of Language Development and Language Disorders," Chapter 8, "Measurement of Amount of Speaking and of the Rate and Disfluency of Speaking and Oral Reading," and Chapter 9, "The Problem of Stuttering." Substantial extensions and refinements of procedure are to be found also in Chapter 3, "General Speech Behavior Evaluation," Chapter 5, "The Speech Mechanism," and Chapter 6, "Examination of Voice Quality Disorders." Chapter 10, "Supplementary Diagnostic Procedures and Referral Principles," consists in large measure of new material.

Although the three authors worked together on the whole book, the division of labor reflects their respective areas of specialization, Darley drafted Chapters 1, 2, 4, 7; Spriestersbach Chapters 3, 5, 6. Darley and Johnson wrote Chapter 11. Johnson wrote Chapters 8, 9, and 10, and as editor prepared the final draft of the manuscript.

Drs. James Hardy, Evan Jordan, Kenneth Moll, Hugh Morris, William Prather, Margaret Stoicheff, and Dean Williams read and made helpful evaluations of various parts of the manuscript. Spencer F. Brown, M.D., Ph.D., commented on the section in Chapter 10 entitled "Referral for Medical Evaluation." Dr. Guy Whitehead, member of the Publications Section, Mayo Clinic, provided editorial assistance with Chapters 1, 2, 6, 7, and 11. Without in any degree committing them to endorsement of statements made in this book, or to responsibility for such error as it may reflect, we are pleased to express our gratitude for the assistance of these colleagues and friends.

Mrs. Varena Wade, with assists from Miss Margaret Seemuth, Mrs. Margaret Bloom, Mrs. Maryann Crew, Miss Joanne McGuire, and Mrs. Frances Niichel, typed the several drafts of the manuscript, and assisted with proofreading, preparing the index, and the many other tasks involved in getting the book from rough draft to bound volume. Miss Lousene Rousseau, Mrs. Georgette Preston, and their associates at Harper & Row were, as always, patient and extraordinarily helpful. Many others have contributed in their respective ways, as students and colleagues, to the making of this book. To all of these we express our warm thanks. They are not, of course, to be held accountable for any of the book's imperfections.

We are pleased to express appreciation for permission to reproduce or adapt material from the following:

1. The University of Minnesota Press
     Davis, Edith A., *The Development of Linguistic Skill in Twins, Singletons with Siblings, and Only Children from Age Five to Ten Years*
     McCarthy, Dorothea A., *The Language Development of the Preschool Child*

Templin, Mildred C., *Certain Language Skills in Children*
Johnson, Wendell, *et al.*, *The Onset of Stuttering*
Johnson, Wendell (ed., with assistance of R. Leutenegger), *Stuttering in Children and Adults*
2. Harper & Row, Publishers, Inc.
Louttit, C. M., *Clinical Psychology*
Fairbanks, G. F., Voice and Articulation Drillbook, 1940
Johnson, Wendell, *People in Quandaries*
Johnson, Wendell, Frederic L. Darley, and D. C. Spriestersbach, *Diagnostic Manual in Speech Correction*
3. University of Iowa, Department of Publications
Scoe, Hjalmar F., *Bladder Control in Infancy and Early Childhood*, University of Iowa Studies in Child Welfare, Vol. 5, No. 4
Templin, Mildred C., and Frederic L. Darley, *The Templin-Darley Tests of Articulation*, University of Iowa, Bureau of Educational Research and Service, Extension Division, 1960.
Wellman, Beth L., Ida Mae Case, Ida G. Mengert, and Dorothy E. Bradbury, *Speech Sounds of Young Children*, University of Iowa Studies in Child Welfare, Vol. 5, No. 2
4. Indiana University, Institute for Sex Research
Kinsey, A. C., W. B. Pomeroy, and C. E. Martin, *Sexual Behavior in the Human Male*, Philadelphia: W. B. Saunders Company, 1948
5. John Wiley & Sons, Inc.
Manual of Child Psychology, Carmichael, L. (ed.)
6. American Speech and Hearing Association
Monograph Supplement 7 of the *Journal of Speech and Hearing Disorders*
Ammons, R., and W. Johnson, "The construction and application of a test of attitude toward stuttering," *Journal of Speech Disorders*, 9, 1944, 39-49.
Bloodstein, Oliver, "The relationship between oral reading rate and severity of stuttering," *Journal of Speech Disorders*, 9, 1944, 161-173
Darley, F. L., and H. Winitz, "Age of first word: review of research," *Journal of Speech and Hearing Disorders*, 26, 1961, 272-290
Tate, Merle W., Walter L. Cullinan, and Ann Ahlstrand, "Measurement of adaptation in stuttering," *Journal of Speech and Hearing Research*, 4, 1961, 321-339.
7. National Society for Crippled Children and Adults, Inc.
Westlake, H., "A system for developing speech with cerebral palsied children," *The Crippled Child Magazine*, 29, 1951, 10-11
8. Holt, Rinehart, and Winston, Inc.
Goodenough, Florence, *Mental Testing*
9. C. V. Mosby Co.
Sandler, H. C., "The eruption of deciduous teeth," *Journal of Pediatrics*, 25, 1944, 140
10. The Journal Press
Anderson, John E., "The limitations of infant and preschool tests in

the measurement of intelligence," *Journal of Psychology*, 8, 1939, p. 376

Smith, Madorah E., "A study of some factors influencing the development of the sentence in preschool children," *Pedagogical Seminary and Journal of Genetic Psychology*, 46, 1935, 182-211

Smith, Mary K., "Measurement of the size of general English vocabulary through the elementary grades and high school," *Genetic Psychology Monographs*, 24, 1941, 311-345

11. Speech Association of America

Travis, L. E., "A point of view in speech correction," *Quarterly Journal of Speech*, 22, 1936, 57-61

12. National Education Association

Davis, Irene P., "The speech aspects of reading readiness," *17th Yearbook of the Department of Elementary School Principals*, NEA, Vol. 17, No. 7, 282-289

13. Abrahams Magazine Service, Inc.

Terman, L. M. and A. Hocking, "The sleep of school children, its distribution according to age and its relation to mental and physical efficiency," *Journal of Educational Psychology*, 4, 1913, 138-147

Johnson, W. and D. Duke, "The dextrality quotients of fifty six-year-olds with regard to hand usage," *Journal of Educational Psychology*, 1936, Vol. 27, 26-36

14. Oberlin College, Publications Department

Stetson, R. H., *Motor Phonetics*, Amsterdam: North-Holland Publishing Co.

15. *Journal of Dentistry for Children*

Hurme, V. O., "Ranges of normalcy in the eruption of permanent teeth," *Journal of Dentistry for Children*, 16, 1949, 11-15

16. American Psychological Association

Irwin, Orvis C., and Han Piao Chen, "Development of speech during infancy: curve of phonemic types," *Journal of Experimental Psychology*, 36, 1946, 431-436

Irwin, Orvis C., "Development of speech during infancy: curve of phonemic frequencies," *Journal of Experimental Psychology*, 37, 1947, 187-193

Malone, A. J., and M. Masseler, "Index of nail biting in children," *Journal of Abnormal and Social Psychology*, 47, 1952, 193-202

17. *Resident Psysician*

Long, P. H., "Editor's Page: On the history and physical examination of the patient," *Resident Psysician*, 7, 1961, 59-62

18. Humanities Press, Inc.

Piaget, Jean, *The Language and Thought of the Child*, New York: Meridian Books (paperback edition), 1955

19. W. Lloyd Warner

Warner, W. Lloyd, M. Meeker and K. Eells, *Social Class in America*, Chicago: Science Research Associates, 1949.

Throughout the text numbers in parentheses refer to sources listed as References at the ends of chapters.

Forms 1-20 may be obtained from the Interstate Printers and Publishers, Inc., 19-27 North Jackson Avenue, Danville, Illinois.

Chapter 5 and certain other parts of this book are concerned in some measure with diagnostic procedures influenced by studies carried out under Grant M 1158 of the National Institute of Mental Health and Grant D 853 of the National Institute of Dental Research. Chapters 8 and 9 reflect in substantial measure the findings of research supported by the Louis W. and Maud Hill Family Foundation and by Grant RD 319 of the Office of Vocational Rehabilitation of the Department of Health, Education, and Welfare of the United States Government.

We are again, as always, particularly grateful to the three co-authors whose first names do not appear on the title page, but whose imprints are to be seen by the knowing on all the other pages of this book.

WENDELL JOHNSON
FREDERIC L. DARLEY
D. C. SPRIESTERSBACH

Iowa City, Iowa
Rochester, Minnesota
October, 1962

DIAGNOSTIC METHODS
IN
SPEECH PATHOLOGY

1 A PHILOSOPHY OF DIAGNOSIS AND APPRAISAL

DEFINITION

The speech clinician seeks to describe adequately any communication problem with which he deals in order to distinguish it from other problems that it may resemble and to determine its distinctive character. He undertakes, that is, to diagnose the problem by making an appropriate examination. On the basis of his findings and his interpretation of them, he proposes a remedial program and attempts to predict its outcome. In carrying out these basic responsibilities he goes through the following steps:

1. He obtains adequate information about the speaker's past development and status. The clinician is interested in finding out how the person came to be what he is today. He is especially interested in the onset of the speech problem. He secures the desired information in a number of ways and from a variety of informants, making use especially of the case history interview (see Chapter 2).

2. The clinician obtains a comprehensive and detailed description of the speaker's problem and of related aspects of his present status. In order to do this he makes considerable use of relevant interview techniques, but he relies also on a variety of tests and observational

1

procedures for identifying and measuring relevant aspects of speech and related behavior.

3. From study of the information gathered, the clinician makes a tentative determination of the causes of the problem. He considers possible hypotheses regarding the conditions and circumstances that could have served to precipitate and maintain it. As he weighs the data, he discards some hypotheses, and retains others for further testing.

4. He uses the facts obtained and the hypotheses drawn from them to formulate an appropriate remedial program.

5. Finally, he attempts a prognosis; that is, given the problem as he sees it with the causes as he understands them, he predicts as best he can the effects of the proposed remedial measures on the future course of the disorder.

You may ask, "When is a diagnosis completed?" or a related question, "Does diagnosis always precede treatment?" For obvious reasons a diagnostic work-up typically precedes remedial steps, which in speech pathology are usually called "therapy." The clinician wants to know with what he is dealing and to have a rationale for doing what he does about it. Nevertheless, it should be understood that there is no absolute division between diagnosis and therapy. Just as the diagnostic procedures employed may have therapeutic effects, so the treatment itself can be diagnostic. In a given case the descriptions of the past and present status may not adequately clarify the causes. Therefore, the clinician prescribes a tentative course of treatment and withholds his diagnosis pending further observation. In speech pathology, as in other "helping professions," it may be necessary for the clinician to embark upon some well-structured experiments in order to arrive at a clear understanding of the nature and scope of the problem with which he is dealing. Furthermore, he may continue to do much of what is called diagnostic, at least at intervals, throughout the period of the activities ordinarily called therapy. Diagnosis is seldom, if ever, completed at one sitting, never to be reviewed. The clinician should continue the critical thinking implied by the term so long as he has any responsibility for the problem.

Although the terms appraisal and diagnosis are often used together, they are not synonymous. When a clinician specifies the presenting aspects of a problem and says something about their relative severity, he is appraising the problem. This appraisal may be an integral part of a diagnostic work-up, or it may be something done by the clinician from time to time in order to chart progress or perhaps to form a basis for prognostic judgments. Appraisal is represented in the second of the five steps presented above. It is not to be thought of as the complete diagnostic process, for in diagnosis the clinician evaluates the description of present status—the appraisal—in the light of what the case history tells him about the past status. He does this with the goal of reaching a conclusion about the characteristics of the person himself or of his environment that may be responsible for the occurrence and continuation of the disorder. Having reached a conclusion regarding etiology, the clinician proceeds to formulate therapy and to make a prognosis, thereby fulfilling—at least for the first round—the responsibility he has undertaken.

The activities involved in diagnosis and appraisal demand critical thinking. A speech clinician is committed to the thoughtful—not perfunctory—application of well-understood and well-practiced methods. He is committed to a thoughtful analysis of the data secured by means of these methods in the endeavor to piece together a coherent picture, to resolve apparent contradictions. He is committed to the thoughtful planning of therapy. This manual is concerned with communicating to students-in-training, working speech clinicians, and other interested readers information basic to the clinical skills necessary for thorough and accurate appraisal and diagnosis in speech pathology.

THE CLINICIAN AS OBSERVER AND REPORTER

The speech clinician is a special kind of observer. As he gathers data by taking case histories and administering tests, he must interact efficiently with his informants and his clients—or patients or students, as he may prefer to refer to them, in accordance with the kind of setting in which he works. His ear must be attuned to detect clinically significant aspects of voice, speech, and language behavior. He must be sensitive to the feelings of those whom he seeks to help and be alert to their subtle as well as obvious expressions of puzzlement, concern, hostility, inquiry, superstition, trust, misgiving, guilt, anxiety, and other relevant feelings. Having made and used his observations, he is responsible for communicating what he has learned to others—judiciously, ethically, in good time, and as required. He is frequently called upon in staffings, clinical conferences, official reports, and in other ways to share his knowledge and his opinions through writing or speaking.

Ideally the clinician should observe impartially, precisely, and reliably. He should observe *enough*, and he should do it by techniques that will permit his information to be compared satisfactorily with that obtained by other observers. It is important that he distinguish between what he observes and what he concludes from his observations. He must distinguish, in other words, between fact and inference. It is not easy to make this kind of distinction and to communicate the results of observation with appropriate objectivity. Without our even recognizing what is happening, our own interests, personal biases, and convictions distort our perceptions, our conclusions, and our reports. We filter all of our sensations through personal filters; and as we report, the filtering process goes on.

It should be the clinician's constant goal to be as objective as possible and to acknowledge and reduce as much as he can the distorting elements in his observations and reports. One of the purposes of this handbook is to help the clinician and the clinician-in-training to minimize distorting personal projections by learning to use certain diagnostic tools designed for precise, detailed, objective, reliable observation.

How can the clinician reduce the undesirable effects of subjectivity in his observations? One helpful way is to recognize the difference between two-valued systems (dichotomies) and multi-valued systems (continua). He can learn early, for example, that children are not either clean or dirty, either bright or backward, either attractive or homely. After he has become acquainted with a number of children, he finds that they vary along the continuum of cleanliness—or of brightness or attractiveness—from "not so very" to "rather" to "quite." As he extends his observations, he discovers that the members of a species practically never can be satisfactorily locked into categories but are dealt with most appropriately by recognizing the subtle differences among them and seeing that they are distributed over an infinite number of degrees of variation.

It is also helpful to the clinician to carry this practice one step further and make use of scaling procedures in comparing individuals with regard to specified characteristics. He finds it useful to get into the habit of assigning numerical values to the extremes of the continua, or graduated scales, that he is dealing with and of thinking about the points along the continua as being equally spaced in the degrees of variation they represent. He finds it useful to think of a five-point scale of hypernasality, for example, or a nine-point scale of severity of stuttering, or other kinds of scales such as "much more than average," "somewhat more than average," "about average," "somewhat less than average," and "much less than average."

Once in the habit of thinking quantitatively and using scaling procedures to nail down his judgment, he becomes sensitive to the need to check his observations and his ratings against his own repeated judgment and against the judgment of others. In other words, he becomes concerned with the *reliability* and *validity* of his observations and judgments. He wants to know how well he agrees with himself on repeated applications of the same test or on repeated judgments of the same behavior. Not only is he interested in his agreement with himself, which is technically referred to as intra-observer reliability, but he is also concerned with how well his judgments agree with those of other equally or more competent observers (inter-observer reliability). And he asks whether the yardstick he is using really measures what it purports to measure. He casts about for outside criteria against which he can measure the effectiveness of his observations and of the tools he is using.

Increasingly the clinician becomes impressed with the need for compiling empirical data, that is, facts derived from experience or experiment, facts that arise from observation. And he learns the necessity of keeping his interpretation of these empirical data quite distinct from the data themselves. More and more the clinician learns to distrust his hunches and intuitive procedures which, because they cannot be communicated to others effectively, cannot, therefore, be adequately subjected to checking and rechecking. Although at times he necessarily relies upon a clinical "hunch" or a clinical impression, he feels duly restrained in drawing conclusions until he is able to check them against the observations of someone else or against his own further data.

Not only does the clinician seek to develop precision, objectivity, and reliability in making observations, but he also attempts to make them comprehensively and in as much detail as possible. The more complex the problem the greater the clinician's need for information about the speaker's past and present status—and no speech disorder can be called simple after thorough scrutiny. In even the simplest case, no one-to-one relationship is found between the speech problem in its entirety and any single causal factor. We have long known, for example, that a description of dentition is by no means adequate in all cases to account for a distorted [s], or that the severity of a client's voice or articulation problem does not parallel exactly the degree to which his cerebral palsy has impaired his motor system.

More than superficial observation is necessary. The clinician has not completed his task when he has noted that a tooth is missing, that a parent is thoughtless and impatient, that a home is broken, that the child has a bilateral hearing loss, or that he cannot get a word in edgewise at home. We are enamored of drawing arrows relating cause to effect, but often we draw too few of them and thereby oversimplify the relationships.

In considering how comprehensive our observations about individuals should be, let us consider an analogy. Do you recall the fable about the six blind men confronted by an elephant for the first time? The one who felt only the trunk visualized the elephant as a snake; the one who felt only a tusk imagined the animal to be shaped like a spear; the one who grasped the ear identified the elephant with a palm leaf; the one who felt of his side pictured him as a stone wall; the massive hind leg suggested to one the dimensions of a tree trunk; and the sixth, upon grasping the tail, identified the elephant as a rope.

In clinical practice, you need to beware of making the mistake of the six blind men. From fragmentary information, considered out of context and without proper perspective, you are likely to draw faulty inferences and reach wrong conclusions.

An elementalistic view—the isolating of a single element in a complex situation and regarding it as sole cause—will not suffice. The speech correctionist, as Cable (*3*) reminds us, must be nonelementalistic and "see the relationships and connections among all things." To oversimplify is to lose something that is needed. Travis (*15*) has directed our attention beyond the speech impairment to the speaker: "A speech disorder is a disorder of the person as well as a disorder in the movements of the speech organs. It is not enough to know what sort of speech defect a person has. In addition, one should know what kind of person has a speech defect. The speech defect has no particular meaning apart from the person who presents the defect."

And it is plain, as Travis (*15*) further suggests, that "every individual is the resultant of the interaction between his original endowment and the environment into which he is thrust." Hence the speech clinician must understand something about the influences that have helped to make the speaker become the person he now is.

If the description of the individual, then, is to be helpful, it must be comprehensive. And the description should make clear the important relationships. The several groups of clinically relevant data and their interrelationships may be formulated diagrammatically in such a way as Johnson has shown in *People in Quandaries* (*9*, p. 411).

Johnson explains the formulation thus:

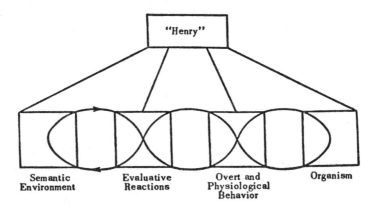

[Fig. A.] Diagram of interrelationships among groups of factors to be taken into account in personality retraining. (From Wendell Johnson, *People in Quandaries*, Harper & Brothers, 1946, p. 411).

In this diagram four general groups of factors are represented, and each is shown as interrelated with all the others. . . . We may regard the four factors as four general kinds of observations that can be made of "Henry" —that is, of any individual. Or for certain purposes we may regard them as four ways of talking about "Henry"—four special languages, as it were. The point of including "Henry" in the diagram is to emphasize that any one factor or point of view represented is partial and incomplete, and that all four, at least, are required for anything resembling a relatively full account. . . .

By *semantic environment* is meant the individual's environment of attitudes, beliefs, assumptions, values, ideals, standards, customs, knowledge, interests, conventions, institutions, etc. . . . It is to be understood that beyond a person's immediate semantic environment is that more extensive environment that we call his culture, the larger social order in which he lives, and in which his parents and teachers live too. . . .

Evaluative reactions include the individual's own attitudes, beliefs, assumptions, values, ideals, etc. Taken all together, they may be regarded as that part of his semantic environment which the individual has interiorized, or adopted. . . .

Under the heading of *overt and physiological behavior* we include generally what the person does—his predominantly nonverbal behavior. . . .

By *organism* is meant not a static unchanging organic structure, but the relatively invariant relationships involved in the processes of growth and deterioration. In the living organism there is no fine line between "physiology" and "anatomy." Roughly speaking, by physiological behavior we mean those bodily changes that can be observed from moment to moment; by the organism we mean those bodily characteristics which change so slowly that from one day, or week, or month, to the next they seem to remain constant (*9*, pp. 411-413).

The clinician extends his observations into all of these matters as far as necessary for clear understanding and reflects in his report as much detail as the reader or the listener can use effectively.

Consider a cerebral palsied child who is brought to the clinic for examination. He is 3½ years of age, but on the Vineland Social Maturity Scale he earns a social age of only 1 year, 9 months. He wears a brace on one foot, and although he moves about fairly well, he is somewhat restricted by his parents in his explorations and in his attempts to show off his physical prowess. He does a great deal of gesturing, but he is using few understandable words. His parents love him and spend some time romping with him, but they have spent little time reading to him or playing games with him, have not encouraged association with other children, and have done little to foster self-help. Instead they have provided a governess who looks after his every need and who protects him from all possible harm. He has never had to pull off his own socks or brush his own teeth, and he has little need to speak and ask for anything because every wish is anticipated.

In considering the cause of the speech problem, one would certainly be mistaken in referring only to impairment in the pyramidal and extrapyramidal tracts of the child's central nervous system. The adequacy of the child's speech mechanism is of interest, but so are the adequacy of the speech stimulation he has received, the need for speech which he has experienced, the reward he has received for his speech efforts, the breadth of experiences to which he has been exposed in the world around him, and the role communication plays in it. His language retardation does not have *a cause* but numerous *causes*.

It is just this point which Brown and Oliver (2) made in their report of a study of 33 cases of cleft palate. It was their purpose to look beyond the function of the palate and to consider the role of other factors in relation to the adequacy of each subject's speech. They made thorough examinations of the oral speech structures of the 33 subjects, rating each of more than 25 different activities or conditions of various structures on a three-point scale. A rating of 1 indicated that the particular condition being rated was judged to have no adverse effect on speech; a rating of 2 suggested a possible adverse effect; a rating of 3 indicated that the particular condition would almost certainly have an adverse effect on speech. They found no subject who did not have some abnormality of the speech mechanism in addition to an abnormality of palatal function itself. Eighty-two percent of the subjects had one or more of the structures rated 3. The median subject had two structures rated 3 and 12 rated 2. Even within the mouths, then, of persons with cleft palates we find multiple causes for any speech deviation we might observe, and we have also to look beyond the speaker's mouths to consider the attitudes of their families and associates, the attitudes of the speakers themselves and their intelligence, the adequacy of their hearing, the amount of speech stimulation they have had, the adequacy of their speech models, their need for speech, their reward for speech attempts, etc.

The further you go in the study of communication disorders, the more likely you are to agree that "the cause of anything is everything." You must be interested in the person who has a speech problem and also in the persons and institutions which help make him what he is and possibly keep him from becoming what he otherwise might be.

All of us do well to remind ourselves that sometimes it is very difficult to distinguish between cause and effect. In our search for the causes of problems, we may be tempted to consider as causal something that is really symptomatic of some more remote cause, and we may consider as "simply a symptom" something that can have tremendous significance as a cause of other clinically significant conditions or behavior. Consider, for example, a child with an articulatory problem who is reported to have done very little babbling as an infant. Does the commonly held view that mastery of speech sounds grows from the matrix of vocal play or babbling point to the cause of this child's articulation difficulty? Or is the lack of babbling simply one symptom of some other more important cause—perhaps a hearing loss, or general parental neglect, or parental lack of understanding of how speech develops and of the importance of the child's pleasure and reward in making sounds like those of some favorite person who loves and fondles him?

As another example, suppose that a child with a cleft palate has very poor articulation and marked hypernasality with speech almost unintelligible at times and a voice scarcely audible. What is the cause here? Have the misarticulations and the possible facial disfigurement themselves brought about personality changes which, in turn, have affected the child's speech behavior? Are the weakness of voice and unintelligibility of speech caused by structural deformities or physiological inadequacies, or rather do they result from the fact that the child has never found talking to be fun and rewarding, has found it instead to be an excruciating and punishing experience which he wishes to avoid as much as possible? Does he as a consequence shrink from speaking out so that he holds his head down, keeps his lips almost closed, and swallows his words? To what extent, that is, have such reactions become causal as well as symptomatic?

As a further illustration of the interaction and blending of cause and consequence, consider the case of a young stutterer who appears to be apprehensive about his speech disfluencies and to seek to avoid them at any cost. He has developed various mannerisms, grimaces, and contortions in his struggle to avoid the stuttering he dreads and, as he puts it, to "help the words come out." His way of speaking has become increasingly tense and his anxieties have mounted instead of subsiding. Are we confronted with symptoms here? If they are symptoms they are obviously also causes. They are ways of reacting which, in turn, make the child's behavior increasingly avoidant and disruptive of the activities essential in speaking. They magnify his unease and discourage him from speaking so that he tends to speak less. In trying to help him, therefore, you would be just as interested in attacking these symptoms as anything else you might regard as causes. Actually you would be dealing with causes in trying to manipulate what you might think of as symptoms. The fact is that the word "reaction" or "response" is in many ways a better term than "symptom" in referring to whatever a speaker does that you regard as stuttering, simply because what the speaker does is behavior. Just as the terms response and reaction are particularly suitable for talking about *behavior*, so symptom is peculiarly appropriate for describing *disease*. And we use the word "stuttering" to refer to something that seems more validly classified as a form of behavior than as a type of disease.

WHY CLASSIFY?

We have seen that the making of a diagnosis involves an investigation which leads to a description by means of which a problem may be classified. This process can be viewed narrowly as "the hanging of a label on a person." Certainly there are dangers implicit in applying diagnostic procedures too superficially and coming up with only a name or label that may serve to delimit an individual's problem too narrowly, or to refer to it too vaguely or ambiguously—or even to contribute needlessly to the aggravation, indeed the very creation, of the problem. There is always a danger in lumping together things which appear to be similar but which are by no means identical. It is hazardous to conclude that a person displays behavior which warrants assignment of a certain label and to assume, then, that certain other things must be true of that person because of the fact that he now bears the label we have given him.

A very crucial consideration is that we all tend to think of other persons and to react to them according to the ways we classify them and the names or labels we give them. Our future perceptions and judgments are influenced by the words we have used in reporting— most fatefully to ourselves as our own most affected listeners—the perceptions and judgments we have already made. In medical dictionaries you will find a dramatic word for the grave consequence of this sort of interaction between what we say and what we do. The word is "iatrogenic." An iatrogenic disorder or disease or problem is one that is caused by the physician—or clinician of any sort—by his way of talking about or to the patient and by his way of dealing with the patient generally.

Consider, for example, some of the problems involved in using the term cerebral palsy. What this term stands for generally is not a readily defined entity with a given set of characteristics invariably distinguishing it. In fact, it encompasses such dissimilar things as spasticity, athetosis, ataxia, rigidity, and tremor. These dissimilar characteristics are lumped together by the neurologist because of his understanding of certain common aspects of the neuropathologies involved: all affect the central nervous system, all occasion motor disfunctions, all involve lesions above a certain point in the central nervous system. But we cannot assume that the term cerebral palsy implies anything in particular about the speech and language behavior of a given child. It is not appropriate, therefore, to speak of cerebral palsied speech. "Stuttering" is another blanket term often inprecisely employed. As is explained in detail in Chapter 8, it is commonly used to refer ambiguously to many kinds of behavior, to many degrees and varieties of personal adjustment, to many different attitudes about

one's self, one's listeners, and the speaking situation, to various
patterns of interaction between the speaker and his listeners, and to
the problem into which all these components are woven.

There is, of course, a proper use to be made of classification in clinical speech work. Certain understandings and implications follow
from an accurate delimitation and naming of a problem. Appropriate
classification can be very useful in helping to decide what to do and to
predict the outcome of one's efforts. For example, we may take five
children severely retarded in speech. One, we shall say, is cerebral
palsied with severe involvement of the speech mechanism; one has a
severe bilateral hearing loss; one is mentally retarded to a marked
degree; one gives evidence of a profound emotional disturbance; the
fifth we find to be an emotionally disturbed, mentally retarded, cerebral palsied child with a profound bilateral hearing loss. What we do
with each of these children and how far we expect him to go in a program of remediation depend importantly upon the conclusions reached
in our diagnostic work-up. If we have been thorough and discriminating we have not merely labeled each child. We have arrived at a kind
of classification which will be useful to us in sorting the children and
assigning them to appropriate sections of our remedial program.
Because the diagnostic classification is to be followed in each case by
constructive management, an accurate and importantly distinctive
classification is essential.

THE CONCEPT OF "NORMAL"

As Johnson (9, pp. 337-342) and others have made clear, there are
several meanings of the word "normal." Johnson distinguishes the
statistical, social, medical, and legal meanings of the term from what
he refers to as the engineering or functional sense of normal, by which
he means essentially that each person has his own par. In this sense
of normal, a performance that is par for you is normal, regardless of
its relation to the average of your group, or to the mores of your
society, the laws of your land, or the standards of your physician. In
most clinical situations we make important use of a sort of combination of these various meanings in which we emphasize especially
statistical norms evaluated with due regard to each individual's personal par.

As a clinician you are, or will be, concerned with the practical evaluation of the persons whom you try to serve to the best of your ability.
When engaged in diagnostic work, for example, you will find yourself
continually making comparisons between the case at hand and other
cases you know about. You will ask questions such as: "Is this child's
behavior to be reasonably expected from a person of his age and sex

and relevant circumstances, or is it in some significant way deviant? Is this child somewhat accelerated in his acquisition of this particular skill, or does he appear to be somewhat retarded?" You will view a given child in the perspective of all the children you have known; and since your experience is always necessarily limited, you must go beyond it and build into your perspective the relevant data compiled by those who have studied many children, whom they have regarded as normal and abnormal. Without exalting mediocrity as an ideal, you must keep in mind statistical information about the average performance in groups of children, and be conscious also of ways in which individual children deviate from the central tendency of an appropriately defined group. All of this means that as a practicing clinician you need to build into your evaluative system a set of norms, compiled carefully and objectively, to which you can refer in sizing up any given child. Only by means of such norms, properly evaluated, can you understand adequately the behavior you observe and decide whether it indicates a need for remedial treatment.

In several of the following chapters, you will find relevant norms. You will want to become familiar with these and other norms and learn to use them with due discrimination. Several important questions are to be asked about any set of norms and among these are the following:

1. *What is the purpose of these norms?* As Meredith (*11*) has indicated, norms are established in different ways and serve various purposes. Some norms are simply *descriptive,* indicating the characteristics or behavior of the groups tested. The data reported tell what the groups were like but present no implicit or explicit value judgments. Most norms for height and weight, development of physical skills, development of speech sound articulation, vocabulary size, age of acquisition of bowel and bladder control, and number of hours of sleep per night tell only what the mean or median performance or characteristic is and the pattern in which subjects are distributed according to the measure applied to them. (See, for example, Table 6, Chapter 2, and Table 11, Chapter 4.) In themselves, such norms do not tell whether a given child is "tall enough," "too heavy," "abnormal," "satisfactory," or "just right."

In the field of speech pathology and audiology we have a few norms designed *for evaluation.* In these instances the descriptive norms are related to some value such as freedom from disorder, intelligibility, or some other criterion essential to the indicated classification. Only when we take the additional step of relating a statistical value to an appropriate value system can we express such judgments as "too," "abnormal," "satisfactory," or "fit." For examples of norms for evaluation, refer to Table 18, Chapter 4, or to the Social Adequacy

Index which is described by Davis and Silverman (*5*, pp. 193-194).

When norms for evaluation are wanting, you may make use of a third type, *screening norms*. These constitute an approach to norms for evaluation and help in the selection of individuals for further scrutiny. They combine descriptions of characteristics in more than one dimension, utilizing jointly two or more sets of descriptive norms in ways suggested by clinical experience. For example, Templin (*14*) used norms on a 176-item diagnostic test of articulation together with scores on a 50-item screening test of articulation in order to arrive at a set of cut-off scores which she proposed as scores separating adequate and inadequate articulation in children. Technically, these cut-off scores do not constitute norms for evaluation, as they do not relate descriptive norms to such values as "intelligibility" and "speaker acceptability." She simply used two sets of descriptive norms in a way suggested by clinical experience to derive a clinically useful screening instrument. In public school hearing surveys use is commonly made of screening tests of hearing acuity; Hirsh (*8*, pp. 278-281) presents a discussion of screening norms as used in audiometry.

2. *Is the population adequately defined?* The compiler of each set of norms has chosen a population for study, out of which he has selected a sample for specific scrutiny (see 3, below). On the basis of his study of the subjects in his sample he makes certain generalizations about the population. It is important to know just how—and especially how precisely—this population is defined. Has the compiler kept in mind all of the important variables that have some bearing upon the measurement being made?

3. *Is the population sample large enough?* How large is the sample of the population studied? Is it large enough to minimize sampling error sufficiently? Is it sufficiently representative of the population as defined?

4. *What is the nature of the data?* Are the data cross-sectional or longitudinal? In longitudinal normative studies the investigator follows a given group over a period of time, taking readings at intervals. He may study a group of children with regard to height and weight when they are 2 years old, and the same children when they are 3 years old, then 4, and again at 5. On the other hand, he may choose to study these four age levels all at once by selecting different groups of children, one group at each of the four age levels. In the latter case the data derived are cross-sectional. Both kinds of norms serve important purposes, and they are especially useful when available to supplement each other.

5. *Are the measures adequately defined?* Having selected his population sample, the investigator elicits a sample of each subject's behavior and analyzes it, using certain specified measures. How precise

is each of the measures which he has applied? What steps has the investigator taken to define each measure distinctively? Was the definition adhered to as the data were compiled? What is known about the reliability and validity of each measure?

6. *Is the behavior sample adequate?* How substantial a sample of each subject's behavior was elicited and evaluated? Was the sample large enough to allow for the deriving of stable values?

7. *In what terms are the data presented?* Are the normative data presented in units that indicate status or in units that indicate progress (increments)? For an example of data presented in terms of both units, see Table 29, Chapter 7.

8. *How comprehensive are the data?* Are measures of dispersion (ranges, standard deviations, Q-values, quartiles or deciles) presented as well as measures of central tendency (means, medians, modes)? Are separate norms provided where variables are judged to warrant such a breakdown—for example, norms for both sexes or norms for various socioeconomic levels? Are observer reliabilities and test-retest reliabilities reported?

9. *How applicable are the data?* How recently were the data collected? The passage of time can make a great difference in the interpretation and usefulness of normative information; in general, other things being equal, the more recent the norms, the better. Are extrapolation or interpolation necessary in using the norms? There are dangers in trying to extend the shapes of distributions beyond the data at hand. We prefer not to have to estimate values intermediate between known values (interpolation), and we should exercise due alertness and caution in guessing—if we feel we must guess—at values beyond those that are presented (extrapolation). Finally, we may ask whether the norms appear to be applicable to our own particular subjects and purposes.

A BASIC ANALYSIS

Communicative oral expression is a multiphasic process, involving the coordination of the following basic functions:

1. *Respiration* provides the energy—the breath—from which speech is made.

2. In *phonation* this energy sets the vocal folds into vibration, producing tones that vary in pitch, loudness, duration, and wave composition.

3. *Resonance* results in the selective amplification of these tones which gives them certain distinctive characteristics. Nasal resonance, for example, characterizes the normal production of the consonants [m], [n], and [ŋ], and occasionally an excess of nasal resonance gives a speaker's voice a distinctive quality called hypernasality. Differences

in oral resonance brought about by adjustments of the shape and size of the oral cavity serve to differentiate the vowels from each other and have some effect on voice quality.

4. In *articulation* the breath stream is interrupted or impeded in certain ways by the articulators (tongue, teeth, and lips). Incidentally, the close relationship between resonance and articulation is pointed up by the term "vowel articulation," which refers to the speech sounds called vowels that result from changes in oral resonance effected by adjustments of jaw opening, tongue position, and lip rounding or retraction.

5. In *pronunciation* the speech sounds are arranged in prescribed sequences of syllables with applications of appropriate syllabic stress.

6. Underlying speech is the *symbolization* process involving the formulation and comprehension of language and other symbolic forms. One must have symbols or symbol systems—languages—and sets of rules, or habits perhaps, for using them, as well as things to say, if one is to speak coherently, or meaningfully, or in conventional and recognizable or acceptable ways.

7. Finally there must be a certain communicative set—a willingness and readiness to speak, a confidence that one can speak well enough, a drive to engage in the kind of interaction we call communication.

As a clinician observing a person speak, to what do you listen? You may listen to the total performance and emerge with a Gestalt impression, but it is not to be expected that as a clinician you would conclude, "That's typical cleft palate speech," or "He's cerebral palsied." Your goal, of course, is to listen analytically. Your basic purpose is to identify the phenomena that constitute the speech impairment or disturbance, to determine the basic process or processes that are involved. Do you hear impairment of respiration, of phonation, or resonance, of articulation, of pronunciation, or of all of these? Or is the problem less one of speech execution than one of language formulation? Or is the problem primarily in the speaker's attitude toward the act of speaking?

In speech and voice problems associated with cleft palate and other palatal anomalies, resonance and articulation are likely to be the processes of major concern to you. In cases of cerebral palsy, the respiration, phonation, resonance, articulation, and pronunciation all may be affected because of motor limitations; and language formulation may be disturbed too, as well as the speaker's adjustment to the speaking situation. The child who is brought to you as a stutterer may have moments of normal speech, while at other moments he refrains from speaking because of his anxiety about stuttering. When he does speak his avoidant behavior tends to interfere with respiration, phonation, and articulation.

As a clinician you are concerned, of course, with the speaker as a person, but you must nevertheless fractionate your observations of his behavior in order to discern adequately the nature of specific deviations and to develop a properly detailed as well as comprehensive plan to remedy them.

A FEW WARNINGS

This section is addressed particularly to the reader who is a student in a professional training program. If you are such a reader you will find it to your advantage to ponder the following words of warning.

1. In diagnostic work, beware of falling into certain careless practices. It is easy to group certain disorders under the general heading "organic" and other disorders under the general heading "functional" or "nonorganic." You will do well to remind yourself periodically that although this dichotomy has a certain usefulness, there is a no-man's land—a range rather than a line—between the two. Of course you will encounter certain speech problems that stem primarily from anatomical or physiological conditions, and other speech problems which clearly result mainly from faulty learning, perseveration of infantile habits, or possibly lack of adequate stimulation or motivation. But you will also find essentially normal speech where substantial organic deviations would seem to militate against it. Occasionally you may see a person who has learned to talk without a tongue, or an individual with an open cleft of the palate speaking with a high degree of intelligibility. You will see speakers with significant anatomical and physiological deviations who compensate for them and produce good speech, whereas others with similar or lesser deviations are apparently unable to compensate for them and as a result produce faulty speech. You will find cerebral palsied children with involvement of certain speech muscles displaying speech errors unrelated to their neuromuscular involvement (16), and you will see aphasic patients with demonstrated neurologic deficits varying in the adequacy of their performance as different kinds of motivating instructions are given to them (13)—undeniable evidence of functional components in clearly organic disorders.

In short, a so-called functional problem may have a heretofore unrecognized organic component, whereas an allegedly organic disorder may have a large functional component. The fact that we can use the words "organic" and "functional" separately does not mean that the processes of speech production and the various speech disorders can be effectively fragmented and classified in terms of these two words. Structure and function interact—so far, that is, as we can determine which is which. Just as matter and energy, or wave and particle, are no longer sharply distinct from one another for the modern physicist, so for the modern clinician structure and function, or, for example, muscle and tension, are by no means always to be clearly differentiated.

2. Another trap into which you could fall if not forewarned is in the words "simple" and "complex" (or "complicated"). Avoid the tendency to think that what are called functional disorders of articulation comprise simpler problems, with which clinicians having minimal training can deal adequately, whereas problems such as are found in cerebral palsy and cleft palate are more involved, or complicated. Obviously there is nothing simple about the problem of a child who has perfect hearing acuity, superior speech-sound discrimination ability, excellent motor control of the speech mechanism, and splendid ability to produce speech sounds in isolation following stimulation, but who, week after week, and month after month, fails to incorporate these correct sounds into his conversational speech.

Thorough consideration of the language process does not lead to the conclusion that it is to be appropriately called simple. It might seem that it would be easier for a young boy with traumatically incurred dysphasia to recall and speak a single noun such as the word "leaf," a single number such as "four," a single verb such as "look" or another noun such as "clover" than it would be for him to put all of these together into some sort of meaningful sentence. But interestingly enough, although the boy cannot speak any of these words individually, he may very well put them all together and sing them with perfect rhythm and melody in the song "I'm Looking over a Four-Leaf Clover." *Calling* a process or a problem simple does not *make* it so. All it does is to make it harder to deal with the problem intelligently.

3. Be particularly aware of the limitations of your clinical procedures and skills in appraising the performance of very young children and in predicting the future course of their problems. Paraphrasing the words of Anderson (1): (a) The earlier your observations, the less reliance you can place upon a single observation in predicting subsequent development. (b) The earlier your observations, the greater care you should take to observe accurately and to record carefully what you see and hear. (c) The earlier your observations, the more weight you should give to the possibility of disturbing factors —negativism, refusals, distractions, fatigue—that operate to introduce error into your conclusions.

4. Nearly everyone seems to admire the clinician who appears to be able to take a quick look at a child and come up with the right answer. But cursory examination can lead easily, of course, to erroneous conclusions and decisions. No law requires you to arrive at a firm conclusion about the nature of any given child's problem before next Tuesday afternoon. A medical dictionary (6) suggests that there is such a thing as a "tentative diagnosis, a diagnosis based upon the available

sources of information but subject to change." You may and should defer the diagnosis if you feel none is warranted at the moment. You serve better those whom you seek to help if you refuse to be defensive, are willing to acknowledge the limits of your knowledge and understanding, and take the time you need to do all you can to insure in each case the best understanding of the problem that you can achieve.

5. You will find your effectiveness as a reporter increased if you keep your reports simple and direct. You probably will communicate more effectively with others, including your fellow clinicians, if you talk about a child's delayed speech rather than his "paralalia prolongata." A few of your professional colleagues may understand what is meant by a child's "hyperrhinolalia" but none will understand less if you record it as "nasal voice quality."

Witness this report furnished by one speech clinic to another: "His speech was severely retarded with all the consonants incorrect or missing completely. There was a mild lingua-labial agnosia and apraxia with some lingua-alveolar apraxia." One cannot tell from this report how the determination of speech retardation was arrived at, since only the status of articulation is reported. And one becomes dubious about the report of articulation when he reads that all of the consonants were either incorrect or missing, since testing that is exhaustive enough nearly always shows that a child can make some of the consonant sounds in some position or in some phonetic context or other. Similarly, it is difficult to know what the child was asked to do or in what way he performed that led to the conclusion that he presented "a lingua-labial agnosia and apraxia," much less one that was only "mild." You should avoid jargon and obscure technical terminology and use descriptive language when your purpose is to communicate effectively about problems involving clinical procedures and classification systems that may differ from clinician to clinician.

ETHICAL CONSIDERATIONS

In diagnostic work as well as in therapy in speech pathology we are bound by the principles embraced in the Code of Ethics of the American Speech and Hearing Association (4). We are reminded by the Code of Ethics that the welfare of those we serve must be paramount; therefore we must become as highly skilled as possible in the use of diagnostic tools and we must refrain from undertaking without adequate supervision diagnostic work for which we are not properly qualified.

The Code of Ethics reminds us that we must use every resource available, including referral to other specialists as needed. We do not depend upon our own skills alone but readily call upon others to counsel and guide us and in fact to take over where we cannot perform effectively.

The Code of Ethics further reminds us that we should "establish harmonious relationships with members of other professions" and should "endeavor to inform others concerning the services that can be rendered by members of the speech and hearing profession, and in turn should seek information from members of related professions." In many cases the otologist and otolaryngologist, the neurologist and neurosurgeon, the psychiatrist and clinical psychologist, the orthopedic surgeon and the physiatrist, the pediatrician and the general practitioner, as well as the teacher, of course, can work very effectively with the speech pathologist and audiologist, and vice versa. Always, moreover, the speech pathologist and audiologist complement each other—indeed, when they are not one and the same person they are fellow members of the same profession, communicology, and share a common concern with the interaction of the speech, language, and hearing functions in the processes and disorders of communication (5, 8).

ASSIGNMENTS

1. Distinguish between the terms "diagnosis" and "appraisal."
2. What is meant by the diagnostic uses of therapy? Suggest some hypothetical cases in connection with which you might wish to make diagnostic use of therapy.
3. Distinguish between the terms "reliability" and "validity." How might you in a specific instance choose the outside criteria for use in evaluating the validity of a testing procedure?
4. Distinguish between the terms "empiricism" and "intuition."
5. Give examples to illustrate how important it may be to understand a person's society and culture in trying to understand him. How might your evaluation of an individual's behavior depend upon the cultural norms to which you are accustomed?
6. What is meant by one's "philosophy of life"? One's "professional philosophy"? Make a list of the principles which might comprise your personal professional philosophy.
7. What is meant by a nonelementalistic approach? Why should you be nonelementalistic in your approach to a person with a spech problem?
8. Suppose that a child severely retarded in speech is brought to you for a diagnosis of his problem and your recommendations for helping him. What does the nonelementalistic approach imply in terms of the testing

procedures you will use and the questions you will ask in the case history interview?

9. To what individuals and groups do you as a person specializing in speech pathology and audiology have responsibilities?

10. If you contemplate specializing in speech pathology and audiology, how should you ready yourself to do an adequate job? What kinds of courses would you consider relevant? What kinds of professional training experiences would best fit you to emerge from a trainee status into the status of an efficient professional worker? If you were tailoring your own curriculum with an eye to how you would want to feel on first being interviewed for a job or on first being confronted with the need for making decisions about policies and practices in a job situation, what would you include in your program of study.

11. With what other professional or nonprofessional groups or agencies or individuals will you be expected to cooperate as a practicing speech clinician? What principles will guide you in your professional relations with them? What boundaries will delimit your areas of responsibility from theirs? To what extent is there likely to be overlapping of responsibility?

12. Secure a copy of the official curriculum or program of the speech pathology and audiology program of your own college or university. What basic philosophy appears to underlie the choice of courses prescribed? What appears to be the rationale for the inclusion of each course? How do the graduate course requirements differ from the undergraduate? What, in your opinion, are the reasons for these differences?

13. Write out your own general definition of "speech problem." How do we know when a speech problem has been eliminated?

14. Suppose that as a practicing speech clinician you read about a new remedial technique that someone has suggested for use with stutterers. How do you decide whether you will adopt the technique in your own work?

15. Secure copies of the *Journal of Speech and Hearing Disorders,* the *Journal of Speech and Hearing Research*, and *Asha*. Who are the individuals and what is the organization responsible for the publication of these journals? What kinds of articles and features are included in each?

16. Secure a copy of *dsh Abstracts* ("dsh" stands for Deafness, Speech and Hearing), published quarterly by Deafness, Speech and Hearing Publications, Inc., sponsored jointly by the American Speech and Hearing Association and Gallaudet College, the national college for the deaf, in Washington, D.C. Note the general character of the abstracts and the system of classification used in the *dsh Abstracts*. Who are the persons responsible for writing, editing, and publishing *dsh Abstracts*? What professional purposes does it serve? What uses can you make of it personally?

17. Make a list of journals other than those listed in assignment 15 which have some bearing on the work you will do as a speech clinician. What kinds of materials do they include which will be of use to you?

18. Secure a recent *Directory* of the American Speech and Hearing Association and study the introductory portions.

  a. What are the purposes of the Association and of the American Speech and Hearing Foundation as given in the By-Laws of the American Speech and Hearing Association?
  b. What are the qualifications for membership in the Association? What requirements must be met by affiliates? How is certification of clinical competency accomplished? What are the requirements for clinical certification?
  c. Read the Code of Ethics of the Association.
    (1) What practices are specifically listed as unethical? Why?
    (2) What are the limits to which the obligation of secrecy can be carried so far as the revelation of confidential information about specific cases is concerned? For what purposes might information in clinic case files be revealed?
    (3) Is critical scrutiny and discussion of the research of other members of the profession unethical?
19. Do you have a regional or state speech and hearing association? Who are its officers? What is the purpose of the organization? When does it meet? Can you belong? How can you join? How can you personally contribute to the greater effectiveness of the organization?

REFERENCES

1. Anderson, J. E., "The limitations of infant and preschool tests in the measurement of intelligence," *Journal of Psychology*, 1939, *8*:351-379.
2. Brown, S. F., and Dorothy Oliver, "A qualitative study of the organic speech mechanism abnormalities associated with cleft palate," *Speech Monographs*, 1939, *6*:127-146.
3. Cable, W. A., "A speech correctionist's professional code," *Journal of Speech Disorders*, 1946, *11*:225-231.
4. *Code of Ethics of the American Speech and Hearing Association*, published in the annual directory, Washington: American Speech and Hearing Association.
5. Davis, Hallowell, and S. R. Silverman, *Hearing and Deafness*, rev. ed., New York: Holt, Rinehart, and Winston, 1960.
6. Dorland, W. A. N., *The American Illustrated Medical Dictionary*, 22nd ed., Philadelphia: Saunders, 1951.
7. Fairbanks, Grant, *Voice and Articulation Drillbook*, 2nd ed., New York: Harper, 1960.
8. Hirsh, I. J., *The Measurement of Hearing*, New York: McGraw-Hill, 1952.
9. Johnson, Wendell, *People in Quandaries: the Semantics of Personal Adjustment*, New York: Harper, 1946.
10. Mayo Clinic Sections of Neurology and Physiology, *Clinical Examinations in Neurology*, Philadelphia and London: Saunders, 1956.

11. Meredith, H. V., "Measuring the growth characteristics of school children," *The Journal of School Health*, 1955, *25*:267-273.
12. Peacher, W. G., "The neurological evaluation of delayed speech," *Journal of Speech and Hearing Disorders*, 1949, *14*:344-352.
13. Stoicheff, Margaret L., "Motivating instructions and language performance of dysphasic subjects," *Journal of Speech and Hearing Research*, 1960, *3*:75-85.
14. Templin, Mildred C., "Norms on a screening test of articulation for ages three through eight," *Journal of Speech and Hearing Disorders*, 1953, *18*:323-331.
15. Travis, L. E., "A point of view in speech correction," *Quarterly Journal of Speech*, 1936, *22*:57-61.
16. Wolfe, W. G., "A comprehensive evaluation of 50 cases of cerebral palsy," *Journal of Speech and Hearing Disorders*, 1950, *15*:234-251.

2 *THE CASE HISTORY*

GATHERING CASE STUDY DATA

In order to help a person with a speech problem effectively, the clinician needs to see him clearly as he is now and describe fully his present problem. The majority of the procedures in this manual are designed as parts of a systematic plan for securing this portrait of the person as he presently is. The meaning of such a portrait can be fully appreciated, however, only when viewed against an adequate background of information about the person's past. In order to determine the etiology of the person's present problem, to estimate its future course with and without remedial attention, and to plan appropriate therapy, you need as a clinician to answer in any given case this basic question: "How did this person come to be what now appears in the portrait of him?"

Among the more useful procedures for answering this question by collecting case study data are the following.

1. The Questionnaire

This device can be very useful for gathering a good deal of information from one person or from many in a brief time, and indeed will serve to collect data from several informants simultaneously. The procedure is economical in providing a record of the answers that is available in usable form without further write-up. You can make a questionnaire as comprehensive or as brief as you wish, and by using it you can cover the same ground in each of a series of cases.

There are also several disadvantages in the use of the questionnaire. Although uniform coverage of the relevant areas is provided for, you cannot be sure that all respondents have interpreted the questions in the same way or even that they have understood the main point of each question. Well do we know that words can mean different things to different people, and that some words mean nothing to some people. Furthermore, the questionnaire method gives only limited guidance in ascertaining the areas to be explored further. Structured as it is, it carries the implication that the areas covered are *the* important ones. Actually some of the areas covered may be almost irrelevant in certain cases.

2. The Autobiography

The autobiography may be a written narrative report or personal document. If the individual under study is old enough and has the necessary ability, you may ask him to write his personal history. It is enlightening to see how the individual sizes up himself as well as his associates and his past and present environments. You may obtain insight into how he perceives the world and his role in it. Also, it may be enlightening to see how he emphasizes or undervalues certain points in his history. You may get a comprehensive and helpful report, for in writing the document the individual may dredge up facts and attitudes that he might not reveal during an oral review. A particularly important consideration is that the autobiography, properly used, tends to have remedial as well as diagnostic value.

Unless due precautions are taken, this procedure can sometimes be unduly time-consuming. It should be noted also that persons vary in ability to reconstruct the past, to remember events, and to relate what they remember. In the preparation of such a document there is also bound to be conscious and unconscious selection of items. Inevitably topics will be omitted which you might want to know about.

3. Spectator Observation

By observing a child or adult in a clinic room through a one-way window, or by watching a group of children at play, or by observing the interactions of parents and children in the clinic or at home, you are able to gain the kind of firsthand knowledge of behavior that is not dependent upon a written report. Through firsthand observation you can obviate some of the biases which enter into any written abstract of what presumably went on in a given situation. You can observe details which are usually lost in verbal reports of observations. You can observe behavior in a specific context with regard to time, space, and participants and thus interpret the meaning of the behavior more readily.

You need to be sensitive, of course, to the fact that if you are seen by those whom you are observing, even though you do not interact with them, you influence their behavior. Furthermore, the range of behavior and the types of social interaction that you can observe are obviously limited in this type of procedure.

4. Participant Observation

You can carry your observations a step further by injecting yourself into the activity of the person whom you are observing. You can structure the situation in certain ways so as to make specific observations. Of course, your presence in the activity makes it different from what it would be if someone else were participating or if no one were present to observe. It might be said that all of the procedures of standardized testing, including those outlined in this manual for making systematic observation of the behavior of persons with speech, voice, and language problems, are special types of participant observation techniques, involving particular kinds of structuring of the situation.

5. The Oral Interview

When you interview an informant you operate in a special kind of interpersonal relationship with him which involves a two-way conversation and a mutual viewing. What the informant sees will determine in large part whether and to what degree rapport develops between the two of you. With rapport, the situation tends to be one of maximum cooperation, confidence, trust, and lack of constriction on the part of the informant. Out of this relationship you can derive at least some of the information needed in order to understand the person and his problems and to bring about desirable changes in his behavior or situation.

THE CASE HISTORY OUTLINE

In order to secure an adequate case history you must explore to some degree all of the areas described on pages 44–49. You may ask,

"How long should the case history be?" Wallin (*54*) stated that as he saw it, case study data must satisfy four conditions: relevancy, sufficiency, representativeness, and reliability. Apparently the question of how long the history should be can be answered in any specific instance only by another question: "How long *must* it be to accomplish its purpose adequately, with reference to Wallin's four conditions, *in this particular case?*" It seems that no single set of questions, such as are listed in typical case history questionnaires with blanks to be filled in, can be adequate for every case, although indeed some are admirably detailed and extremely useful to study—for example, see that of Van Riper (*51*, pp. 545-566). The reason is that a question irrelevant in some cases may only begin to delve into matters of crucial importance in other cases. And what of the myriad questions not included in the questionnaire simply because there had to be a stopping place somewhere? Every case is unique. No inflexible case-history questionnaire will do the job; and even though the questionnaire may be intended to be flexible, "fill-in-the-blanks" thinking tends to be inflexible.

The case history outline included here has been developed through many years of clinical work and is in current use at the University of Iowa Speech Clinic. As presented in this handbook, it represents a slight modification of the particular form of the outline prepared by Brown (*27*, Appendix 4). The headings and questions are suggestive rather than exhaustive. Since the outline cannot be complete, it has been made brief intentionally; it represents a skeleton outline and it is up to you as the user of it to put the flesh on the bones. In the mutual exchange of words that characterizes the particular type of interpersonal relationship which we call a case-history interview, you as interviewer need to be alert to hints of fruitful areas for exploration, interesting cues to follow up, unsuspected relationships to scrutinize. You will not be able as a rule to follow the outline carefully as you pursue the conversation in which you are engaged, but it will help to look at it from time to time, and your prior study of it will go far to guarantee adequate coverage.

You will find the outline particularly useful in organizing your information in order to make a written record of the completed interview. It provides a way to systematize and order a chaos of data. In preparing your report you can assign to each part the weight you think it should be given in pointing up the particular problems of the individual. You are sure to find sometimes that sections of the interview overlap and need to be combined. Properly employed, the outline does make it possible for you to arrive at a balanced account of a given problem in which many interacting variables are to be seen in perspective.

Before attempting to use such an outline, you should understand clearly why such questions are to be asked. You should understand not only what the words themselves mean but how each question relates to other questions and to the presenting problem. For example, ask yourself, "Why am I questioning the mother of this stuttering boy about his childhood diseases?" Is it because a direct causal relationship is known to exist between a reported illness and the problem of stuttering? Or is it rather because a *supposed* causal relationship in the thinking of the parents is likely to affect their evaluation of the child and his problem? Or is it because of psychological factors associated with the specific illness, such as the concern and solicitousness of the parents shown at the time of the illness, and their consequent effects? Or is it for some other reason?

You may wonder particularly about the use you are expected to make of certain kinds of medical information which we suggest you ask questions about. We are, of course, not suggesting that you play doctor and independently diagnose medical conditions to which some of the suggested questions relate. The basic point is that you need to be aware of the kinds of information which medical personnel use in arriving at certain diagnoses, which serve to clarify the nature of specific disorders of communication and to indicate the needs and possibilities for particular kinds of improvement in speech, language, or hearing. You have a responsibility to be sensitive to the possible significance of these kinds of information in relation to the communication problems with which you are professionally concerned.

Just to be sure that you do not mistake this outline for a complete list of questions (as a case-history questionnaire too often is mistakenly supposed to contain blanks about *all* the important questions), it would be well for you to take time to ask yourself about the implications of some of the listed questions. For example, if you were to try to obtain a picture of the parent, parent-child, and sibling relationships as suggested under *Social History*, what would be the first 30 or 50 or 100 questions you would like to ask in order to obtain the details needed to clarify the rather general answers most informants give to such questions? When you have filled several pages, you can remind yourself, "This list is only a beginning. And even when I've supplemented these questions with scores of others, the data I might obtain could not be more than an abstract of all that conceivably could be secured."

Following the basic case-history outline presented at the close of this chapter, you will find several supplementary case-history outlines. These present additional topics of inquiry and specific questions that you may use in order to obtain more nearly adequate special information that is needed in cases of cerebral palsy or other brain damage, dysphasia, cleft palate, laryngectomy, and stuttering. In order to make the relevance of these additional questions clear, we have included certain information about each of the disorders. Not all of the questions you might ask have been listed. The questions that are presented will indicate to you which areas deserve particular scrutiny, but it will be up to you to explore each such area in sufficient detail for your specific purposes. In Chapters 5, 6, 7, 8, and 10 additional information is given concerning articulatory disorders, voice disorders, problems of speech and language development, dysphasia, and the stuttering problem, together with implied and explicit suggestions regarding case history interviewing.

You may sometimes be at a loss to interpret some of the data you obtain from your informants. The normative information presented in this and other chapters of this manual will help you to understand whether the individual whose history you are securing is generally average or accelerated or retarded in certain aspects of development. The relative incidence of various birth conditions is summarized in Table 1. You will need to be familiar with the definitions of certain of the terms used in this table. For example, the criterion for prematurity that seems to be most generally used is a birth weight of less than 2500 grams (5.5 pounds); sometimes the definition includes also a birth length of less than 44.9 centimeters (17.7 inches), but usually the duration of the pregnancy is not considered in the definition of prematurity. As another example, Odell, Randall, and Scott (41), like other researchers in this area, have defined precipitate labor as labor lasting less than 3 hours and prolonged labor as that lasting more than 30 hours.

Tables 2 and 3 present the mean heights and weights of American boys and girls between the ages of 2 and 18. Table 4 summarizes the results from 11 studies concerning the ages at which boys and girls acquire certain motor skills. Tables 5 and 6 provide normative information about the sleeping times of children. Tables 7 through 9 summarize information obtained in a questionnaire study of the attainment of bowel and bladder control by children. Table 10 provides normative information about the incidence of nail biting in children between the ages of 5 and 18. To derive maximum usefulness from these and other tables of normative data, you must become familiar with the studies upon which they are based. Definitions and procedures used by investigators in compiling specific sets of normative data are crucial in interpreting them for specific purposes.

THE HOW OF INTERVIEWING

A subject that many books cannot exhaust is impossible to cover fully in these pages. Here are simply a few suggestions that should serve as practical guides to most case history taking, together with a list of some of the more useful books on the techniques of effective interviewing.

1. Set the Right Tone

Experienced interviewers have learned and repeatedly confirmed that the atmosphere most conducive to successful elicitation of information is one of mutual respect. You and the informant are by no means on equal grounds, for he has come for help which you are in a position to give. It is to be expected that most of the questions and the guidance of the interview will issue from you, while most of the information will come from the informant. And yet you as the interviewer cannot afford to be aloof, superior, critical, moralistic, God-like, rigid, intolerant, disdainful, or amused. You must show a liking for the person and sincerely try to understand his behavior and his problems. You must certainly refrain from ridicule or condemnation. Rapport grows only as you show the informant that you still will like him and respect him and do your best to help him no matter what he says. You do this largely by accepting and acknowledging (not necessarily approving outwardly) what he tells you, by trying to fit together in a meaningful pattern the various bits of information he provides, and by making obvious that you want, above all else, to understand him and his problem as well as you possibly can. Kinsey, Pomeroy, and Martin have stated it this way:

One is not likely to win the sort of rapport which brings a full and frank confession from a human subject unless he can convince the subject that he is desperately anxious to comprehend what his experience has meant to him. . . . Histories often involve a record of things that have hurt, of frustrations, of pain, of unsatisfied longings, of disappointments, of desperately tragic situations, and of complete catastrophe. The subject feels that the investigator who asks merely routine questions has no right to know about such things in another's history. The interviewer who senses what these things can mean, who at least momentarily shares something of the satisfaction, pain, or bewilderment which was the subject's, who shares something of the subject's hope that things will, somehow, work out all right, is more effective though he may not be altogether neutral (29, p. 42).

2. Get the Interview Off to a Good Start

Do not assume that the person you are questioning understands the purpose of the interview without having it explained to him. When a parent comes to a clinic or speech pathologist for help, he may be unprepared for the kind of questioning he will experience. Tell him the purpose of the interview, the use that will be made of the information,

to whom it will—and will not—be revealed, why information is needed
in such detail, even who you are and the function you serve. The informant will submit readily to a great deal of questioning if he is convinced that the answers are needed and will be handled responsibly.

See that the informant is comfortable. Be alert to conditions of
temperature and ventilation; invite the informant to smoke if he
wishes (and provide an ashtray) ; see that he doesn't have to face the
light; and in other ways arrange a comfortable, relaxed interviewing
situation.

In all cases it is desirable to encourage the person who has come for
help to talk as freely as possible about his problem or his child's
problem, as the case may seem to be. With an attitude and posture
that suggest that you have all the time in the world, let the person put
into his own words the feelings, the questions, the beliefs and curios-
ities, the anxiety and sense of guilt perhaps, the hope and the doubt
that he has to express before you begin to ask questions. In some
cases the person will want, and may deeply need, to talk quite a long
while. In most cases, however, you will sense fairly soon that the informant rather expects to be questioned or perhaps tested and examined in some way. If he does not seem to have any particular need to
"get talked out," at least a few minutes of friendly conversation at the
beginning without the intrusion of note taking may be helpful in establishing rapport early. Usually you can get down to the business at
hand fairly soon. If the informant obviously is ready to cooperate,
don't waste time.

3. Learn to Listen

Generally informants find it annoying to be asked a question, provide the answer, and then be asked the question once or perhaps even
more times subsequently. Such a sequence indicates to them that the
interviewer simply did not listen the first time. You should become
sufficiently familiar with your interviewing procedures and the particular sequence of questions you are likely to use so that as the interview progresses you need not be worried about how you are doing or
what question you will be asking next; rather you should be concerned
about the feelings and replies of the person you are interviewing.
Although you probably will be making notes on what you hear (see
Section 8 below), you will need to absorb the information even as you
are obtaining it. Do not let the process of questioning become automatic. Keep it vital, and listen actively. As Long (*31*) has written
concerning the way medical students should take histories, "The
eager beaver who knows all the questions and gives his patients little
opportunity to say anything but 'yes' and 'no' rarely gets a decent

history. Once we missed a diagnosis of late syphilis from the patient because we talked too much, and did not let the patient give us this final confidence about himself. So be easy and take it easy."

You will find it easier to listen if you have allowed yourself plenty of time for taking the case history. Quoting again from Long, "One can't rush through a history and do anyone justice. . . . A relaxed patient and doctor result in the most satisfactory histories" (*31*, p. 61). You will want to work your way rather rapidly through the case history (see Section 6 below), but the informant should not get the impression that you are in a big hurry.

4. Frame Questions Clearly, Economically, Neutrally

Although the general atmosphere you establish is more important than the specific way you frame any given question, you can learn a lesson from the experienced public opinion poll-taker and word your questions carefully. If you do, you will save yourself much time and will secure more reliable information.

a. First of all, make sure you understand why you are asking each question. What is the main point of it? Now state it briefly in words of one syllable if you can. It makes sense to use the sort of vocabulary your informant seems to be in the habit of using; if you err in any direction, err in the direction of underestimating the informant's sophistication.

Avoid starting a question, then qualifying part of it, then going back and reframing it, ending lamely with an ambiguous set of incoherent ideas and multiple queries for the informant to sort out. *Not this*: "How old was your child when you began to teach him habits of—uh, well, letting him know that he should go to the bathroom— you know, control his bladder—and then when did he attain control for the most part?" *But perhaps this*: "When did you begin Eddie's toilet training?" *Then*: "How old was he when he learned to stay dry during the day? During the night?"

In clarifying the point of a question, you may need to define some terms, even fairly common ones. For example, if you want to find out how often a child is punished at home, you will need clearly to differentiate punishment from reprimands or scolding and even give some examples of each so you and the informant will mean essentially the same things by the terms you are using.

b. Avoid yes-no questions which, when they are answered, still will need to be supplemented with further questions to clarify the response. Instead ask questions requiring factual answers, placing more of a burden upon the informant. For example, "What illnesses has John had?" is a more efficient question than the more general "Has

John been sick much?" The latter, whatever the answer, will need to be followed up with other questions framed to elicit details.

c. Avoid wording your question in a way that will bias the answer. If you ask the parent of a stuttering child, "You didn't tell Tommy to stop and start over, did you?" you will often get "Oh, no!" for a reply. A less slanted question such as "What have you done to help Tommy talk better?" or "Have you sometimes suggested that Tommy stop and start over?" is likely to elicit a more valid reply. Avoid putting answers in the informant's mouth. Avoid suggesting how his answers will be received.

d. In order to expedite answers to some questions, you may find it helpful to provide the informant with a set of possible answers or a rating scale for making a judgment. For instance, it may help a parent to describe how he handles his child if you suggest that some parents reprimand their children by hollering at them, others by threatening. Then: "What do you mostly do in reprimanding your child?" Again, statement of the frequency of parental reprimands may be more easily secured by suggesting various possible frequencies—25 times a day, or once a week, or once a day, or ten times a day—avoiding any particular sequence in the suggested answers and avoiding making the last of the suggested answers seem to be the most appropriate or expected answer.

We sometimes want parents to evaluate their children with regard to particular types of behavior or personality traits. A useful tool to offer them—partially to objectify their evaluations in terms of what they know of other children (their own or somebody else's)—is the following 5-point scale: In comparison with other children of his age, would you rate the amount of talking your child does as much more than average, somewhat more than average, about average, somewhat less than average, or much less than average? If you want a parent to rate the severity of his child's stuttering, you may want to suggest to him a scale such as is given in Form 14, page 281.

5. Adjust the Sequence of Topics to the Anxiety of the Informant

Some anxiety on the part of the informant is implicit in the interviewing situation. The fact that he has come for help means that he is more or less concerned about something. It has been said that if the informant feels no anxiety, he won't talk—indeed, he probably will not have come to the clinic at all. But if he feels too much anxiety, the course of the interview may be seriously impeded. Arrange the sequence of topics so as to allow time for gradual building of rapport without introducing too shocking, too emotion-laden matter too early.

6. Move Rapidly Through the Interview

In many areas of questioning a rapid-fire technique probably results in greater reliability, for it allows the informant less time to study his answer and to compare it with some presumably ideal answer and therefore modify it or try to justify it. Yet some questioning must be almost exhaustingly slow if certain subtle details of etiological significance are to be dredged up and clarified.

7. Maintain Appropriate Visual Relationship

It is important to look at the informant in a way that encourages him to talk freely. It is not good to look at him constantly, of course, as though staring him down, nor should you eye him as though you were doubtful of the truth of his statements. It is not good either always to look down at your notes or to look past him or in other ways to seem to avoid looking directly at him. Much of the time your eyes should meet his. As Kinsey, Pomeroy, and Martin have stated, "People understand each other when they look directly at each other" (*29*, p. 48).

8. Record Information During the Interview

Take notes as expeditiously as possible, using a shorthand system, or telegraphic English, or some system of codes to avoid either long silences after answers while you catch up in your notes or inhibition of the flow of important material from the informant by asking him to wait while you catch up. Probably less harm is done to rapport than one might suppose by note taking; some informants actually find it reassuring to have the interviewer making an accurate record as the questioning progresses. Some seem to feel more at ease if the interviewer is doing something. But note taking must be kept within reasonable limits and should be done on a clip-board or pad that can be maneuvered easily so the informant cannot read the notes.

You may want to consider tape recording your interviews. The tape recorder is being used more and more in clinical situations. It is probably used more, however, in counseling and therapy than in case history taking. If you tape record your case study interviews, you then must have each recording transcribed in order to abstract the transcription, or else work directly from the tape, taking notes as you listen to it. In either case the extra time consumed will be considerable. If you do use a tape recorder you would be well advised, in our judgment, to be open and aboveboard with the informant, making clear at the outset in each instance that you are going to tape record the interview, that this will make it unnecessary for you to take notes and so you will be able to give your undivided attention to the interview, and that the informant can best cooperate by speaking up and staying in a proper relationship to the microphone. In our experience most persons accept the microphone and recorder as tools of the clinician's trade, and after the first few moments they seem to pay no attention to them and to talk as freely as they would without them. In fact, if you ask permission to make educational and scientific use of the tape recordings at a later time very few, if any, interviewees will refuse permission.

9. Ask Ticklish Questions Straightforwardly

Inevitably you will get around to matters that are intimate, emotion-laden, socially involved. How shall questions about parental relations be asked—questions about sources of conflict in the home, separations, divorces—or questions about causes of death, reasons why breast feeding was abandoned, mental disorders in the family history, home disciplinary practices, parental estimates of the intelligence of the child, and the like?

The best practice, though it takes most beginning interviewers a while to recognize this and boldly try it out, is to be matter-of-fact. Having laid a solid foundation of rapport, mutual understanding, and respect, ask the questions in a direct manner—as Kinsey, Pomeroy, and Martin have said, "without hesitancy and without apology." They add, "If the interviewer shows any uncertainty or embarrassment, it is not to be expected that the subject will do better in his answers. . . . Evasive terms invite dishonest answers" (*29*, p. 53).

Sometimes the posing of a ticklish question will result in a long painful pause while the informant wrestles with the problem of deciding how best to answer or evade it. Resist the impulse to ease the tension by interposing a too-ready "I understand" or an equivalent expression. If you have properly laid the groundwork for a profitable discussion of some vital question, don't throw your work away by unwisely doing the informant's thinking and deciding for him.

10. Attempt to Get Beneath Superficial Answers

An informant may not realize the importance of a question or, trying to take the easy way out and evade a crucial subject, may dismiss a question hurriedly. You may ask: "Did you ever do anything to correct your son's stuttering?" "No," is an easy but seldom accurate answer. Dig under that too-ready "No." Ask additional specific questions. Ask questions that put the burden of denial on the informant, such as, "How many times a day do you ask him to slow down?"

Parents often have a hard time recalling details of events remote in time, such as the age of first steps, the kinds of approval and disapproval they expressed during the child's early toilet training, the times and details of early illnesses, the nature of first so-called stuttering reactions and the specific situation in which they were first noticed. Here is a tremendous and very important challenge to your ingenuity. Suggest to the informant ways of pinning down an event. Help him establish certain milestones such as family moves from one community to another, changes in employment, visits to or from relatives, entrance into school, births, deaths, marriages, memorable trips, fires, accidents, and so on; and then relate to these markers the incidents about which you are asking. Frame a question in various ways, suggesting details you wish recalled, and don't give up too readily in your search for these details.

Unless you can establish a reasonably clear relationship in time and place between two events, you cannot conclude that they are, in fact, related. For example, parents will often say something like, "The stuttering started at the time Arthur had a ruptured appendix and had such a bad time in the hospital." Such a statement is by no means to be taken at face value. Get both events, the rupturing of the appendix and the onset of the stuttering, dated with pin-point precision, or as accurately as you possibly can, by relating them to other clear family time-markers. It is impressive how often such pin-point questioning of time relationships results in the disclosure that the two events actually occurred several months apart. We all feel the need to explain to ourselves and to others the important events in our lives or in the lives of our children. Sometimes in trying to work out the needed explanations we put close together in memory events that were far apart in reality. This is such a strong and common tendency among people that as a clinical interviewer you need to cultivate a very keen sensitivity to it.

Even in cases in which it is established that events did occur together, or nearly so, *in time*, it must still be established that they were related *in space*. This may seem a strange way to put it, but a moment's reflection will probably make it seem very sensible. For example, having established that an appendix ruptured in an organism at about the same time that a listener first decided that stuttering was beginning to occur in that organism, you must somehow get from the appendix to the mouth, as it were. Indeed, in such a case as this one, you would first have to determine whether the child had, in fact, begun to speak in some new and different way or his parents had begun to pay attention to and wonder about something the child had been doing all along (see Chapter 8). Assuming that the child had begun to speak in some unusual way, then it has to be determined what *relevant* events inside the organism took place between the rupturing of the appendix and the uttering of, possibly, "Wh-wh-wh-where is my c-c-c-cap?" a few hours later, or even within the next minute—to saying nothing of four weeks later. Even when such questions clearly cannot be answered, you should ask them of yourself, and often of the informant. It is essential that everyone concerned understand as thoroughly as possible that a causal relationship between two events is necessarily a relationship between them not only in time but also, and necessarily, in space.

Very often the answer "I don't know" is most revealing and important. A parent who comes to the clinic convinced that a child's cerebral palsy is due to the use of instruments at time of birth, or that a youngster's stuttering was caused by a bad fright, takes a basic step toward better understanding of the problem in recognizing a lack of precise and sufficient supporting information, if such recognition is in order. Usually it will enable the parent to consider, at least, other and more sound and helpful interpretations than those he had previously made.

One specific problem in this connection is worthy of special mention. Quite often you will find that the parents of a stuttering child, when asked how long the child has stuttered, will reply, "From the beginning," or "All his life," or "From the time he first began to talk." Of course such an answer is not to be accepted at face value. A moment's reflection can only lead to genuine questioning about what such a statement could possibly mean. On the basis of what specific standards or norms of speech development might you conclude that a child has "always" stuttered?

Moreover, you must recognize the need to visualize or imagine as vividly as possible just what, if anything, is being described when a parent says, for example, that a child *suddenly* "could not say a word," or "was blocked," presumably at some exact time by the clock such as 9:15 of a particular Tuesday forenoon—after two or three or even more years of evidently normal functioning of the speech mechanism and, on top of that, in the absence of any apparent cause, or "just after a fall," or "when he had the measles," or "when he started to school," or some other circumstance under which a sudden failure of normal neuromuscular functioning would not usually be expected and no explanation for it is apparent. The onset of stuttering—or of any other problem, for that matter, although there are special difficulties in describing the beginnings of stuttering—is a matter to be investigated with the keenest possible sensitivity to vagueness, memory fashioned to accord with "what must have happened," and confusions of fact and unexamined assumption, not only on the part of the informant but of yourself as well. In general, you should consistently take care to have the informant *describe* quite exactly what he allegedly has observed, to distinguish at all times between vague or generalized family legends and actual memories of specific events, and to relate everything as closely as possible to times, places, and persons. This kind of interviewing takes much more time than routine questioning, of course, and often it cannot possibly be carried as far as you would like. Even so, it is to be kept in mind as a standard, and general information obtained hurriedly and without thorough pin-pointing and evaluating is to be weighed and discounted accordingly.[1]

11. Note Discrepancies in the Account and Check Them

The longer the interview, the greater its reliability, for the chances of your including interlocking questions are greater and there is greater likelihood that a given item will be touched on more than once by the informant. As the informant expresses more and more attitudes and adds more details, you may recognize inconsistencies. These may be accidental and unimportant or they may suggest uncertainty, evasion, ambivalence, or untruth somewhere along the line.

Do not ignore these inconsistencies as probably trivial or due to an error on your part; likewise do not simply let them stand for someone else to puzzle out and interpret. Rather check the point concerning which the discrepancy was noted in each instance. Do it unobtrusively later in the interview, avoiding a blunt challenge to the informant's veracity.

12. Handle Emotional Scenes Tactfully

You can expect some proportion of the persons you interview to become upset and weep as their feelings of anxiety find an outlet, as they recall earlier moments of sorrow or anxiety, or as feelings of guilt or shame overwhelm them. One possible way to handle the situation is to excuse yourself until the informant has had an opportunity to reestablish his composure. Or you may immediately express understanding and then present a new question that leads off in a quite different and more neutral direction. The emotion expressed by the informant may be anger; he may become hostile, resentful, or aggressive. In such a case reassurance should be offered, a mistake in judgment acknowledged, and a new tack taken if possible.

[1] The sorts of problems discussed in this section are illustrated particularly well in parts of tape recorded interviews, reproduced with comments and explanations, in Wendell Johnson, *Stuttering and What You Can Do About It*, Minneapolis: University of Minnesota Press, 1961 (New York: Doubleday Dolphin, 1962), chap. 2.

13. Obtain the Informant's Interpretation of the Events He Narrates

As a clinician you are interested in what the informant and the child or other person in question have done and the things that have happened to them, but you are also very much interested in their own evaluations of these happenings. It may be important for you to know that the child first walked at 15 months of age; it may be equally important for you to know whether the parents considered the child retarded, average, or advanced with regard to this aspect of development. It is good to see the child's report cards and to know that his grade average is B; it is also valuable to know whether his family approves or disapproves of such a record. It is important to know not only what it is a child does in speaking that his parents classify as stuttering, but also whether the child's parents believe that he does this sort of thing because of nervousness, fatigue, a change of handedness, a serious illness, a fall, a burn, tongue-tie, being tickled, thinking faster than he can talk, talking faster than he can think, imitation, faulty school handling, or their own mismanagement of the child. It is important, moreover, to know how well they understand such explanations, how they defend them and feel about them.

Consideration of how an informant interprets the significance of the things he relates will often remind you that the narrative of events cannot always be taken at face value, and will give you valuable insights into the whole situation with which you must grapple as a speech clinican working not just with speech problems but also with the people who are caught up in them. You will see repeatedly that ignorance, motivated or even innocent forgetting, the desire to explain things simply, and a need for approval, as well as feelings of resentment, anxiety, guilt, and shame can color and even render invalid an apparently factual report.

14. Encourage Free Expression of Opinion and Emotion, But Keep in Mind the Limitations of the Interview Situation

Your primary goal in the case history interview is to compile the data necessary for a properly balanced understanding of the current situation. It is not primarily to foster catharsis; it is not primarily therapeutic. An informant may experience welcome relief in unburdening himself to you as a sympathetic listener, and you should not inhibit the outpouring of his feelings unless you have to. Receive with interest what he says, keeping alert, empathic, and spontaneous in your reactions. But occasionally in this type of interviewing you may have to stem the flow in order to accomplish your task of thorough coverage in a limited time. Do it tactfully, suggesting that there are other matters you need information about which may prove equally important to both of you.

15. Be Prepared for Questions from the Informant

If you have succeeded in establishing a warm relationship with the informant, it is natural for him to feel like asking you a question now and then, too—especially a question that has been bothering him and about which he needs reassurance. How you handle a question should depend upon your role in the clinic routine and upon what your answer will mean in terms of helping or hindering the progress of the interview.

If someone else is in charge of the final disposition of the case and of the counseling that normally follows the clinical routine of examination and history taking, you might well refer the informant to that person. For example, a mother says to you, "I'm so worried about Sue's not talking. What do you think is the basis of her problem?" You as interviewer can avoid a long and useless, if not harmful, discussion of your ideas by telling the parent that your function is to get as full a picture as possible of the child and the myriad influences that have molded her, and that Mr. Jones, the clinic supervisor, will review the history and the examination results later and will discuss them with her.

In some cases a truthful answer will jeopardize the relationship you have labored to build. A parent says, "Whenever Freddie stuttered, I just told him to wait until he could say it clearly and then to speak. That's all right, isn't it?" If you say "Yes" in order to get yourself off the hook, you are giving questionable advice and very possibly doing harm. If you say, "No, you shouldn't have done that," you may put the parent on the defensive and spoil to some degree the rapport already established. It is better to refer the question to the person responsible for counseling the parent, or, if it is up to you to give the answer, better to postpone it until a more favorable time.

Some questions may be handled simply by responding to the emotion expressed in the question rather than to the question itself. An answer such as, "It certainly is hard to know what to do," or "Children surely are a problem," or "I can see why you would feel that way," often satisfies the questioner. At other times a direct truthful answer should be given the informant so as to direct his thinking elsewhere as soon as possible.

16. Record Your Observations of the Characteristics of the Informant

The behavior, the speech, the attitudes of the informant are just as much grist for your mill as are the facts he relates to you. Report these in the *Comments* section at the close of the history. Some of the observations you might make are these:

Development of Rapport: Was the informant friendly and open? Or indifferent or nonchalant, parrying your questions? Or overtly hostile, refusing to answer or answering only cryptically?

Language Behavior: What does his language suggest about the informant's intellectual or educational level? Is he critical, specific, clear, careful in qualifying his answers, extensional (showing a feeling for validity of report, as indicated by due emphasis on the who, what, where, when fundamentals of his account)? Or does he use a "lumpy" language, speaking in general terms, using emotionally colored words, confusing fact with opinion? Is he glib in using labels, catchwords, and cliches, rigidly either-orish in his orientation? Is there a recurrent theme song that runs through his conversation, repeated allusions to some topic?

Expressive Movements: What do the informant's handshake, gait, posture, directness or shiftiness of gaze, quality of voice, rate of speech, and facial expressions suggest to you?

Emotional Reactions: What significant reactions to specific questions do you notice—flushing, pausing, speeding up, weeping, anger?

Insight: How well does the informant see into the heart of the problem, recognize the interrelationships of various aspects in the history and present situation, and how clearly does he see his own role in the problem?

Rationalizing: Does the informant strive to justify his acts and behavior, explain away things that might be unfavorably interpreted, give "good" reasons instead of the real reasons?

Unconscious Projection: Does the informant blame someone or something else, or attribute to others the emotions, attitudes, or behavior he sees in himself but cannot admit? Does he talk about people and events as though they were in fact what he takes for granted they are, not seeming to be aware of the degree to which he is projecting his unexamined assumptions and preconceptions about them?

Ambivalence: Does the informant seem to harbor conflicting feelings about the child, about himself, about the speech problem, or even about you?

17. Bring the Interview to a Close Gracefully

Explain that you have asked the questions which you have considered most important and express your appreciation to the informant for his cooperation in answering them. Ask him if there is anything further which he feels might have some important bearing on the problem. Explain when he will have an opportunity to discuss the decisions and recommendations with the person responsible for case disposition. Thank him again and say goodbye.

18. Write a Functional Report

In writing your report of a case study interview, your fundamental purpose is to communicate effectively the fruits of your questioning. The following few suggestions will help you do an effective job.

a. Come to the point—whatever it may be—clearly, quickly, precisely. Use the simple expression, the direct phrase. You don't have to be fancy in your writing.

b. Quote exactly (and if you are to do it *exactly,* you can't quote at length) those statements which are so unusual, questionable, or revealing that a paraphrase of them would lack something important.

c. Use a question mark in parentheses (?) to indicate that the information immediately preceding is questionable as furnished. If the reason why it is questionable is not obvious, explain.

d. List all informants in the heading of the case history report. If there are more than one, ascribe to each the information whose source it is important to know.

e. Use complete sentences, composing a readable, flowing narrative, not merely the jerky outline for a narrative.

f. Vary sentence structure and sentence length, avoiding monotony.

g. Be factual. Distinguish fact from inference. The statement "His grades are good" is somebody's inference. What are the actual grades —A's, B's, or C's? The sentence "Home discipline is strict" describes an attitude, either yours or the informant's; tell instead what disciplinary measures are used, by whom, for what offenses, with what frequency. "The child started to stutter when he was five" refers to a classification made by you or the informant of something the child did "when he was five." What exactly did the child do that was so classified? And just when did he do it "when he was five"? What facts show that he wasn't four instead of five, or three, or six?

h. Adhere to accepted usage of capitals and punctuation marks; and if you aren't sure, consult a reliable guidebook.

i. Don't be reluctant to check doubtful spellings, using an ordinary or special (for example, medical) dictionary as necessary.

j. Be professional, serious, sincere in tone, but not pedantic or overly formal. Avoid "asides," frequent underlining for emphasis, and excessive exclamation points.

k. Be human and informal enough to refer by name to the person the history is about rather than to refer monotonously (and depressingly) to the case, the subject, or the client.

l. Follow a uniform format throughout the history with regard to spacing, indentation, capitalization, underlining, and punctuation of headings. The form of the outline presented at the end of this chapter is suggested as a model.

m. See that the sources of what you record are properly indicated. Use first-person reference to yourself to indicate clearly, especially in the *Comments* section, the evaluations or observations reported that are your own rather than the informant's. Do not use first-person reference to yourself in recording observations and opinions of the informant or someone else.

n. Form careful habits of signing and dating reports. In writing dates include day, month, *and year*. See that the names of the client, the parents, informants, siblings, physicians, and other persons involved are written legibly and in full. Include adequate addresses of parents, physicians, teachers, and others to whom you or your supervisor might want to write. Write your own name and the full date carefully on all reports and papers bearing interview notes.

Listed below are four sources of further information about interviewing procedure, all of which should prove helpful to you:

Bingham, Walter V., and Bruce V. Moore, *How to Interview,* rev. ed., New York: Harper, 1941. This is perhaps the best-known general treatment, a standard work. Of special interest should be Chapters 1, 2, 11, 12, and 15.

Fenlason, Anne F., *Essentials in Interviewing: For the Interviewer Offering Professional Services*, New York: Harper, 1952. This book is especially useful in showing how background knowledge in the social sciences—anthropology, psychology, sociology—can help you in understanding and working effectively with people during interviews. Sample case studies and interviews are included.

Garrett, Annette, *Interviewing: Its Principles and Methods*, New York: Family Welfare Association of America, 1942. A brief treatment, especially suited to clinical purposes, providing insight into psychological determinants of what happens in interviewing and offering clear answers to practical questions of procedure in questioning, avoidance of pitfalls, and interpretation of information and observations. Nine selected interviews illustrate the process.

Kinsey, Alfred C., Wardell B. Pomeroy, and Clyde E. Martin, *Sexual Behavior in the Human Male*, Philadelphia: Saunders, 1948. Chapter 2 is a rich source of information concerning the interview as a research instrument; it can help any interviewer do a better job. Special light is thrown upon the importance of the personal relationship in interviewing (establishing rapport), manipulating the anxiety level of the informant, and increasing the reliability of data obtained by interviewing.

ASSIGNMENTS

1. Interview another member of the class, using the case history outline at
   the end of this chapter. If the person you interview does not have a generally recognized type of speech problem, ask him to describe his most
   important shortcoming or difficulty in speech and language behavior—
   stagefright perhaps, or a feeling of uneasiness in conversing with certain
   persons or kinds of persons, or uncertainty about grammar or pronunciation, unsureness or distress in using the telephone, or some other defin-
   able problem in oral communication. In most cases this will not be a speech
   disorder, as this term is ordinarily used, but it might well be a problem
   that is important to the person who is concerned with it. Prepare a case
   history report.
2. Interview the mother of a preschool child in order to get practice in asking questions especially pertaining to younger children. Prepare a case
   history report. If the child in question has no speech problem, the section
   in the case history entitled "History of Speech Problem" may be designated "History of Speech Development."
3. The point has been emphasized that the case history outline presented in
   this chapter does not include all the questions that might be asked. Make
   a list of some of the specific questions you might ask in securing adequate
   information about each of the following areas:
   a. Early speech stimulation and need for speech
   b. Feeding practices and problems
   c. Child's school relations
   d. Family discipline practices
   e. Child's personality

Name: _____ Date History Taken: _____

Birthdate: _____ Interviewer: _____

Address: _____ Informant: (Full name and relationship to
                                     speaker) _____

Complaint: State in informant's own words, if possible. Is this the only problem?

Referral: Full name of individual or agency making referral. Indicate relationship.

History of Speech Problem: Age of speaker when first regarded as having a speech problem? Who first so regarded him? Under what circumstances? What sort of treatment has been attempted? By whom? Have parents made any effort to correct problem at home? Exactly what have they done? What results from treatment? Has speaker made any effort to improve his speech? If so, what has he done? What results? What has been the general course of the problem—has it become better or worse? Parents' estimate of present severity. Speaker's own estimate of present severity. What things have seemed to affect the severity of the problem? Anyone else in family or among friends with similar problem or other speech problem? Did problem cause any adverse comment from relatives and others? Were such comments made in speaker's presence?

Speaker's attitude toward speech problem. Has he withdrawn from speech or other situations because of it? Attitude of parents, siblings, and other relatives. Variations in attitude with different situations.

(If problem has been present since first speech or began to develop soon afterward, include such items as are mentioned in following paragraph. If problem began long after first speech, include these items under Developmental History.)

Did speaker babble during infancy (3-12 months) and after? How much? Age at first words. Age at two-word combinations. Age at combinations of three or more words. Amount and type of early speech stimulation. Need as a child for speech. Reward for speaking. When a child, did speaker talk much or little? Was he taught to speak pieces and perform for strangers? If so, how did he react to such situations? Bilingualism in home?

Developmental History: Health of mother during pregnancy. Length of pregnancy. Delivery—difficult or easy, length of labor, type of presentation, etc. Was labor induced? Drugs used? Were instruments used? Evidence of birth injury? Birth weight and length. Any cyanosis, difficulty in initiating breathing? Breast or bottle fed? If not breast fed, why not? If breast fed, for how long? Any feeding difficulties? Ages of sitting up, first steps, bowel and bladder control. Describe toilet training techniques. Amount of constipation. Handedness, manual dexterity, bodily coordination.

Medical History: Illnesses—age of speaker at each illness, degree of severity, duration, amount of fever, any complications or sequelae. Care provided when ill. Were parents overly concerned or solicitous or matter of fact? Same for all injuries and operations. Condition of tonsils and adenoids. History of mouth breathing? Ever worn glasses? If so, why? Parents' or speaker's own estimate of hearing and vision.

School History: Age when entered school. Ever failed or skipped a grade? Present grade placement. Kind of grades child makes. Any special difficulties with school subjects? How has speaker gotten along with teachers and schoolmates? Amount of education completed. If speaker is a child, parents' estimate of his intelligence.

Social History: Estimate of family socioeconomic status, based upon parents' occupations, amount of education, source of income, house size and type.* Leisure-time activities of family and of speaker, community activity participation, group membership. Parental, parent-child, and sibling relationships. Discipline practices of parents when speaker was a child; present relationship between speaker and his parents. Personality characteristics of speaker. Behavior abnormalities as a child—thumb sucking, temper tantrums, destructiveness, overactivity, nail biting, etc.; present adjustment problems. Age of speaker's associates, especially in childhood. If speaker is an adult, include work history and estimate of his own socioeconomic status.

Family History: Age and health of parents and siblings. Any family health problems? Speech abilities and disabilities in the family background, and family reactions to them.

Comments on Interview: Development of rapport, nature of informant's language behavior, expressive movements, emotional reactions, insight, evidence of rationalization, of unconscious projection. Any other important observations.

  * See pages 305-307, Chapter 10, for information about indexes of socioeconomic status which you may find useful.

SUPPLEMENTARY CASE HISTORY OUTLINE: CEREBRAL PALSY

GENERAL INFORMATION ABOUT THE DISORDER

The brain consists of a number of parts which do not act independently of one another but interact with each other in a complex fashion. Certain parts of the brain control the voluntary movements of parts of the body which are used in such acts as walking, speaking, and writing. The muscles concerned move as a result of impulses coming from what are called the motor projection areas of the brain. These impulses do not pass directly from the motor areas of the brain to the muscles but are subject to modification enroute by the activity of other parts of the central nervous system and pass through certain relay stations of the brain and brain stem before they arrive at the muscles.

When these motor control centers, modification areas, or relay centers do not function properly because they have been damaged or have not developed normally, control of bodily movements is impaired. This result and its causes, taken together, are designated cerebral palsy. Cerebral palsy is not a result of damage to the spinal cord or the peripheral nerves leading from the spinal cord or brain stem but is due entirely to impairment of the brain's motor control centers, modification areas, or relay stations.

The disturbance of motor control may be very widespread and affect all four limbs, the muscles of speech and breathing, the muscles of the trunk, head, shoulders, etc., or it may be limited to one or more specific sets of muscles. If the cerebral palsy involves the muscles employed in producing speech, then speech will not be normal. Articulation may be disturbed because of the slow or jerky or uncoordinated action of the articulators. Various aspects of voice may be affected: pitch may be too high or low, markedly monotonous, or perhaps uncontrolled; rate will very possibly be slower than average; the voice may be louder than normal; impaired voice quality such as harshness or breathiness may appear; rhythm may be disturbed. Breathing may be shallow and exhalation may be poorly controlled, with consequent gasping, attempts to speak on residual air, and faulty phrasing and rhythm.

Associated with the motor disability implied by the term cerebral palsy there may be other problems, some of them being concomitant results of the brain damage, while others are the result of the speaker's reaction to his condition or to his treatment by others. Some of the physical and psychological problems of persons with cerebral palsy are these: convulsions, mental retardation, visual impairments, hearing loss (especially in persons with athetoid cerebral palsy), other impairments of sensation, strong fears and adjustment difficulties, perseveration, forced responsiveness to stimuli, distractibility, and hyperactivity.

The great majority of cases of cerebral palsy fall into four main clinical types.

46

These categories are somewhat arbitrary, since many cases represent mixed types. (1) Spastic cerebral palsy: characterized by an impairment of voluntary move-ment, an increase in deep reflexes, increased muscle tone (tenseness), resistance to manipulation, and an exaggerated stretch reflex (elicited when a muscle is sud-denly stretched, with a consequent blocking of the movement because of the reflex contraction of the antagonistic muscle). (2) Athetosis: the essential characteristic of which is the presence of unpatterned, unrhythmical, involuntary wriggling and writhing movements overlaid on voluntary bodily movements and interfering with them. (3) Ataxia: characterized by incoordination, the individual being unable to control the magnitude or direction of voluntary movements. (4) Rigidity: char-acterized by a more continual and more pronounced degree of tenseness than is found in spastic cerebral palsy.

SOME POINTS TO BE EMPHASIZED

1. Some speech-retarded children have been disagnosed as cerebral palsied before coming to the speech examination. In such cases, you should determine from parents or medical records the clinical type and the probable etiological factors.

2. In undiagnosed cases of speech retardation with suspected physical basis for the problem, you should obtain full details concerning past and present speech and physical symptoms, the birth and developmental history, and the medical history. Minimal cues picked up from a detailed history may prompt a referral for a neurological examination which in turn may indicate whether a clear diagnosis of brain damage is warranted.

3. The social history should indicate how the speaker feels about himself and how he is being treated by his family and associates. Scrutinize closely the speaker's semantic environment and his semantic reactions. Explore here particularly, as well as in the developmental history, for indications of what the family has done to develop independence in the speaker as a child, and consider what this manner of treatment suggests concerning the family attitude toward the speaker and his problem.

4. Most cerebral palsied persons have multiple handicaps; and it is necessary, therefore, to determine the nature of the many obstacles that confront each such person and his potential for overcoming them.

SUPPLEMENTARY QUESTIONS

History of Speech Problem: Describe the speech problem. If the speaker is a child, when he wishes something, does he ask for it by using words or does he simply point? Can others understand what he means? Does the family make an effort to require him to speak when he wants something? In the opinion of the parents, did he begin to speak at the same age as the other children in the family? As the child grew older, did his speech improve, become worse, or remain the same? Does the child's speech become worse at certain times? Under what circumstances? Have the parents tried to help the child with his speech? Does he like to be read to? Can the parents hold his attention in reading, conversation, and game-playing? Does he usually seem to understand what is being said to him? (If the speaker is an older child or adult, these questions are to be modified accordingly.)

DEVELOPMENTAL HISTORY

Pregnancy: During pregnancy did the mother have any of the following: severe nausea and vomiting; toxemia; hypertension; any acute disease (especially virus infections such as German measles); anemia; bleeding; X-ray treatments in pelvic region; nutritional deficiency; metabolic disturbance? Did she take insulin, thyroid, drugs? Specify during what part of the pregnancy the above conditions, if any, occurred. Is there a parental Rh incompatibility? Any family history of syphilis?

Birth and Neonatal Period: Duration of labor. Labor induced? Breech delivery? Cesarean section? Forceps used? Placenta previa? Was there a drop in maternal blood pressure during delivery? Was the mother given morphine or barbiturates? Did she have spinal or caudal analgesia?

Concerning the baby, is there a report of jaundice; blueness; pallor; weak cry; convulsions; twitchings; drowsiness; listlessness? Was he considered premature? Was there evidence of head trauma; kinking of umbilical cord; strangulation by cord; blockage of respiratory tract by mucus or fluid? Was blood transfusion necessary; administration of oxygen; incubator? Birth weight. (Birth weights of other children in family and of the parents themselves.)

Physical Growth and Development: At what age was the physical incapacity noticed? Was there a persistence of the tonic neck reflex? Was baby hypertonic? Was there excessive crying; trouble swallowing or sucking; vomiting; refusal to nurse? Was baby a feeding problem; a "colic" baby; a "tongue-pusher"? How were eating and drinking problems handled? Describe present diet. Appetite at first and now? Much drooling; when ended?

Was the baby a "back-archer"? Did he resist a slow pull upward from supine to sitting position? Was he able to hold head up when supine; when prone? Age of sitting; of standing? Age when rolled over? Age, manner, and distance of creeping or crawling?

Age when he stood with support; stood alone; walked with support; walked alone? Did he fall much? Was he able to move easily from lying to sitting or standing? How is his sitting balance; kneeling balance; standing balance? Does he stand wide-based? Position of knees while standing (flexed, hyperextended)? Does he climb stairs? How? Does he walk on toes; have scissors gait? Does he have more trouble with hands or feet? How much time has been spent in teaching him to walk?

What is speaker's handedness? Any left-handedness in family? At what age did child develop grasp and release? Can he turn pages; write with crayons or pencils; use scissors?

What degree of self-help has speaker developed? Is he able to feed self; use spoon, fork, knife; wash; dress; button; tie shoe laces; brush teeth; go to bathroom unaided; comb hair? What articles can't he handle? If certain skills have not been developed, to what extent have opportunities been afforded the speaker to develop them? How much time has been spent in teaching him self-help?

Medical History: Secure full details concerning each early serious illness: duration; high fever; diagnosis; known sequelae; any headaches associated with illness? Has speaker suffered any violence to head; possible skull fractures; convulsions? Give age at each, sequelae, and medication.

Has speaker had any operations? Have braces ever been recommended or fitted? How successful were they? Are eyes involved? How? Impression of hearing. How has hearing been tested? Does speaker startle easily? Does he respond to loud noises; soft noises; loud voices; soft voices; whispering? Does he attempt to localize sounds?

Have tremors been noted; nervous movements in tongue or extremities; rhythmical or unrhythmical involuntary movements; tenseness of muscles; muscle weakness; paralysis? Has speaker ever been described as spastic, athetoid, or ataxic? Has anyone suspected or diagnosed cerebral palsy?

Social History: What does the speaker do during the course of the day? How much freedom does he have to choose his activities? If speaker is a child does the mother consider him to be more trouble to her than the other children? Is he more disobedient, dependent, quiet, withdrawn, irritable, impulsive, distractible, hyperactive? Does he have a shorter attention span?

How is the child punished when he misbehaves? Does he play with his siblings or other children very much? Does he get around the neighborhood alone or accompanied to meet other children? Do the parents take the child with them when they go to church or the movies or visiting friends? Does he enjoy going places and meeting people? Do other children ever make fun of him because of the way he speaks, walks, or acts? If so, how have the parents handled such incidents? Does the child seem motivated to improve in walking, self-help, speech? (If the speaker is an older child or adult, these questions are to be modified accordingly.)

What do the parents think is wrong with the speaker? If they have heard of cerebral palsy, what do they think causes it? What reading have they done on the subject? Do they feel that they are in any way responsible for the speaker's problems? Do they seem to have guilt feelings about his condition? Are they ashamed of him or of themselves? Are they oversolicitous; rejecting? What do they think will be the probable outcome of the problem? Are they optimistic; pessimistic?

SUPPLEMENTARY CASE HISTORY OUTLINE: CLEFT PALATE

GENERAL INFORMATION ABOUT THE DISORDER

Cleft palate and cleft lip are the result of some factor or factors which interfere with the normal development of the mouth and face during early embryonic life. The exact nature and mode of operation of these factors is not yet fully known, but they must be in operation by the third month of fetal life because by the end of the third month the lips, upper dental arch, and palate have been completely formed. Generally the severity of the cleft condition depends upon how extensively these factors are operating during the part of the fetal period when the facial and palatal structures are undergoing particularly rapid growth.

The speech problems encountered with cleft palate vary from case to case. The most frequent cause of the speech problems is velopharyngeal incompetence. When this is true the speech is usually characterized by slighted, omitted, distorted, or substituted fricatives and plosives, and by nasal voice quality. Sometimes a nasal snort or a glottal stop is substituted for a fricative or plosive. The person with a cleft palate may produce facial contortions in his attempts to build up sufficient intraoral breath pressure and to compensate in other ways for difficulties in phonation and articulation. In addition, the speech problem may be complicated by other abnormalities of the articulators that may be associated with cleft palate. Moreover, the speaker may misarticulate for reasons that are nonorganic as well as organic.

A child with a cleft palate may have difficulty in eating. Soft food and liquid may pass up into the nose during swallowing. Sucking may be difficult. In some cases teeth are missing or misaligned, causing problems in mastication and digestion, as well as distortions in articulaton.

Hearing also is frequently impaired. One possible reason for the high incidence of hearing problems in cases of cleft palate is that the mechanism for opening the pharyngeal orifice of the eustachian tube may be faulty, with a resulting impairment of the aeration or ventilation of the tube and increased danger of infection within the tube and middle ear. Another possible reason is that, in the abscence of a normally functioning palate, the eustachian tube is unusually susceptible to infection because of undue exposure to foreign bodies and bacteria.

Obviously a facial disfigurement or a severe speech problem can result in emotional disturbances and special problems of adjustment for the child and the parents as well. Parental rejection and overprotection may result. The child may find it hard to accept his problems and to live happily in spite of associates who do not understand and accept him, and he may gradually withdraw from social relationships. Manifestations of such withdrawal may be obvious (refusal to meet new people or to participate in social activities, or reduction of verbal output) or more
50

subtle (failure to speak loudly enough, or reduction in activity of the articulators in speaking). Adjustment problems may be intensified during adolescence, and in adulthood they may take on importance in relation to vocational development and marriage.

SOME POINTS TO BE EMPHASIZED

1. For diagnostic purposes and also in the interests of long-term research objectives it is advantageous to obtain a record of any etiological factors possibly related to heredity or events occurring during the first trimester of pregnancy.

2. Some of the information to be included in the History of the Speech Problem is obtained by examination of the speech mechanism or by consulting medical records rather than by questioning the parents. Whatever sources you use, you should obtain (a) a description of the cleft and any associated abnormalities, (b) an account of any surgery that has been performed and an evaluation of its effectiveness, and (c) essential information about the nature and suitability of any prosthetic appliances with which the person has been fitted.

3. The Social History should indicate how the speaker feels about himself and how he is being treated by his parents, his siblings, and his associates. You should give special attention to his semantic environment and his own semantic reactions.

SUPPLEMENTARY QUESTIONS

History of Speech Problem: When was the cleft discovered? Specify which of the following structures the cleft involved: the lip, alveolar ridge, hard palate, soft palate. Was the cleft unilateral or bilateral?

What surgery has been performed? Specify which of the following structures it involved: the lip, alveolar ridge, hard palate, soft palate. Did it include a pharyngeal flap operation for improving velopharyngeal competence? Has any plastic surgery been done? At what age was each operation performed?

Has the speaker been examined by a prosthodontist or orthodontist? Has he ever been fitted with a prosthetic device ("speech appliance," obturator)? If so, does it consist of a palatal bulb, a replacement for missing teeth, or both? How successful have the operations and prosthetic appliance been in assisting the person with his eating and speaking?

Describe the speech problem. If the speaker is a child can the parents usually understand what he is saying? Do the other members of the family understand the child when he speaks? When the child wishes something, does he ask for it by using words or does he simply point? In the opinion of the parents, did he begin to speak at the same time as the other children in the family? Did he at first and does he now speak as much as the other children? As the child grew older, did his speech improve, become worse, or remain the same? Does he speak loudly enough? How have the parents tried to help him with his speech? Has the child received any outside help with his speech? Does the child realize that the speaks differently from other children? How has he shown this realization? (If the speaker is an older child or adult, these questions are to be modified accordingly.)

Developmental History: Describe any unusual things that happened during the pregnancy: Did the mother have any illness such as German measles; have any X-ray therapy directed to the pelvic region; take any drugs during pregnancy; suffer any bleeding?

What difficulties were there in nursing the child? How were these handled? Did the child have difficulty in eating solid foods? How was this handled? Does the person at present have any difficulty in eating? Does he have a normal diet?

Social History: What does the child do during the course of the day? Does the mother consider this child to be more trouble to her than the other children; more dependent? How is the child punished when he misbehaves? Does the child play much with his brothers and sisters or other children? Do the parents take the child with them when they go to church or the movies? Do they take the child with them when they visit their friends? Does he enjoy going places and meeting people? Do the other children ever make fun of him because of the way in which he speaks or looks? If so, how have the parents handled such incidents?

What do the parents think caused the child's problem? Are they concerned about having more children? If so, is the concern the result of the care required by this child or because of the possibility that subsequent children may also have clefts? Do they think that clefts tend to "run in families"? What reading have they done on the subject of cleft palate? Do they feel that they are in any way responsible for the child's problems? Do they have guilt feelings about them? Are they oversolicitous; rejecting? What do they think will be the probable outcome of the child's problem? (If the speaker is an older child or adult, these questions are to be modified accordingly.)

If the speaker is an older child or adult are there problems concerning the selection of a vocation? Are the vocational goals realistic? Has the speaker's choice been influenced by the attitudes of others concerning the place of individuals with clefts; by the attitudes of the speaker concerning his "place"? Does the speaker feel that his cleft will make it difficult for him to get married? If married, does he feel that his cleft has affected his marriage in any way?

SUPPLEMENTARY CASE HISTORY OUTLINE: DYSPHASIA

GENERAL INFORMATION ABOUT THE DISORDER

Dysphasia is a disorder of language function—a disturbance of the ability to recognize and use the symbols by means of which we relate to our surroundings and to other people. It is not the result of paralysis of the speech musculature nor of deafness or other sensory loss. It is a specific dysfunction in the recognition or expression—or both—of language symbols. It results from damage to the brain. The damage (whether the result of a hemorrhage, thrombosis, embolism, infection, tumor, bullet wound, concussion, or other cause) involves part of the so-called association areas of the brain, which constitute complex cortical mechanisms by means of which sensory complexes are correlated, integrated, and resolved into motor complexes. When the damage results in a complete loss of language, the condition is known as aphasia. The more usual effect is a less than complete impairment of language function, and so the more appropriate term for most cases is dysphasia.

Dysphasia is not only a disorder of language but may also involve one or more of a large number of nonlanguage effects, including physical and personality changes. No one statement can describe dysphasia adequately; not only is each dysphasic person different originally from every other, but also the changes that result from brain injury are numerous and assume a variety of patterns. However, in the following paragraphs we offer, for purposes of general orientation to the problem, a greatly oversimplified description of some of the principal changes recognized in the language, personality, and physical behavior of persons who have become dysphasic.

Language Disturbances: Sufficiently detailed questioning and testing will probably reveal that the langauge difficulty is both receptive and expressive in nature.

The dysphasic person may not be able to express himself adequately. For example, he may wish to say, "I want a glass of water," and be unable to say "water"; or he may substitute another word for "water," such as "butter"; or his sentence may be incomplete or incorrectly organized. This inability to express himself may be so severe that his speaking vocabulary is limited to a few automatic expressions or to a few meaningfully used words such as "yes" and "no." In some cases the person may be unable to produce voluntarily even the speech sounds of the language. Difficulty in expression may extend to disability in writing the language.

The dysphasic person may have difficulty in understanding what is said to him. For example, if he is told to point to a pencil, he may point to some other object or in some other way respond incorrectly. He is likely to manifest increasing difficulty in responding as the instructions increase in length and complexity. Difficulty

53

in comprehension may extend to understanding written or printed language.

These are only a few examples of the ways in which language behavior may be affected. It should be remembered that dysphasic patients typically have some degree of difficulty in many areas of language and that these disabilities are present in varying degrees of severity in different persons.

Personality Changes: These changes may be extreme or comparatively mild. A person whose family would have described him formerly as generally complacent may come to exhibit extreme irritation and anger on slight provocation. On the other hand, a tense, driving individual may become passive.

Since the dysphasic person is less able to do certain things that he formerly could do with ease, he is likely to experience repeated frustration. For example, he may be unable to understand clearly what is said to him, to speak his name or the names of his family, to ask or answer questions, to name objects, to do simple arithmetic, to read the newspaper, or to write even his own name. It is not difficult to understand, therefore, why emotional outbursts may occur in dysphasic individuals.

Some dysphasic persons become depressed or anxious as a result of their condition. Tearfulness, discouragement, and worry are not uncommon reactions. Other patients, however, show an abnormal unconcern and even cheerfulness (euphoria). The patient's ability to concentrate his attention on a particular task for a given period of time may also be reduced; his memory may be poor; his judgment, initiative, and organizing ability may be impaired; and the patient may become withdrawn, impulsive, or even infantile.

Physical Disturbances: There may be motor and sensory impairments associated with the purely dysphasic difficulties. The person may be paralyzed, for example; if the paralysis involves the speech and breathing musculature, the resulting speech disturbance is called dysarthria. Vision may be impaired. The patient is likely to tire easily. He may experience feelings of dizziness, fainting, severe headaches, and sudden losses of consciousness. He may be subject to convulsive seizures.

SOME POINTS TO BE EMPHASIZED

1. Prognosis in dysphasia depends upon a number of physical and psychological factors. Therefore, in order to plan a program of therapy and estimate its probable success, you need a full description of the patient's premorbid abilities and personality characteristics, together with an account of the changes noted in his language, personality, and physical behavior.

2. A dysphasic patient may be expected to progress faster in therapy if the clinician uses materials related to his former occupation, interests, and hobbies and in line with his educational background. Therefore, it is desirable to obtain information about these matters.

3. The environmental aspects of the dysphasic person's life are crucial. His progress may be determined by the reactions of the persons with whom he is in

daily contact. Find out what his associates know about his problems and what insights they have into them. Get a clear picture of whether their everyday, moment-by-moment treatment of him is such as to facilitate or to hinder his recovery. His semantic environment and his semantic reactions deserve close scrutiny.

4. The term dysphasia does not denote disturbed sensory or motor function, but associated incidentally with dysphasia there may be either sensory or motor impairments or both. It is necessary to determine the nature of all the obstacles that confront each patient and his potential for overcoming them.

SUPPLEMENTARY QUESTIONS

History of Speech Disorder: What has been regarded as the cause of the patient's dysphasic condition? When did the accident (operation, illness, etc.) occur? Obtain details of the subsequent course of events: initial symptoms or behavior, "spontaneous recovery," nature and rate of changes noted.

Secure as much detail as possible concerning the initial language behavior and the reactions to this behavior by physicians, nurses, and members of the family. Were these people eager to have him start talking? Did they talk to him or at him but without asking or expecting a response? Did they urge him to answer them? Did they show concern or impatience if he failed to answer adequately? How did they handle fragmentary and incorrect answers? Similarly describe current practices and expectations.

Has he had any speech help? What kind? Results? Is speech therapy currently available? Has medical clearance been given for speech therapy?

Expressive Aspects: Does the patient try to use words? Sentences? When he wants something, does he ask for it in words (or try to ask) or does he just point? Does he use the right words? Does the family understand what he is saying or is he difficult to understand because he mixes up the words? If he speaks in sentences, does he leave out the little words such as "if," "of," "the," and "and"? Can he recall the names of persons and things? Can he use nouns; verbs; adjectives; prepositions; conjunctions; articles?

Does he say greetings and farewells such as "Hello," "How are you?" "Hi," "Good-bye"? How well can he repeat the alphabet; count; say the days of the week; swear? Does he remember parts of prayers or poems or scripture passages? Is he able to sing? What songs or parts of songs does he sing?

Does the family include him in their conversation as much as possible or, as a rule, pay little attention to him? Does the family let him talk for himself as much as possible or do they try to talk for him? (For example, when someone asks him a question, is he allowed to answer it as best he can or is the answer supplied for him?) Does the family try to help him by supplying words when he encounters difficulty in expressing himself? Does the family anticipate his needs and wishes or try to guess what he wants? (For example, at meals are dishes passed to him at his request or in anticipation of his request?) Do his associates correct him when he says the wrong word?

Does he begin conversations himself without first being addressed by someone else? Does he do as much talking now as he did before his accident (operation, illness, etc.)? How well is he able to write? What special disabilities in writing does he show?

Receptive Aspects: Can he follow simple requests and instructions (for example, "Turn on the radio") or does he seem not to understand what is said to him? Can he carry out more complicated instructions? Does he understand when someone tells him of some incident or of something in the paper? How does the informant know he understands?

How much does he read? What does he read? How well does he apparently grasp what he reads? How well does he grasp what he hears on radio and TV?

Does he know what the different table utensils are (for example, does he distinguish between a knife and a fork)? Can he recognize parts of the body; colors; forms? Can he make change?

Medical History: Who is the physician in charge of the case? Does the patient have any paralysis? What parts of his body are paralyzed? What treatment is being used for the paralysis? With what results?

Has he had any operations? What? When? Has he ever had a plate inserted in his head? Were any changes noted after insertion of plate? Does he ever complain of headaches? Severity? Frequency? Does he ever complain of faintness? Dizziness? Does he ever lose consciousness? Does he ever have convulsive seizures? What kind? What medication has been prescribed for them? Results of medication?

Does he seem unusually fatigable? How much sleep does he get daily? Does he spend most of his day resting or is he usually active? How much walking does he do? How is his appetite? Does he have any difficulty in eating; in dressing himself? Does he have a sense of direction? Does he distinguish between right and left?

Does he ever complain that he cannot see, hear, or feel things properly? Estimate his auditory and visual acuity.

School History: How far did he go in school? What kind of grades did he make in school? Has he ever studied any particular subject since he left school? Has he maintained an interest in intellectual pursuits?

Social History: What is or was his occupation? Did he like his work? Would he like to return to it? Does he expect to? Is he worried that he may not be able to? Are the members of his family worried that he may cease to be their breadwinner? Have they discussed this matter with him? Has he changed jobs often? What hobbies and other interests has he had outside of his job? Does he still show an interest in these? What did he formerly do for recreation? What clubs, fraternal organizations, or other groups did he belong to? How active has he been in them? How active is he now?

What kind of movies did he formerly like to go to? Does he go now? What did he formerly like to read in the newspaper? Does he read papers now? Did he and does he now like to read books and magazines or to be read to? Describe his radio and TV listening habits.

Did he formerly take a great deal of interest in his family—spend much time with them? Does he now take an interest in the family? (For example, if he has children or grandchildren, does he play with them quite often?)

Does he like card games? Which ones? How frequently does he play them now? Is he interested in his friends? Does he like to see them? How often does he see them? Has he indicated that he would like them to visit him? When there are visitors in the home, does he seem interested in them and what they are saying? Does he understand and laugh at jokes? Does he try to carry on conversations? How well does he succeed?

Has his personality changed? How? Describe his present personality. Does he ever lose his temper suddenly or become very angry or highly emotional? If so, does the informant know of any reasons why he should become upset as he does? Does he become angry when members of the family try to help him with something? Is he depressed or anxious about his condition, or perhaps too cheerful and unconcerned about it? Has he ever indicated in any way that he desires to do something about his problem? Does he trust his ability and judgment?

When he has difficulty in doing something such as dressing himself, does the family help him as much as possible or allow him to do it for himself and assist him only when he asks for help? Do they think it would be a good idea to allow him to do as many things as possible for himself? Are they oversolicitous?

Has anyone ever explained aphasia or dysphasia to the family? Have they read about it? How do the members of the family feel about the patient? Have they ever expressed any opinions about his condition and his present characteristics? What opinions? Were they expressed in his presence? Do members of the family become angry or impatient with him or criticize him in any way? How do they act when he becomes angry or upset? Do they try to reason with him or scold him, or do they leave him alone and hope he will soon get over it? Do they or does he for any reason feel guilty about his condition or the causes of it? Do they seem to want to spend time with him and try to help him? Are they optimistic or pessimistic about the outcome?

GENERAL INFORMATION ABOUT THE PROBLEM

Total removal of the larynx is commonly resorted to in cases of cancer of the larynx. The problem occurs most often among persons over 50 years of age and more often in men than in women. In learning to speak without a larynx, a person must, of course, learn to speak in a manner somewhat different from that in which normal speech is produced. He can no longer use the air from the lungs to set the vocal folds into vibration. He may be taught to take air (most appropriately called an "air charge") into the esophagus and then to expel it in such a way that certain structures near the top of the esophagus at approximately the level of the cricoid cartilage are set into vibration. The sound produced is then articulated. Because of X-ray burns on the tissues of the neck, or the reactions of the patient to the use of the air charge, or his inability to control the air charge, it may be necessary for him to use an artificial larynx of some type. In such instances tone is produced by an electrically powered vibrator, and the articulators are used in the normal way to form the speech sounds.

SOME POINTS TO BE EMPHASIZED

1. Determine the period of time that has elapsed since surgery. Has medical clearance for the starting of speech therapy been given?

2. Determine how much information the person has about his condition. Does he understand why it was necessary to have his larynx removed? Does he have some idea of how speech is produced? Does he realize that the vibrators that normally produce the sound necessary for speech have been removed? Does he know that it is possible to produce speech even though the larynx has been removed? Was any information given to him about alternative methods of speech production before the operation? Did he have the proper information and opportunity to practice the production of esophageal tones before the operation? Has he talked to any other laryngectomized person?

3. Success in mastering a wholly new way of speaking depends to a considerable degree upon certain personality factors. Successful acquisition of skill in using esophageal speech requires much experimentation on the part of the patient. How willing is he to devote time and effort to experimenting in an effort to master a new skill? How likely is he to be discouraged by initial failure? Is he apt to be easily embarrassed while attempting to learn esophageal speech? Before his operation how talkative was he, how socially inclined, how extrovertive? Is he currently disturbed by insecurity regarding future employment or by fears of the

recurrence of cancer? What information has he been given about his physical condition? Is he able to continue doing the same work that he was doing before the operation? Does he have other problems of readjustment?

4. Have his wife and other members of his family been counseled concerning the effects of his laryngectomy on his speech? Are they encouraging, impatient, over-protective, solicitous, matter-of-fact, embarrassed, optimistic, pessimistic? How has the person's laryngectomy changed their relationship with him?

5. Does the speaker have information about groups and agencies that will be interested in helping him, such as the local division of the American Cancer Society, or The International Association of Laryngectomees (521 W. 57th Street, New York 19, New York)? Does he know about *IAL News* which will be mailed to him by the Association upon request? Does he know about the existence of Lost Chord Clubs? Has he tried to find out if one exists in his locality?

SUPPLEMENTARY CASE HISTORY OUTLINE: THE STUTTERING PROBLEM

In adapting the basic case study interview methods described in this chapter to the study of the stuttering problem, it is important that you keep clearly in mind the three major uses of the term "stuttering" that are discussed in Chapter 9. By doing so you will minimize confusion and bring into focus the three main aspects of the problem: (1) the ways in which the speaker's important listeners evaluate and react to his speech disfluencies; (2) the ways in which the speaker evaluates and reacts to his own speech disfluencies and to the reactions made to them by his listeners; and (3) the speaker's disfluencies and related tensings and other reactions, together with such factors, other than (1) and (2), as may seem to be associated with them.

SUPPLEMENTARY QUESTIONS AND CONSIDERATIONS

Interviewing and counseling methods provide the major approaches to the first two of the three aspects of the problem referred to in the preceding paragraph. In taking the case history of a stutterer you should be at special pains to obtain essential information concerning the following aspects of the problem.

Onset and Early Development of Speech Problem: You should make a reasonably thorough, but considerate, effort to find out from the informant— whether this is the stutterer himself or some other person—if his account of the onset and early development of the problem is (1) about his own personal observations, his own clear and detailed memory, or is (2) mostly or wholly a secondhand account told to him by others, or is (3) essentially a family legend without documented reference to dates, places, or other relevant particulars. You will seldom be able to obtain a clear and detailed firsthand account documented as to specific time and place. What the stutterer, or other informant, however, believes the facts were is quite as important as the facts themselves, whatever they may have been. What a person believes to be true affects his attitudes, feelings, and actions. As a clinician you have this question to ask of yourself: "If I were to believe the facts to be what the informant thinks they are, and if I were to view the nature and causes of the problem as he does, how would I be most likely to feel about it and what would I probably try to do about it?" Your answer will hardly be exactly like that of the informant, of course, but if you appreciate this fact, your conscientious effort to answer the question should serve to expand somewhat your understanding of the problem.

Speaker's Experience with the Problem: Cover the highlights of the speaker's experience with the problem. At what times and in what places have there been marked changes in his speech behavior for the worse or the better. If the stutterer is old enough to cooperate, use Form 1 to obtain a graphic summary of his account of the ups and downs in the severity of the problem and of the changes in his situation or other conditions that were, either in fact or in his belief or supposition, associated with them. If the speaker is a child and the problem is one that is to be defined chiefly in terms descriptive of the feelings and assumptions and overt reactions of the parents, you should try to get from them an account of their own main experiences with the problem. Although Form 1 will hardly be suitable in such a case, you should find out what you can about the circumstances associated with the waxings and wanings of the parents' concern about the child's speech.

Social Aspects: What differences has the problem made to the speaker socially, educationally, vocationally, and in more deeply personal ways, provided he is old enough for the problem to have made such differences? Again, what the stutterer believes the facts to have been is quite as important as the actual facts, if indeed these might ever be known.

Outlook: What is the informant's outlook on the future? If the speaker is a young child, do the parents seem to expect him to get better as he gets older, or are they inclined to worry about the future course of the problem? If the speaker is old enough to have taken on the problem himself, is he hopeful of improving his speech? Or has past experience with clinical treatment, or with do-it-yourself speech correction, left him with a degree of discouragement, and perhaps with certain unfortunate ideas about himself and his problem, that must now be counteracted if he is to make a sustained effort to improve?

You can sometimes find out a great deal about the significance of the problem, as the speaker himself feels it, by asking him, "If you were to awaken in the morning and find yourself able to speak normally, what difference would it make? What would you do that you have not been doing? What have you been doing that you would stop doing?" The stutterer's answers to these questions can suggest to you much about the way he understands his problem, how he feels about it, and just how it is important to him. His answers will also indicate what significance normal speech or "becoming a normal speaker" holds for him. They will give you a clue as to what, if anything, improvement means to him, or whether—as may well be the case—he recognizes no middle ground for *improvement* between stuttering and normal speech. Finally, on the basis of what he says, it may be possible for you to gauge the strength of his motivation or determination to work for improvement.

Language Used in Talking About Problem: What language does the informant use in talking about the problem? If the speaker is an older child or adult, does he talk about "his stuttering" as though he personally has nothing to do with "it," except to contend with "it," to endure "it," to fear and regret "it," Or does he at least now and then or in a few respects, talk as though the aspects of his speaking that he calls stuttering were something that he himself does, rather than some alien thing that happens to him? Does he talk a "do" language ("I *do* certain things that interfere with my speaking; I *hold my breath,* for example, *I press my lips together,* and I *do* other things like that instead of *doing* the things anyone else would *do* in talking")? Or does he talk instead a "have and am" language ("I *have* a tendency to *have* blocks when I talk because I *am* a stutterer and I *am* nervous, and I *have* trouble talking because I don't *have* confidence and so I don't *have* good speech because, after all, I *am* not a normal speaker")?

The basic question is this: To what extent does the speaker take personal responsibility for doing the hesitating, tensing, and other activities that he refers to as stuttering, and to what extent does he talk as though these activities or goings-on were none of his doings? In general, the more he talks about stuttering as something he does, the more likely he is to take personal responsibility for doing it—and so for doing something different in order to talk better or as well as possible. On the other hand, the more he talks about stuttering as something that happens to him, the more likely he is to exert effort to try to avoid it or control it. He may even pretend he doesn't know about it or that he is not speaking in any unusual way, because he doesn't see anything he can do about it and so he acts as though he were telling himself that nothing is the matter at all. And there are other ways in which he may contend with "it" as though with some mysterious and unnerving assailant or external force. Moreover, if he believes that ' it" is something beyond his control he will be inclined to take for granted that someone else must cure him because he will feel that there is nothing he can do about "it" himself. The language the speaker uses in talking about the problem is, therefore, an important part of the problem, and modification of it from a "have and am" to a "do" language—from a language that is largely animistic and vague and disowning of personal responsibility to one that is appropriately descriptive and clear and acknowledging of personal responsiblity—is an important aspect of therapy.

If the informants are the parents, you will want to note whether they talk about the stuttering as though it were a disorder, or affliction, or impediment, or defect visited upon the child, or as though it were an activity performed by the child. Do they refer to stuttering as a *symptom of* something or as the child's *response to* something? Do the parents recognize or acknowledge a personal role of any sort in creating or maintaining the problem, or in affecting it in any way? Do the parents talk as though they wonder if the child, in doing what they refer to as stuttering, is reacting to them? If so, to what about themselves in particular do they seem to think the child is reacting? Do the parents take personal responsibility in any sense for the problem and, if so, in what sense? If they do not, what specifically do they seem to be talking about when they answer the question, "What is the problem?"

TABLE 1. Incidence of Various Birth Conditions of Children as Reported in Specified Sources Indicated by Reference Numbers

Birth Condition	Incidence Percent[a]	Reference Number
Entirely normal	38.9	7
Premature	6.1	2
	2.4	40
	3.0	14
Postmature	24.1	36
Cesarean delivery	3.8	7
	2.7	30
	2.4	42
	5.0	15
	2.0	17
Instrumental delivery	33.6	7
Operative delivery	29.3	41
Breech delivery	1.8	7
	4.8	45
	3.9	55
	2.8	39
	3.2	12
	2.6	23
Cyanosis; asphyxia neonatorum	5.6	6
Induced labor	30.0	38
Precipitate labor	11.5	41
Prolonged labor	2.7	41
Postpartum fever	25.5	41
Maternal deaths	0.7	41
Infant deaths	10.4	41

[a] Rounded to one decimal point.

TABLE 2. Mean Height and Weight of American Boys, Aged 2 to 18 Years, as Reported in Four Studies

	(1)		(2)		(3)		(4)	
Age yrs.	Height cm.	Weight kg.	Height cm.	Weight kg.	Height cm.	Weight kg.	Height in.	Weight lb.
2	84.9	11.7			86.8	12.7		
2½	88.6	12.8			91.4	13.8		
3	92.8	13.7	97.84[a]	15.63[a]	94.8	14.7		
3½	96.3	14.6	101.66[a]	16.71[a]	98.5	15.6		
4	100.1	15.5	104.99[a]	17.47[a]	102.5	16.6	40.9	38.2
4½	102.7	16.3	108.48[a]	18.44[a]	105.8	17.4		
5	105.8	16.9	111.40[a]	19.48[a]	108.9	18.6	43.9	43.2
5½	108.8	17.7	114.49[a]	20.45[a]	112.4	19.7		
6	112.0	18.6	117.41[a]	21.50[a]	115.6	20.6	46.1	47.6
6½	119.1	20.3			118.7	21.7		
7	120.7	21.3	121.91	23.52	121.5	23.3	48.2	52.5
7½	125.0	23.3			124.1	23.9		
8	127.8	24.6	128.13	26.34	127.4	25.3	50.4	58.2
8½	130.8	25.4			129.6	26.3		. .
9	131.1	27.4	133.71	28.98	131.9	27.7	52.4	64.4
9½	133.9	28.2			134.7	30.3		
10	135.9	30.4	138.94	32.53	137.0	31.0	54.3	70.7
10½	138.9	32.3						
11	138.9	33.3	143.20	35.29			56.2	77.6
11½	142.0	34.3						
12	145.0	36.7	147.81	38.66			58.2	85.6
12½	147.1	38.4						
13	149.9	40.6	153.31	43.64			60.5	95.6
13½	151.9	39.8						
14	154.7	43.1	159.39	48.62			63.0	107.9
14½	159.0	44.9						
15	163.8	47.6	165.15	54.94			65.6	121.7
15½	164.3	52.6						
16	166.9	53.9	169.73	58.36			67.3	131.9
16½	166.4	57.7						
17	168.9	58.3	173.51	62.42			68.2	138.3
17½	168.9	57.6						
18	168.9	58.5	174.15	64.67				

[a] The midpoint of the range of ages represented by these mean values is the age indicated plus 3 months; e.g., the value for age 3 represents the mean of all values within the age range from 3 years 0 months to 3 years 5 months 30 days, with a midpoint of 3 years 3 months. The remaining values in this study pertain to age ranges with a midpoint as indicated; e.g., the value for age 7 represents the mean of all values within an age range of 6 years 6 months to 7 years 5 months 30 days, with 7 years 0 months as the midpoint.

SOURCE: (1) Baldwin, 3; (2) Meredith, 37; (3) Vickers and Stuart, 52; (4) Martin, 34.

TABLE 3. Mean Height and Weight of American Girls, Aged 2 to 18 Years, as Reported in Four Studies

	(1)		(2)		(3)		(4)	
Age yrs.	Height cm.	Weight kg.	Height cm.	Weight kg.	Height cm.	Weight kg.	Height in.	Weight lb.
2	83.5	11.1	86.94	12.32	85.9	12.4		
2½	87.9	12.2	91.47	13.33	90.8	13.6		
3	91.5	13.1	95.57	14.46	94.6	14.5		
3½	95.3	14.1	98.94	15.62	98.4	15.7		
4	98.4	14.6	102.48	16.63	101.0	16.7	40.9	37.3
4½	101.7	15.4	105.68	17.44	104.6	17.8		
5	105.1	16.4	108.93	18.19	108.0	18.8	43.6	42.0
5½	107.4	17.1	112.39	19.51	111.5	19.7		
6	109.7	18.1	115.02	20.56	113.9	20.5	45.8	46.4
6½	117.4	21.2			116.8	21.6		
7	120.9	21.9	120.94	22.90	119.5	22.8	47.9	51.2
7½	122.9	22.2			122.5	24.0		
8	125.0	23.3	126.74	25.65	124.9	25.4	50.0	56.9
8½	126.2	25.2			127.0	26.9		
9	130.8	26.4	132.54	28.47	130.9	27.7	52.0	63.0
9½	130.8	26.9			132.3	28.6		
10	134.6	29.7	137.65	31.63	136.5	32.0	54.2	70.3
10½	137.7	29.8						
11	140.0	30.3	143.62	35.83			56.5	79.0
11½	143.8	32.9						
12	145.6	34.2	150.28	40.70			59.0	89.7
12½	147.6	37.7						
13	152.9	43.0	155.96	45.52			60.6	100.3
13½	154.7	43.1						
14	157.0	46.5	159.45	50.32			62.3	108.5
14½	157.5	47.0						
15	159.0	50.8	160.73	53.62			63.2	115.0
15½	159.0	50.4						
16	159.8	49.4	161.35	54.42			63.5	117.6
16½	160.0	51.0						
17	159.8	51.4	161.40	54.31			63.6	119.0
17½	161.8	52.9						
18	162.1	52.5	160.97	54.59				

SOURCE: (1) Baldwin, *3*; (2) Boynton, *8*; (3) Vickers and Stuart, *52*; (4) Martin, *34*.

TABLE 4. Ages at Which Children (Boys and Girls Combined) Have Been Observed to Acquire Eight Motor Skills

Skill	Class of Population Sampled											
	Middle N=107	Middle N=12+	Middle & Upper N=25	All N=61	All N=215	Representative N=100+	Normal N=98	Upper Middle N=45	Upper Normal N=30	Gifted Children N=643	Well Children N=[a,b,c]	Severely Ill Children N=81
	Median Wks.	First Sign Wks.	Median Wks.	Median Mos.	Average Mos.	Average Mos.	Median Mos.	100% Achievement Yrs.	Earliest Age Yrs.	Mean Mos.	Mean Mos.	Mean Mos.
	(1)	(2)	(3)	(4)	(5)	(6)	(7)	(8)	(9)	(10)	(11)	(12)
Sitting	24		31	6.2	6.2					5.96	5.3[a]	5.8
Creeping	48		44.5	9.2	7.3						8.4[b]	9.4
Standing	56		64	10.5	10.7							
Walking	56		64	13.0	12.0	18				13.10[f]	12.8[c]	14.4
Grasping	28[d]	24[e]	64	4.1	8.1					12.87[g]		
Self-feeding	72											
Self-dressing	260							5.0-5.5	2.5-3.0			
Throwing ball	56					36	29[h] 30[i]					

[a] N=619.
[b] N=583.
[c] N=831.
[d] Median age of release varied from 40 to 52 weeks depending upon degree of volition involved in release.
[e] Release was also observed at age of 24 weeks.
[f] Boys.
[g] Girls.
[h] Small ball.
[i] Large ball.

SOURCE: (1) Garrett, 21; (2) Halverson, 24; (3) Shirley, 47; (4) Bayley, 4; (5) Aldrich and Norval, 1; (6) Cunningham, 13; (7) McCaskill and Wellman, 35; (8) Key et al., 28; (9) Wagoner and Armstrong, 53; (10) Terman, 49; Smith, 48; (11) Smith, 48; (12) Smith, 48.

Age	Estimates by Authorities Hours (1)	(2)	(3)	(4)	(5)	Observations Hours: Minutes (6) N=2692	(7) N=78	(8) N=5558	(9) N=102	(10) N=1186	(11) N=34	Summary
0-1		16-18		16	16-22		15:05			14:45		15.00
1-2		12-13	12-14	15	16		13:20		13:42	13:14		13.50
2-3		12-13	12-14	13-14	15		12:49		12:45	12:43	12:30	12.75
3-4		10-11	12-14	13-14	14		12:30		12:52	12:07	11:23	12.25
4-5		10-11	12-14	13-14	13		12:00		12:07	11:43	10:57	11.75
5-6			11-12	13-14	12-13		11:21		11:30	11:18		11.25
6-7	13.5		11-12		12	11:14		9:55	11:16	11:04		11.00
7-8	13		11-12		12	10:41		10:04	11:03	10:58		10.75
8-9	12.5		11-12		11.5	10:42		9:49	10:35			10.50
9-10	12		11-12		11	10:13		9:44	10:42			10.25
10-11	11.5		10		11	9:58		9:15	10:32			10.00

SOURCE: Adapted from Louttit, 32, p. 343. (1) Dukes, 16; (2) Hess, 26; (3) Birnham, 10; (4) Brown, 9; (5) Seham and Seham, 46; (6) Terman and Hocking, 50; (7) Flemming, 20; (8) Hayashi, 25; (9) Chant and Blatz, 11; (10) Faegre and Anderson, 18; (11) Reynolds and Mallay, 43.

TABLE 6. Amount of Time Reportedly Spent in Bed by Children Between 11 and 18

Age	Hours:Minutes
11-12	10:00
12-13	9:36
13-14	9:31
14-15	9:06
15-16	8:54
16-17	8:30
17-18	8:46

SOURCE: Terman and Hocking (50).

TABLE 7. Percentages of Children Whose Parents Considered Them to Have Attained Reliable Bowel and Bladder Control

Age months	Bladder		Bowel	
	Boys	Girls	Boys	Girls
0–8	00.0	00.0	10.4	14.3
9–14	4.8	43.9	31.2	51.2
15–20	45.2	34.2	39.8	22.5
21–26	40.5	17.1	16.6	6.1
27 plus	9.5	4.8	2.0	6.1

SOURCE: Scoe, 44.

TABLE 8. Ages in Months at Which Children Were Reported by Their Parents to Have Attained Reliable Bowel and Bladder Control

	Boys			Girls		
	N	Median	Range	N	Median	Range
Bowel	41	16	6–30	49	12	6–30
Bladder	42	21	12–30	42	16	9–35

SOURCE: Scoe, 44.

TABLE 9. Ages in Months at Which Parents Reported Having Started Toilet Training Their Children

	Boys			Girls		
	N	Median	Range	N	Median	Range
Bowel	71	7	3–24	61	6	1–24
Bladder	65	12	3–24	56	9	1–24

SOURCE: Scoe, 44.

TABLE 10.　Incidence of Nail Biting in Children Aged 5 to 18

Age in Years	Males		Females	
	Number of Cases	Percentage Biting Nails	Number of Cases	Percentage Biting Nails
5	81	42.0	87	34.4
6	155	40.5	137	50.5
7	84	41.6	105	48.5
8	105	63.7	93	59.2
9	75	57.5	75	62.7
10	88	60.2	100	61.0
11	78	64.1	78	51.5
12	88	58.0	78	43.6
13	84	56.0	89	42.6
14	219	53.8	410	36.6
15	317	44.4	443	35.1
16	341	37.8	353	27.1
17	335	38.2	354	18.3
18	80	31.3	55	23.7
Total	2130	46.1	2457	36.7

SOURCE:　Malone and Massler. *33*.

FORM 1.

CHART OF SIGNIFICANT VARIATIONS IN SEVERITY OF THE STUTTERING PROBLEM SINCE ONSET

Name _____ Age _____ Sex _____

Examiner _____ Date _____

As severe as the prob-
lem has ever been

The average severity
of the problem

As slight as the prob-
lem has ever been

No problem (indicate
periods)

1 2 3 4 5 6 7 8 9 10 11 12 13 14 15 16 17 18 19 20 21 22 23 24 25

Years Since Onset

Onset
Year: 19___

Trace the variations in the severity of your stuttering problem by drawing a continuous line from the point representing the onset of the problem (lower left-hand corner of the chart) to the point representing the present time. Write the number 1 beside the first major rise or fall in the line you draw representing a change. Write the number 2 beside the second major change represented, the number 3 beside the third indicated change, and so on, numbering each important turning point in the line, up or down, that represents an increase or a decrease in severity of the problem. Either on the face or on the back of the chart write beside each of the numbers a brief description of the circumstances associated with the change in the problem represented by the number.

Additional copies of this form may be obtained from the Interstate Printers and Publishers, 19-27 North Jackson Street, Danville, Illinois.

REFERENCES

1. Aldrich, C. A., and Mildred A. Norval, "A developmental graph for the first year of life," *Journal of Pediatrics*, 1946, *29*:304-308.
2. Bain, K., J. P. Hubbard, and M. Y. Pennell, "Hospital fatality rates for premature infants," *Pediatrics*, 1949, *4*:454-460.
3. Baldwin, B. T., "The physical growth of children from birth to maturity," *University of Iowa Studies in Child Welfare*, 1921, *1*:1.
4. Bayley, Nancy, "The development of motor abilities during the first three years," *Monographs of the Society for Research in Child Development*, 1935, *1*.
5. Bingham, W. V., and B. V. Moore, *How to Interview*, 3rd rev. ed., New York: Harper, 1941.
6. Blossom, A., "Asphyxia neonatorum, a new method of resuscitation," *Journal of the American Medical Association*, 1951, *146*:1120-1124.
7. Bolduan, C. F., and N. W. Bolduan, *Public Health and Hygiene*, 4th ed., Philadelphia: Saunders, 1949.
8. Boynton, Bernice, "The physical growth of girls," *University of Iowa Studies in Child Welfare*, 1939, *12*, No. 4.
9. Brown, A., *The Normal Child: Its Care and Feeding*, Toronto: McClelland and Stewart, 1926.
10. Burnham, W. H., "The hygiene of sleep," *Pedagogical Seminary*, 1920, *27*:1-35.
11. Chant, Nellie, and W. E. Blatz, "A study of sleeping habits of children," *Genetic Psychology Monographs*, 1928, *4*:13-43.
12. Cummings, W. G., "Breech presentation and delivery," *Quarterly Bulletin of Northwestern University Medical School*, 1951, *25*:304-309.
13. Cunningham, Bess V., "An experiment in measuring gross motor development of infants and young children," *Journal of Educational Psychology*, 1927, *18*:458-464.
14. Dana, E. S., "Premature delivery, causes and results," *American Journal of Obstetrics and Gynecology*, 1946, *51*:329-342.
15. Davis, M. E., "Complete cesarean hysterectomy," *American Journal of Obstetrics and Gynecology*, 1951, *62*:838-853.
16. Dukes, C., *Remedies for the Needless Injury to Children Involved in the Present System of School Education*, London: Rivington, 1899.
17. Eastman, N. J., *William's Obstetrics*, 10th ed., New York: Appleton-Century-Crofts, 1950.
18. Faegre, Marian L., and J. E. Anderson, *Child Care and Training*, Minneapolis: University of Minnesota Press, 1929.
19. Fenlason, Anne F., *Essentials in Interviewing: For the Interviewer Offering Professional Services*, New York: Harper, 1952.
20. Flemming, B. M., "A study of sleep of young children," *Journal of the American Association of University Women*, 1925, *19*:25-27.

21. Garrett, Annette, *Interviewing: Its Principles and Methods*, Family Welfare Association of America, 1942.
22. Gesell, A. L., and C. S. Amatruda, *Developmental Diagnosis*, New York: Hoeber, 1941.
23. Grimes, W. H., R. A. Bartholomew, E. D. Colvin, J. S. Fish, and W. M. Lester, "Management of breech presentation in pregnancy and labor," *Journal of the American Medical Association*, 1952, *148*:788-793.
24. Halverson, H. M., "An experimental study of prehension in infants by means of systematic cinema records," *Genetic Psychology Monographs*, 1931, *10*:107-286.
25. Hayashi, Y., "On the sleeping hours of school children from six to 20 years," *Jido Jatshi (Child's Journal)*, 1925, p. 296. (*Psychological Abstracts*, 1927, *1*:1926.)
26. Hess, J. H., *Principles and Practice of Infant Feeding*, 2nd ed., Philadelphia: Davis, 1918.
27. Johnson, W., S. F. Brown, J. F. Curtis, D. Edney, and Jacqueline Keaster, *Speech Handicapped School Children*, 1st ed., New York: Harper, 1948.
28. Key, Cora P., M. R. White, M. P. Honzik, A. B. Heiney, and Doris Erwin, "The process of learning to dress among nursery-school children," *Genetic Psychology Monographs*, 1936, *18*:67-163.
29. Kinsey, A. C., W. B. Pomeroy, and C. E. Martin, *Sexual Behavior in the Human Male*, Philadelphia: Saunders, 1948.
30. Levine, W., and S. Zeichner, "Rising incidence of cesarean section and effect on maternal and infant mortality," *New York State Journal of Medicine*, 1950, *50*:2707-2713.
31. Long, P. H., "Editor's page: On the history and physical examination of the patient," *Resident Physician*, 1961, *7*:59-62.
32. Louttit, C. M., *Clinical Psychology of Children's Behavior Problems*, New York: Harper, 1947, p. 343.
33. Malone, A. J., and Maury Massler, "Index of nailbiting in children," *Journal of Abnormal and Social Psychology*, 1952, *47*:193-202.
34. Martin, W. E., *Basic Body Measurement of School Age Children*, Washington: U.S. Department of Health, Education and Welfare, Office of Education, 1953.
35. McCaskill, C. L., and Beth Wellman, "A study of common motor achievements at the preschool ages," *Child Development*, 1938, *9*:141-150.
36. McKiddie, J. M., "Foetal mortality in postmaturity," *Journal of Obstetrics and Gynecology of the British Empire*, 1949, *56*:386-392.
37. Meredith, H. V., "The rhythm of physical growth," *University of Iowa Studies in Child Welfare*, 1935, *11*, No. 3.
38. Miles, L. M., "Elective induction of labor at term," *American Journal of Obstetrics and Gynecology*, 1951, *62*:649-653.
39. Moore, W. T., and P. P. Steptoe, Jr., "The experience of John Hopkins Hospital with breech presentation; analysis of 1444 cases," *Southern Medical Journal*, 1943, *36*:295-302.
40. O'Connell, W. T., "The premature infant: A study of one hundred

seventy-three liveborn premature infants," *American Journal of Obstetrics and Gynecology*, 1948, *56*:765-769.

41. Odell, L. D., J. H. Randall, and G. W. Scott, "Prolonged labor, with special reference to post-partum hemorrhage," *Journal of the American Medical Association*, 1947, *133*:735-739.

42. Quigley, J. K., "A ten-year study of cesarean section in Rochester and Monroe County, 1937 to 1946," *American Journal of Obstetrics and Gynecology*, 1949, *58*:41-50.

43. Reynolds, Martha M., and Helena Mallay, "The sleep of young children," *Journal of Genetic Psychology*, 1933, *43*:322-351.

44. Scoe, H. F., "Bladder control in infancy and early childhood," *University of Iowa Studies in Child Welfare*, 1933, 5, No. 4.

45. Seeley, W. F., "Fetal Mortality in breech deliveries," *American Journal of Obstetrics and Gynecology*, 1949, *57*:113-121.

46. Seham, M., and G. Seham, *The Tired Child*, Philadelphia: Lippincott, 1926.

47. Shirley, M. M., *The First Two Years; A Study of Twenty-Five Babies:* Vol. 1. *Postural and Locomotor Development*, Minneapolis: University of Minnesota Press, 1931-1933.

48. Smith, S., "Influence of illness during the first two years on infant development," *Journal of Genetic Psychology*, 1931, *39*:284-287.

49. Terman, L. M., *Genetic Studies of Genius 1. Mental and Physical Traits of 1000 Gifted Children*. Stanford: Stanford University Press, 1925.

50. Terman, L. M., and A. Hocking, "The sleep of school children, its distribution according to age and its relation to physical and mental efficiency," *Journal of Educational Psychology*, 1913, *4*:138-147.

51. Van Riper, C., *Speech Correction: Principles and Methods*, 3rd ed., New York: Prentice-Hall, 1954.

52. Vickers, V. S., and H. C. Stuart, "Anthropometry in the pediatrician's office: norms for selected body measurements based on studies of children of North European stock," *Journal of Pediatrics*, 1943, *22*:155-170.

53. Wagoner, L. C., and E. M. Armstrong, "The motor control of children as involved in the dressing process," *Journal of Genetic Psychology*, 1928, *35*:84-97.

54. Wallin, P., "The prediction of individual behavior from case studies." In P. Horst, *The Prediction of Personal Adjustment*, New York: Social Science Research Council, 1943, pp. 183-239.

55. Zacharias, L. F., and Ralph Heery, "An evaluation of breech presentation and vaginal delivery," *American Journal of Obstetrics and Gynecology*, 1950, *60*:1352-1355.

3 GENERAL SPEECH BEHAVIOR EVALUATION

There are situations in which you may wish to make a quick general assessment of the attributes of a speaker's voice and his ability to articulate sounds and use language in oral expression. For instance, you may wish to identify those members of a school or college class who have speech problems which need to be observed more extensively. A screening procedure of the kind you would use for such purposes gives an indication of the gross clinical needs of groups of speakers and provides a basis for the important initial stages of program planning.

In other situations, persons with speech problems will be referred to you. In these instances you will not only wish to study more extensively the specific problems for which the referral was made but will also wish to evaluate the speaker's entire complex of attributes of oral expression in order to view the complaint in proper perspective. You will need to identify those attributes that are satisfactory as well as those that are deviant. You will want to make some preliminary observations concerning any possible relationships that may exist between such attributes as pitch level and harshness. Finally, and perhaps most important, you will want to evaluate the speaker's oral expression in a relatively unstructured speaking situation. The way one typically speaks is, in the final analysis, the "proof of the pudding."

Finally, having completed your first examination of a problem, you may wish to summarize your various observations by means of a rating sheet. You may also wish to compare your initial observations with those which you will make following a period of remedial work.

The General Speech Behavior Rating (see Form 2) can be used for all of these purposes. It should be noted, however, that the set of ratings involved is designed for speakers who have developed some proficiency in the use of language. While no minimal age limits have been established, it is unlikely that the General Speech Behavior Rating would be used with speakers below the age level of the first grade. The rating procedure is most commonly employed in screening adult speakers.

The following procedure for making a general speech behavior evaluation is recommended.

1. Obtain a Speech Sample

a. If the speaker is old enough to read, observe him while he reads aloud some nonemotional prose. Also observe his extemporaneous and conversational speaking. You are interested in describing the person's typical speaking behavior rather than his ability to read aloud, per se.

b. If the speaker is a nonreader, elicit a speech sample by having him talk about some pictures, tell what he did yesterday, etc.

c. If it suits your purposes, you may, of course, use the procedure described in Chapter 7 for obtaining samples of speech and oral reading.

2. Record Your Observations and Evaluations on Form 2

a. Remember that you are making a record not only for your own future reference, but also for other interested individuals who will not have heard the speaker. Your observations and impressions must therefore be recorded clearly and fully enough to be meaningful and useful to others.

b. Rate each of the speakers on each of the eight attributes represented on the form. Circle one of the numbers for each attribute, using the following definitions of the four categories: 1—adequate, within the normal range, 2—a deviation which does not make for a communicative handicap, 3—a deviation which occasions a moderate communicative handicap that should be given clinical attention, 4—a deviation which results in a serious communicative handicap that requires immediate clinical attention. Rate each stutterer twice, once on the basis of his typical speech behavior including stuttering, and once on the basis of his fluent or nearly fluent speech. In the first instance place the letter S over your ratings and in the second instance place the letters *NS* over your ratings. The two ratings of the stutterer are required if you are to observe not only the nature of his speech behavior while stuttering but also the nature of his speech when he does not stutter. If the speaker stutters sufficiently to make it difficult to obtain an adequate sample of nonstuttered speech, you may instruct him to read in chorus with you or, preferably, with a third person. He will be able to do this with little or no stuttering. The use of chorus reading may distort, of course, certain aspects of his speech behavior. However, under this condition you should be able to make a reasonably valid assessment of voice quality, articulation, and those aspects of pitch and volume not influenced by the speech pattern employed.

You may, as you prefer, rate the speaker by tentatively judging each of the attributes separately as you go along or attempt to complete the ratings when you have finished observing the complete speech sample. If you find it difficult to categorize the articulation errors as you go along, you may wish to make informal marginal notes of observed articulation errors and categorize them at the end of the period of observation.

c. Substantiate your over-all ratings of the various attributes by checking the appropriate items listed below the main headings. Refer to the appropriate chapters in this manual for discussions of attributes and items listed on the form that you do not understand. Whenever you rate an individual above 1 on any attribute you should check at least one of the listed items, or after the word *Other* write in one or more things that were observed but not listed on the form. The point is that if you feel that a speaker is deviant in some respect, you must have a reason. To rate a speaker as 3 or 4 on an attribute without providing substantiating information is to cast doubt on the validity of your rating.

Listed under the attributes are such wordings as "too high," "too low," "too weak," "too loud," "too rapid," and "too slow." These terms are to be used in evaluating the usual or modal performance of the speaker. Thus, if you rate a speaker's pitch as "too high," you are saying that in your judgment his usual pitch level is inappropriate for his sex and age and the speaking occasion, and is likely, therefore, to interfere with his general effectiveness as a speaker.

See Chapter 7 for definitions of the terms listed under *Fluency*. See Chapter 5 for background information that you will find useful in making the judgments called for under *Language*.

d. In rating the *General Adequacy* of a speaker, represent the overall impression which he makes on you. This rating is not an average of the ratings you have given the various attributes. In this instance the meaning of each of the numbers on the scale will depend upon the use you propose to make of the results, and therefore each number must be defined in terms of the practical decisions to be made on the basis of your findings. For example, a rating of 4 might signify that you recommend intensive clinical instruction for the individual, and 3 might mean that the individual is recommended for assignment to a class or section in which attention will be given to the correction of the deviation but in which intensive remedial work will not be provided, etc. The meanings of the various numbers in this rating scale will be determined, therefore, by the nature of the instructional and clinical programs to be provided, and these will vary more or less from one situation to another.

e. Use the *Remarks* section to note any assets of the speaker which may be profitably exploited in trying to bring about improvement; diagram any patterns of speaking, such as rising inflections, that you observe; describe affectations, facial or bodily mannerisms, faulty usage of emphasis and stress; note mispronunciations; specify any regional or foreign dialect observed; describe the circumstances under which a voice quality deviation or any other fault is particularly noticeable or diminished; indicate whether the speaker appears to be a stutterer, or has a cleft palate, or has some other notable condition of clinical significance; suggest further particular tests that you feel are needed, etc.

f. Indicate possible relationships among the deviations you have observed. For example, if you have noted a jerky rate and you feel that it is due to part-word repetitions, draw an arrow between these two items to show the suspected relationship. Or, if there is breathiness that seems to be associated with a low loudness level, again use an arrow to relate these two variables.

g. Finally, remember that this set of ratings is frequently done to summarize momentary impressions that may be based upon inadequate observations. Obviously, then, the ratings may and often should be changed as you observe the speaker more systematically in additional and varied speaking situations. As a first careful approach to an understanding of an individual's problems, however, this rating procedure will provide you with valuable cues for diagnosis and important leads for the first stages of remedial work.

ASSIGNMENTS

1. Complete the General Speech Behavior Rating for three female and three male adult speakers, at least two of whom have speech deviations.
2. Complete the General Speech Behavior Rating for yourself, serving as your own listener and making use of a mirror and a tape recorder. Ask a classmate or friend to rate you also, and compare your ratings with those of the other observer.

FORM 2. GENERAL SPEECH BEHAVIOR RATING

Name _____   Age _____ Sex _____

Examiner _____   Date _____

PITCH: 1 2 3 4
_____Too high
_____Too low
_____Pitch pattern
_____Monotonous
_____Pitch breaks
_____Other

LOUDNESS: 1 2 3 4
_____Too loud
_____Too soft
_____Monotonous
_____Loudness pattern
_____Other

RATE: 1 2 3 4
_____Too rapid
_____Too slow
_____Rate pattern
_____Monotonous
_____Jerkiness
_____Other

VOICE QUALITY: 1 2 3 4
Laryngeal Function:
_____Breathiness
_____Harshness
_____Hoarseness
_____Glottal attack
_____Other
Resonance:
_____Hypernasality
_____Hyponasality

ARTICULATION: 1 2 3 4
_____General misarticulations
_____Plosives misarticulated
_____Fricatives misarticulated
_____Semivowels misarticulated
_____Nasals misarticulated
_____Glides misarticulated
_____Vowels misarticulated
_____Dipthongs misarticulated
_____Substitutions
_____Distortions
_____Omissions
_____Voicing errors
_____Other

LANGUAGE: 1 2 3 4
_____No response to examiner
_____Brief responses
_____Responses grammatically incom-
        plete
_____Responses slow
_____Responses irrelevant
_____Lack of spontaneity in verbaliza-
        tion
_____Limited vocabulary
_____Incorrect use of case of pronouns
_____Incorrect use of verb tense
_____Responses vague or ambiguous
_____Responses seemingly invalid, in-
        consistent, implausible, bizarre,
        incoherent
_____Excessive verbal output
_____Glib use of platitudes and cliches

FLUENCY: 1 2 3 4

_____Interjection of sounds, syllables, words or phrases
_____Part-word repetitions
_____Word repetitions
_____Phrase repetitions
_____Revisions
_____Incomplete phrases
_____Broken words
_____Prolonged sounds
_____Unvocalized intervals
_____Other

REACTION TO SELF AND SITUATION:
    1 2 3 4

_____Apparent tension and strain
_____Visual evasiveness
_____Distracting postures
_____Distracting bodily movements
_____Apparent uneasiness or embar-
    rassment
_____Distracting laughter or giggling
_____Blandness
_____Other

GENERAL ADEQUACY: 1 2 3 4
REMARKS:

Additional copies of this form may be obtained from the Interstate Printers and Publishers, 19-27 North Jackson Street, Danville, Illinois.

4 *TESTING ARTICULATION*

There are several aspects of speech, voice, and language that engage your attention as a clinician. These include vocal pitch, time, loudness, and quality; such dimensions of language behavior as vocabulary size, length of response, complexity of sentence structure, or relative frequency of use of the various parts of speech; and the rate and fluency, or disfluency, of speech. Of all the attributes of communicative behavior, the one that you are likely to examine and evaluate in the greatest proportion of cases is that of articulation, the ways in which the speaker produces the speech sounds of his language. In this chapter we present essential information about the development of speech sound articulation, together with a number of procedures for examining and describing a person's articulation patterns.

A recent nation-wide sampling of public school speech clincians reported that children with functional articulation problems constituted 81 percent of their average current caseload (*18*, pp. 37-38). It is very likely that a considerable proportion of the remaining children in the average caseload also present articulation problems—children with delayed speech development (4.5 per cent), hearing loss, (2.5 percent), clefts of the palate (1.5 percent), and cerebral palsy (1.0 percent) swell the total percentage of children with articulation problems in the average current caseload to 90.5 percent. It is clear that testing procedures which can help you define the problems of these children and point the way to economical and effective remedial services for them are highly important.

HOW SPEECH SOUND ARTICULATION DEVELOPS

There are between 45 and 50 different speech sounds used in the three main dialects of English spoken in the United States. The way in which children acquire these sounds has been the subject of considerable research, some of the most enlightening of which has been reported by Irwin and his associates (9, 10, 11, 12, 13, 14, 15, 36). They studied 30-breath speech (phonation and articulation) samples obtained at monthly intervals from a sizable group of infants from birth to age 2½ years. Analyzing the 30-breath samples in terms of two main measures, the number of different sounds produced on the average in the samples (phoneme type) and the total number of sounds produced during the thirty breaths (phoneme frequency), Irwin derived curves indicating an impressive orderliness in the appearance of speech sounds in the babbling and speech of infants. Figure 1, based upon data presented in Table 11, indicates that at the first age level (months 1 and 2 combined) the average child produces seven different sounds in a sample of 30 breaths. By the 15th age level (months 29 and 30) the average child is producing 27 different sounds. This is a decelerating curve, with the faster acquisition of new sounds being demonstrated at the earlier ages. The child begins with a meager repertory of sounds, gradually adding sounds which he hears about him. Figure 2, based upon data in Table 12, shows that the growth in total number of sounds produced in the 30-breath period accelerates with increase in age.

For each of the measures mentioned above there is considerable variability among children (10). Data based upon groups of children are highly stable, but it has been reported by Winitz and Irwin (36) that the individuals studied did not consistently maintain their positional standings in the group with respect to the two measures of speech-sound development.

Most parents and speech clinicians, wanting to determine whether a child's speech sound usage is satisfactory for one of his age or whether he has an articulation problem, are less interested in the number of phonemes the child can produce in his babbling and connected speech than they are in the correctness of his articulation of the phonemes. Three well-known studies give a picture of the sequence in which chil-

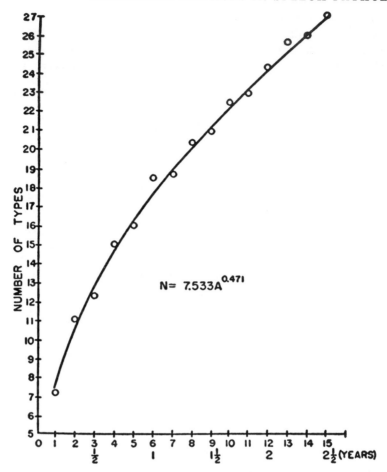

FIGURE 1. Curve of development derived from mean numbers of different phonemes (types) produced during 1622 observation periods of 30 breaths each by a total of 95 infants at the designated age levels. Circles represent the obtained values and the solid curve is described by the indicated equation. Reprinted by permission of the American Psychological Association, publisher of the *Journal of Experimental Psychology*, and the authors, Orvis C. Irwin and Han Piao Chen (*15*).

dren master speech sounds in context. Wellman *et al.* (*34*) studied the ability of 204 children ranging in age from 2 to 6 years to produce 133 items in an articulation test. Table 13 indicates the earliest ages at which various sounds and consonant blends were correctly produced by 75 percent of the children tested. Davis (*4*), having administered an articulation test to more than 20,000 preschool and school-age children, reported on the ability of children to articulate 23 different consonant sounds. Table 14 shows the earliest age levels at which 100 percent of the children tested were able to produce them correctly.

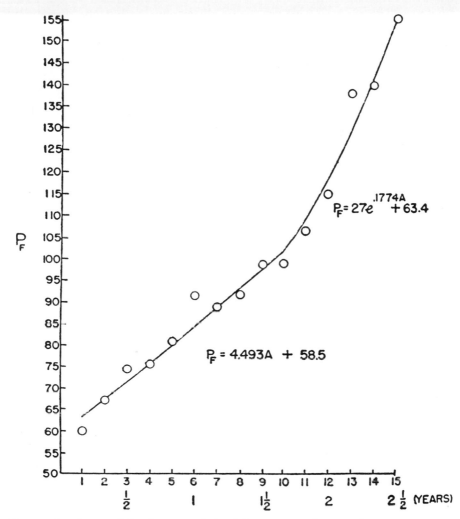

FIGURE 2. Curve of development derived from mean phoneme frequencies (numbers of speech sounds of all types produced) during 1622 observation periods of 30 breaths each by a total of 95 infants at the designated age levels. Circles represent the obtained values and the solid curve is described in its lower and upper portions, respectively, by the indicated equations. Reprinted by permission of the American Psychological Association, publisher of the *Journal of Experimental Psychology*, and the author, Orvis C. Irwin (*9*).

Templin (*26*) administered a 176-item articulation test to a total of 480 children, of whom 60 (30 boys and 30 girls) were at each of eight age levels. Table 15 indicates the earliest age levels at which 75 percent of the children tested produced correctly the consonant sounds indicated.

Comparing these three sets of data, Templin (*26*, pp. 53-54) reported: "There are, of course, some discrepancies but the agreement is substantial, especially if the differences in the samples are taken into account. . . . There is complete agreement in the age placement on five of the 17 sounds reported in all three investigations, a spread of one year on six sounds, and a spread of two or more on six sounds. . . . There is an essential similarity in the sequence of sounds reported in these three studies." There is similar agreement in a series of studies by Roe and Milisen (21), Sayler (22), Barnes (2), and Hall (7) with regard to the sounds most often misarticulated by both children and adults. Table 16 lists the ten consonant sounds most frequently reported to be in error by each of the above-named investigators.

THE SPEECH SAMPLE

As in any other type of speech test, a sample of speech is necessary in a test of articulation. The nature of the sample depends upon the purpose of the testing.

Usually we wish either to assess the general adequacy of a child's articulation or to obtain a detailed description and evaluation of it. In the first instance we are using a screening test. Such a test is used frequently in speech surveys or other initial contacts with children to detect those who need speech correction because their articulation is inadequate for their age. It need test only those sounds and sound combinations which are associated with significant progress in the development of articulation. In the second instance we use a diagnostic test. Such a test may be used in deciding whether a child needs speech correction, but more frequently it is used with children already identified as having articulatory problems to aid in prescribing the nature of speech correction. It provides detailed information about a child's ability to produce a wide range of speech sounds in a variety of positions and phonetic contexts (Templin and Darley, 29, p. 1).

However sketchy or detailed your examination of articulation is to be, you must have a method of eliciting the desired sounds and a systematic method of recording what you hear when the speaker attempts to produce these sounds. You may elicit the sounds in any one of several ways. You may hold a conversation with the individual you are testing and note the correctness of his production of the various sounds as they occur in his speech. Obviously, however, this procedure is inefficient and time consuming. You may have to wait a long time for some of the less common sounds to appear. At best the observations would not be systematic and probably the conclusions drawn from them would lack precision.

You may ask the subject to read sentences prepared to contain specific sounds in specific positions and phonetic contexts. The procedure will prove highly satisfactory and efficient in the case of sufficiently good readers, but many of the individuals given articulation tests read poorly if at all.

With most preschool children or those in early elementary grades you probably will resort to one of two other methods. In one, pictures are used to elicit as spontaneous speech responses words containing the desired sounds in given positions and contexts. Such a procedure is fairly interesting to most children and is fairly economical of time. With the other method you have the child repeat after you words containing the desired sounds. This procedure is even more economical of time, but it is likely to become rather boring to young children. Templin and Darley (29, pp. 4-6) have reviewed research done on the relative merits of these two methods, which may be called the "spontaneous" and the "imitative," respectively. They concluded that when what is desired is the most typical response of the subject—that is, a response influenced as little as possible by any prior stimulation—the spontaneous method is probably better.

In the following paragraphs we present procedures designed to elicit either a brief sample of speech for screening purposes or a more detailed sample for diagnostic purposes, to record the results of the articulation testing, to make use of International Phonetic Alphabet symbols, and to analyze the results for precise appraisal of the problem and cues for therapy. Frequent reference is made to the work of Templin (26), whose normative research findings give meaning to the results obtained in clinical use of the procedures, and to the test manual developed by Templin and Darley (29), in which a more detailed presentation of the rationale for each step of the procedure is presented.

A word of warning: It is well to remind yourself periodically that the results you have derived from your articulation testing are based upon a small sample of speech behavior. You cannot generalize safely from one such brief sample to a person's total performance at all times and in all situations. You will want to be alert to the possibility of two important kinds of variation.

1. The subject may vary in articulatory performance from time to time and from day to day in relation to his mood; degree of fatigue; interest in communicating; security in the speaking situation; and other factors pertaining to his physical, motivational, and emotional conditions.

2. The observer or examiner fluctuates, too, in how critical he is and how discerningly he listens. We have all too little information about the temporal (day to day or time to time) reliability of the examiner or observer in articulation testing, but what we do know indicates that at different times the observer listens differently depending upon how

hurried he is, or how tired, or what he is tuned to listen for, etc. It is essential that you appreciate the fact that these statements apply to you as they do to other clinical observers. Depending upon your perceptual set, everyone may seem to have a hissing [s] or everyone may sound just fine.

As a careful examiner, then, you will beware of over-interpreting your data and drawing conclusions that are too sweeping or final about what a speaker can or cannot do.

PREPARATION OF PICTURE TEST

You may use the printed picture test developed by Templin and Darley (*29*), or you may prepare your own picture materials for eliciting the speech responses of the children you are to test. Your broadest purpose in any instance is to test the speaker's production of a total of 176 items. These items are listed in the Articulation Test Form (Form 3). The form contains 176 blanks, each blank representing one item on the diagnostic test. Fifty of the items, indicated by double lines on the Articulation Test Form, comprise the screening test of articulation.

1. General

You are to construct a diagnostic articulation test with a built-in screening portion. This test can provide a practical starting point for the several kinds of more detailed testing instruments that speech clinicians personally develop on the job.

2. Material Comprising the Test

The test will consist of 63 cards of convenient size (3" x 5" or 5" x 7"), each of which will carry two, three, or four pictures. Each picture is designed to elicit a given sound as a single or one blend, each in one position. The items to be tested by each card are indicated in Chart A on p. 87.

3. Key for Each Picture

a. On the face of the appropriate cards place a line beneath each picture designed to elicit one of the 50 items of the screening test.
b. On the back of each card make the following entries:
    (1) The number of the card
    (2) The numbers of the items on the Articulation Test Form which the pictures on the card are designed to test

CHART A. Arrangement of Items in Picture Test

Card	Pictures	Test Items[a]				Card	Pictures	Test Items[a]			
1	3	1,	2,	3		33	3	50,	51,	52	
2	3	4,	5,	6		34	2	53,	54		
3	2	7,	8			35	2	55,	56		
4	4	9,	10,	11,	12	36	2	57,	58		
5	3	13,	14,	15,		37	2	59,	60		
6	3	16,	17,	18		38	3	61,	62,	63	
7	3	19				39	4	64,	65,	66,	67
8	3	20				40	4	68,	69,	70,	71
9	2	21				41	4	72,	73,	74,	75
10	3	22				42	2	76,	77		
11	3	23				43	3	78,	79,	80	
12	3	24				44	2	81,	82		
13	3	25				45	3	83,	84,	85	
14	3	26				46	2	86,	87		
15	3	27				47	4	88,	89,	90,	91
16	2	28				48	3	92,	93,	94	
17	3	29				49	3	95,	96		
18	3	30				50	2	97			
19	3	31				51	2	98			
20	3	32				52	3	99			
21	3	33				53	2	100,	101		
22	3	34				54	2	102,	103		
23	3	35				55	2	104,	105		
24	3	36				56	3	106,	107,	108	
25	2	37				57	2	109,	110		
26	2	38				58	3	111,	112,	113	
27	4	39,	40			59	3	114,	115,	116	
28	2	41				60	3	117,	118,	119	
29	3	42				61	2	120,	121		
30	3	43				62	3	122,	123,	124	
31	3	44,	45,	46		63	4	125,	126,	127,	128
32	3	47,	48,	49							

[a] Items numbered as in Articulation Test Form 3.

(3) The phonetic symbols representing these items
(4) The words which the pictures are designed to elicit
(5) A simple starter question or statement for each item which (if possible) should not contain the sound the picture is designed to elicit.

For example, entries such as the following would be entered on the back of card number 4:

9.	ɑ	clock.	We tell time by the _____.
10.	ɔ	ball.	We throw the _____.
11.	ʊ	book.	It's fun to read a _____.
12.	u	soup.	We eat _____.

Entries such as the following would be entered on the back of card number 52:

99.	sk-	skate.	The little girl likes to _____.
	-sk	mask.	On Halloween you wear a _____.
	-ks	books.	These are _____.

You should vary the starter questions or statements throughout the test in order to avoid a monotonous repetition of the question, "What's this?"

4. Subject Matter of the Pictures

The words you select for use in the test should be appropriate to the vocabulary level of preschool children; they should be words one would reasonably expect young children to know, for this is to be a speech examination and not an intelligence test. To find out what words occur in the vocabularies of children you may refer to relevant studies (*3, 5, 8, 19, 20, 31, 32, 33, 35*).

Select pictures that are simple in subject matter, clear in detail, and colorful. A common error is that of selecting a picture containing several items of interest or representing a complex and possibly confusing collection of things, thus providing distractions from the one item to which a response is desired. A picture of one simple object is to be preferred. Colored pictures should be used in preference to black and white. You may get them, of course, from magazines, catalogues, children's dictionaries, and other common sources.

5. Suggestions

a. You can handle a group of test cards more easily if you orient all the pictures toward either an end or a side than you can if you mix them up with some lengthwise and others sidewise of the card.

b. A neat paste job adds greatly to the appearance.

c. Uniformity of design of the pictures (for example, all colored photographs, all colored drawings, all water-colored cutouts from paint books, etc.) is preferable.

d. If you like, you may "animate" the test with actual objects (for example, a feather, a button, a miniature knife) which can be affixed flat on the card. You should not use bulkier objects (toy cars, miniature furniture) which make the repeated and hasty handling of a single pack of cards unwieldy.

e. When you submit the completed test to your instructor for grading, divide the cards into two groups, putting in one group in numerical order the 26 cards containing items in the screening test and placing in the other group the remaining 37 cards, also arranged in numerical order.

Although you will use the norms developed by Templin (*26*) with this 176-item diagnostic test, it is not necessary that your test employ the same words Templin used in her normative study. In an earlier investigation Templin (*28*) found that "there is little difference in measured articulation when the same sound is tested in different words. . . . The measure of a specific sound is a measure of the general ability to produce that sound and not to articulate it in a specific word." Hence you are justified in choosing words that you find easily pictured and highly suitable for the age level of the children.

FORM FOR RECORDING AND ANALYZING RESULTS OF ARTICULATION TEST

1. Recording

Form 3, the Articulation Test, is a standard form for recording the results from the diagnostic and the screening tests of articulation. On the record sheet of the Articulation Test Form, space is provided after each test item for you to record the subject's response. Three common types of error are the following:

Substitution: The use of one speech sound in place of another, as of [w] for [r] in the pronunciation of "wabbit" for "rabbit," or of [n] for [ŋ] in "singin" for "singing."

Distortion: The faulty production of a speech sound, although the sound produced is recognized as being an example of the desired phoneme. For example, a whistled or lateral [s] may be considered a distortion of the [s] sound.

Omission: The failure to produce a sound in the position where it should occur and the failure to insert any other sound in its place. For example, an omission of final [t] is noted in the pronunciation of "ca" for "cat."

You will note that the Articulation Test Form provides for entries derived from the testing of the single consonant sounds in three positions—initial, medial, and final. We recognize that the traditional concept of three positions of consonants in words is artificial—an artifact growing out of orthography in disregard of the dynamics of speech production. We recognize that a more meaningful phonetic analysis would be one related to the findings of Stetson (*25*), who showed that the syllable is "the smallest indivisible phonetic unit." He demonstrated that "the syllable is a puff of air forced upward through the vocal canal by a compression stroke of the intercostal muscles. It is usually modulated by the actions of the vocal folds. It is accompanied by accessory movements (syllable factors) which characterize it. These are the *release* (by the action of either the chest muscles or the releasing consonant), the *vowel shaping* movements of the vocal canal, and the *arrest* (by the action of either chest muscles or the arresting consonant)" (*25*, p. 200). Consonants are properly understood, then, as serving a releasing function, initiating the syllable pulse, or an arresting function, bringing the syllable pulse to a close.

In spite of our conviction that this classification of consonants is meaningful and descriptive of the dynamics of speech *as spoken,* we have retained the traditional classification of consonants with regard to their position in the written word—initial, medial, final—in the articulation testing here to be described. We have done this in order to permit you to relate your test findings to available yardsticks, especially the normative data reported by Templin. We anticipate, however, that before long these normative data will be revised in recognition of the more dynamic concepts of release and arrest, and when that day comes testing procedures can be modernized. Until then, adherence to the traditional positional classification scheme seems warranted.

Make entries on the Articulation Test Form as follows for each vowel, diphthong, and single consonant[1] (items 1 through 43):

    a. If the subject articulates the sound correctly, enter a check mark (✔).

    b. If the subject substitutes another phoneme, enter the phonetic symbol representing the phoneme produced.

    c. If the subject omits the test sound in pronouncing the test word, indicate the omission with a dash (—).

    d. If the subject distorts a sound, enter an (x).

To illustrate, part of the Atriculation Test Form might be completed as follows:

		I	M	F				
24.	t	✔	✔	—		44.	pr-	pw
28.	r	w	w			121.	spr-	xpw
34.	s	x	x	x		125.	-kst	kx-

These symbols would be interpreted as follows: the single consonant [t] was correctly produced in the initial and medial positions but was omitted in the final position. The consonant [w] was substituted for the single consonant [r] in both the initial and medial positions. The

---

[1] See the Manual for the Templin-Darley Tests of Articulation (*29*, p. 2) for an explanation of the classification of sounds, particularly the [r] and [l] sounds.

production of the single consonant [s] was distorted in all positions. In the consonant blend [pr-] the consonant [p] was correctly articulated but [w] was substituted for [r]. In the three-consonant blend [spr-] the [s] was distorted, the [p] was produced correctly, and the consonant [w] was substituted for the consonant [r]. In the three-consonant blend [kst] the consonant [k] was correctly produced, the consonant [s] was distorted, and the consonant [t] was omitted.

2. Analyzing

Analysis is accomplished through use of the analysis-sheet portion of the Articulation Test Form. Such an analysis indicates patterns within the speaker's articulation responses, from which cues may be derived for the planning and implementation of a speech correction program. You are to carry out three main steps: compare the speaker's performance with appropriate norms; analyze the misarticulations with regard to type of error, consistency of the error, and the speaker's response to stimulation by you on sounds he makes incorrectly; and look for any possible common factors related to the patterns of misarticulation observed.

Comparison with Norms: If you administered only the 50 screening test items (items indicated by double lines), count up the number of correctly produced sounds and enter the total on the Analysis Sheet in the space provided after *1a*. Refer to Tables 17 and 18 for information to enter in the spaces provided after *1b* and *1c*. Table 17 contains information about the mean performance of groups of girls and boys in the normative sample on the 50-item screening test. Table 18 presents cut-off scores developed by Templin (*27*) for eight designated age levels to indicate the boundary between adequate and inadequate performance on the screening test.

If you administered the entire 176-item diagnostic test, count up the number of sounds produced correctly and enter this total in the space provided after *1d*. Consult Table 19 to find the mean number correctly produced by other children of the age and sex of the subject and enter this value in the space after *1e*. Finally, count up the number of single sounds (items 1 to 43) that were misarticulated *in any position* as tested; enter the total of these misarticulated singles in the space provided after *1f*. Both the total score of the diagnostic test and the number of faulty singles produced in it have been found to be valid indicators of severity of articulation impairment, being significantly related to the judgments made by listeners who rated the misarticulations of children in connected speech (*16*).

Grouping by Types: Enter all errors recorded in the first 43 items in section *2a* in the appropriate column as omissions, substitutions, or distortions. Research findings of Wellman and associates (*34*), Roe and Milisen (*21*), Snow and Milisen (*23*), Templin (*26*), and Jordan (*16*) indicate that omission is the articulation error consistently associated with the most immaturity and a good predictor of judged severity of articulation impairment. The data suggest that children who have difficulty in articulation may progress from errors of the omission type to substitution errors and then to distortion errors on their way toward mastery of the speech sounds. It is important, then, to determine the sounds on which the child makes errors and the type of error he is making on these sounds. Analysis of a child's errors according to this system indicates something of the severity of his problem and helps in deciding on what sounds to begin working in therapy.

Completion of parts *2b* and *2c* of the Articulation Test Form indicates the consistency with which the child made the errors noticed during the articulation test. Sometimes an error on a single sound is noted in one position but not in another, and often a child misarticulates a sound as a single but produces it correctly in certain consonant blends. Investigations summarized by Spriestersbach and Curtis (*24*) have shown that when children misarticulate certain consonant sounds, they tend to misarticulate them inconsistently. That is, sometimes a child produces a correct [r] or [s] sound while at other times he does not. Given a large enough sample of speech, an examiner would presumably find that almost any child sometimes articulates correctly the sounds which he usually misarticulates. The inconsistency appears to depend in part upon the phonetic context of the sounds in question; for example, a child may produce the [r] sound correctly when it follows the consonant [t] in the blend [tr-], as in the word "tree," but not when it occurs as a single, as in the word "Mary." Possibly the inconsistency also depends partly on the child's ability to discriminate between incorrect and correct forms of a given sound.

In testing a speaker's articulation performance, you will be interested in determining the ease with which he can correct his incorrect sounds following intensive auditory stimulation. After recording in parts *2a, 2b,* and *2c* of the analysis sheet those sounds which the speaker has produced incorrectly throughout the tests, go back over each of these sounds with him. Present each of them five times in isolation (for example, t-t-t-t-t) slowly and distinctly, and ask him to imitate your production of the sound as closely as possible. Then present the sound in a syllable, in a word, and in a consonant blend in a word. List in the appropriate column the sounds that are produced correctly after the specified type of auditory stimulation.

It will pay you in several ways to make such an examination of a subject's ability to produce his faulty sounds. For one thing, if the subject is producing the sound correctly a considerable part of the time or if he can produce it rather easily following stimulation, you can be reasonably certain that his speech mechanism is structurally adequate for production of the sound, at least in those contexts. (You should not assume, however, that his speech mechanism is physiologically capable of producing the sound at all possible rates at which he might speak. The articulation skills of dysarthric individuals and persons with cleft palates may indeed be found adequate at certain slow rates and markedly inadequate at higher rates.) Then, too, other things being equal (and excepting particularly the influence of mental subnormality), the prognosis should be more favorable for a speaker whose misarticulations are not consistent or who can produce the sounds correctly following a limited amount of stimulation than for one who is consistent in his misarticulations. The speaker who is inconsistent must at least be aware of the phoneme which he has misarticulated in some contexts, but not in others, and so he should not require as much ear training as a person who never produces the faulty sounds correctly. With a view to economy in subsequent retraining, it is worthwhile to determine the phonetic contexts in which a speaker correctly produces the sounds that he sometimes misarticulates. You may find, for example, that you need not teach the [r] sound "from scratch." After showing the person that he does produce the sound correctly in saying certain words, you can more readily and quickly motivate him to go from the correct productions to attempts at producing the sound in other phonetic contexts.

List any sounds not produced correctly during the test or following stimulation in the space provided under *2e*. These are probably sounds which the speaker consistently misarticulates.

All sounds listed in *2a* because they were misarticulated as singles should appear once and once only in sections *2b, 2c, 2d*, and *2e*. You have not completed the analysis you are to do in Part 2 until you have accounted for each error among items 1 to 43 in one of the latter four subsections. For example, here is a sample listing of entries in the analysis section:

2a.	Omissions	Substitutions	Distortions
	t (*F*)	*w/r* (*I, M*)	*s* (*I, M, F*)
	k (*F*)	*t/k* (*I, M*)	
2b.	*t*		
2c.	*s*		

As a Single

2d.			
	In Isolation	*In a Syllable*	*In a Word*
	k		

2e.   *r*

These entries indicate that the single consonant [t] was omitted in the final position but was correctly produced in the initial and medial positions. The single consonant [s] was distorted in all positions (initial, medial, and final) but the [s] sound was correctly produced in at least one blend later in the test (2c). The single [k] sound was omitted in the final position and the phoneme [t] was substituted for it in the initial and medial positions, but a correct [k] sound was produced as a single in isolation following intensive stimulation. A substitition of [w] for the single consonant [r] was noted in both positions (initial and medial) ; [r] was never produced correctly in a blend, nor was it produced correctly following stimulation. It is the only consistently misarticulated sound on this test for this subject.

Search for Patterns: At the conclusion of the test, review the subject's performance in a search for patterns among the errors noted. On the basis of what you find, you may hypothesize that the errors noted are due to a problem in impounding intraoral breath pressure, or to faulty dentition, or perhaps to a high-frequency hearing loss.

You will find it helpful also to make notes of these additional observations : (1) The types of distortion errors noted in the articulation of the consonant sounds during the test. (2) Any omissions, substitutions, and distortions which you noted in connected speech that were not apparent in the speaker's pronunciation of single words in the articulation test. It is quite possible for a person to produce correctly given sounds in single words but to fail to maintain this degree of articulatory competence in rapid conversation. For example, a cerebral palsied child or a dysarthric adult may be able to attain correct placement of his articulators and impound adequate amounts of intraoral breath pressure for satisfactory articulation of fricative and plosive sounds in single words but rapid speech with its requirements of quick adjustments of the articulators may place excessive demands upon muscles limited in precision, speed, and extent of movement. You may note a marked discrepancy between such a speaker's intelligibility in saying words and his intelligibility in speaking sentences. (3) Significant features of the testing situation and of the behavior of the speaker tested.

SUGGESTIONS FOR ADMINISTERING THE ARTICULATION TEST

Certain problems are sometimes encountered in testing young children. The professional workers who probably know most about testing children are psychologists, who have had years of experience in administering standardized intelligence tests that require a sampling of various behaviors in attempting assigned tasks. You have much to gain from their observations and suggestions. Goodenough (*6*, pp. 297-304) and Terman and Merrill (*30*, pp. 69-71) are especially good sources, and some of the remarks that follow are in part paraphrases of the comments of these writers:

1. A child does not easily become absorbed in an externally imposed task. He is easily distracted and quickly fatigued. If you are to keep him attentive, cooperative, and talkative you must remember Goodenough's statement that the child "can be allured but not coerced" (*6*, p. 297).

2. Conduct the test with no observers present, if possible. If the child requires the presence of a parent, ask the parent to be unobtrusive and never to prompt a response; the parent may be called upon to interpret if necessary.

3. Don't work too fast. Let the child become accustomed to the testing situation. Direct his attention away from himself; ignore him perhaps for a time; interest him initially in things other than the picture cards—for example, toys, blocks, etc. Goodenough warns, "Do not urge the child to respond before he is ready. Let the child make the advances when he is ready" (*6*, p. 300). Of course when you are ready to present the test stimuli you will remove the play materials, which otherwise might continue to distract him.

4. Respond to every remark made by the child. Praise him liberally. Keep him motivated, using his desire for approval and his curiosity.

5. Remember that you are in charge: don't let the child take over, dominate the testing session, or play with or destroy the test materials. It is possible for you to be friendly and participate in the game without surrendering the leadership.

6. Some examiners appear to believe that to make the child feel at home and interested they must descend to the child's level. The resulting foolishness, effusiveness, and childishness sometimes become excruciating and ridiculous, even to the youngster. Other examiners, remembering that they must maintain control, mistakenly assume an air that is too austere and aloof, to which the child reacts with cold withdrawal. Others are so conscientious about their task that they hover eagerly over the youngster, like overhanging trees smothering a young sapling, tensely awaiting each response and overwhelming the child.

You will usually find that the best approach is a straightforward, man-to-man naturalness, quietly communicating to the child a feeling that you like him, consider him your friend, and have some fascinating pictures to show him.

7. Some children are curious about why the examiner writes things down during the articulation test. If a young child quizzes you about this, you can explain that the two of you are going for a walk through

the Magic Woods and you are Mr. Pencil and have to write down everything you see. "So you tell me what to write down." Such an explanation usually provides rationale enough for the child. For older children you can provide less fanciful explanations, in the main saying simply that you need to keep track of the observations that you want to make use of later.

8. You may not always catch the child's response the first time. Ask him to repeat, but avoid asking for too much repetition or you may meet rebellion. It is better to go back later and recheck doubtful responses.

9. The picture articulation test cards constitute a tool, and the tool may prove inappropriate for use with a given child. With younger children and those with short attention spans, small objects which the child may manipulate often prove more successful in stimulating speech responses. Most speech clinicians who work with children collect a set of dime-store objects for use in testing or for rapport building.

10. The child, not the test, must be central. Don't be afraid to abandon a routine and adjust to circumstances. It is better not to use the test materials at all and just play and talk if that is the only way you can obtain a speech sample.

TESTING SPEECH-SOUND DISCRIMINATION

If a speaker's articulation problem warrants clinical attention, you will try to determine its causes. Your investigation will cover the structural and physiological adequacy of the person's oral speech mechanism (Chapter 5), his intelligence (Chapter 10), his hearing acuity (Chapter 10), the amount and type of speech stimulation he has received, the adequacy of his speech models, the rewards provided for his speaking endeavors, and his need for speech (Chapter 2). Since, as suggested above, one reason children vary in their ability to produce certain speech sounds is that they vary in ability to discriminate between incorrect and correct forms of sounds, you should include a test of speech-sound discrimination ability among your articulation-testing procedures.

Templin (26, pp. 61-63) has reviewed methods developed for testing the ability to discriminate between speech sounds. Studying groups of children ranging in age from 3 to 8 years, she found that "sound discrimination ability shows a consistent increase with age, but its rate of growth is decelerated at about 4.5 to 5 years of age" (26, p. 72). About 25 years ago several investigators reported that individuals with so-called functional articulatory problems were inferior to normal speakers in the general ability to hear differences between speech sounds. More recent investigators, such as Hall (7) and Mase (17), using more systematically matched groups of normal and non-normal speakers and testing under more rigorously controlled conditions, have found that speakers with articulation problems who do not have associated organic impairments of the speech mechanism do not show a general inferiority in discriminating one speech sound from another.

Considering the way in which we learn to produce speech sounds, we should expect to find what Hall and Mase have reported. It is to be appreciated, for example, that the error sounds produced by most speakers with articulation problems are few compared to the sounds they produce satisfactorily. If such speakers have learned to speak, as presumably we all do, primarily as the result of auditory stimulation, then obviously they have learned to discriminate one sound from another, at least so far as their correctly articulated sounds are concerned.

You should not interpret the foregoing discussion to mean that you have no need to examine the ability of a child with an articulation problem to discriminate between speech sounds. Even though the child is generally able to discriminate among the sounds he produces correctly, he may have difficulty singling out the auditory characteristics of the sounds he always or sometimes misarticulates. See the discussion by Spriestersbach and Curtis (24) for a more detailed examination of this problem. In all probability, you will find that most individuals with articulation problems can discriminate between their own incorrect sounds and the correct sounds. Nevertheless, you will find it worthwhile to test speech-sound discrimination because (1) the occasional failures in discrimination that may be revealed are likely to be of some importance in connection with the planning and use of remedial procedures and (2) it is important to rule out definitely the factor of nondiscrimination as a consideration in those cases in which normal speech sound discrimination is found.

Procedures: The testing procedure to be described here is a modification of one devised by Anderson (1) and described by Spriestersbach and Curtis (24). The test is relatively gross, but the more refined and perhaps more valid measuring techniques are too elaborate in procedure and equipment to be practical in the day-to-day work of the average clinician. The test described here can be given by anyone who will take the time to prepare the required word lists. The test yields information that is helpful in many cases in planning therapy.

1. On the basis of the results from the diagnostic test of articulation, select the sound that seems the most consistently misarticulated.
2. Prepare at least 50 items that include this sound to serve as a specific test of its articulation.

3. Have the subject repeat the test words after you. Keep a record of his responses to the stimulus words, indicating the nature of the error, if any, in each response.
4. Use the same word list as a basis for a speech-bound discrimination test. Seat the subject with his back to you at a distance of 8 to 10 feet. Provide him with a pencil and an answer sheet numbered for each item, and tell him that as you pronounce each word four times, he is to mark *R* (for right) when you say it correctly and *W* (for wrong) when you say it incorrectly. Then, speaking with a loudness level characteristic of ordinary conversation, pronounce each word correctly three times and incorrectly once, applying the suggestions that follow. Keep your own record of whether the words pronounced by you were right or wrong.
   a. If the subject misarticulated the sound being tested when he pronounced the word during step 3, imitate this particular error in your incorrect presentation. If he did not misarticulate the sound in this word, simulate an error commonly made in articulating the sound being tested.
   b. From test word to test word, randomize the position of the faulty presentation within the series of four.
   c. To avoid introducing extraneous cues that might assist the subject in identifying the correct and incorrect responses, keep the pitch, rate, and loudness of the four presentations of the test word as nearly uniform as possible.
5. Appraise the results from both parts of the test. Some of the following questions may be helpful:
   a. What percentage of the words tested were misarticulated?
   b. What percentage of the words tested which were misarticulated were also missed in the discrimination test?
   c. Do there appear to be more discrimination errors when the misarticulations are omissions? Substitutions? Distortions?
   d. Does the frequency of the discrimination errors appear to be related to the position of the sound in the word?
   e. What evidence do you find that the inability to discriminate a given speech sound is related to the phonetic context in which the sound occurs, rather than to a general inability to discriminate sounds?
   f. What cues, if any, do you get from your test data that might be helpful in giving direction to your remedial instruction?

ASSIGNMENTS

1. Administer your articulation test to five children of preschool or early elementary school age, recording the results of each test on Form 3.
2. On the basis of your administrations of the test, write a brief evaluation

of your test cards, indicating which pictures prove ambiguous or consistently elicit some response other than the desired one, and suggesting desirable changes. Make alterations in your test in accordance with your evaluation.

3. Summarize the impressions you gained from administering the test to five children. What mistakes did you make? What did you do that appeared to foster rapport and make for maximum interest and cooperation on the part of the children? What other approaches will you use next time?

4. Consider the data presented in Tables 13, 14, and 15, which show the sequence in which the articulation of consonant sounds is mastered by children. What factors can you think of that might account for this sequence? Consider sensory and motor aspects of speech production and the relative frequency of occurrence of the various consonant sounds in English. Does any single factor adequately account for the sequence or does a summation of several possible factors provide a more reasonable explanation?

5. Study the results you have obtained in administering the articulation tests. On the basis of your findings, which sounds might you logically select to start work on in a remedial program with each of the children you tested? Why?

TABLE 11. Mean Frequencies of Phoneme Types Uttered in
30-Breath Samples by Young Children

Age Groups (Months)	Boys N=10–18	Girls N=9–17	Both Sexes N=19–80	Laboring Parents N=6–18	Non-laboring Parents N=13–62	With Siblings N=9–36	Only Children N=10–44
1–2	7.2	7.7	7.2	7.1	7.2	7.5	6.8
3–4	11.2	11.1	11.1	11.4	11.1	11.0	11.2
5–6	12.5	12.1	12.3	12.9	12.1	12.2	12.3
7–8	15.2	15.5	15.1	15.7	14.9	15.9	14.6
9–10	16.6	17.6	16.0	14.1	16.6	16.0	15.9
11–12	18.7	20.1	18.6	16.4	19.3	18.1	19.1
13–14	19.9	19.2	18.8	19.1	18.8	17.8	19.6
15–16	21.6	21.6	20.4	19.8	20.6	20.3	20.6
17–18	21.8	20.8	21.0	20.2	21.3	20.6	21.3
19–20	21.8	25.0	22.5	20.4	23.3	22.7	22.4
21–22	22.5	24.4	23.0	21.6	23.4	23.2	22.9
23–24	24.4	21.1	24.4	23.0	24.9	23.4	25.2
25–26	26.6	24.8	25.8	23.9	26.5	25.2	26.3
27–28	24.0	28.5	26.1	25.4	26.4	27.4	24.8
29–30	27.2	27.1	27.2	25.2	28.1	26.1	28.1

SOURCE: Irwin, *13*, *14*; and Irwin and Chen, *15*.

TABLE 12. Mean Totals of Phonemes Uttered in
30-Breath Samples by Young Children

Age Groups (Months)	Boys N=10–18	Girls N=9–17	Both Sexes N=19–80	Laboring Parents N=6–18	Non-laboring Parents N=13–62	With Siblings N=9–36	Only Children N=10–44
1–2	64.4	59.1	60.3	57.9	61.1	58.8	61.7
3–4	71.3	62.0	67.1	70.0	66.2	64.8	69.0
5–6	74.7	71.5	73.9	74.6	73.7	71.1	75.8
7–8	79.9	71.5	76.4	77.1	76.2	74.8	77.5
9–10	80.4	80.4	81.1	78.3	81.9	76.2	84.8
11–12	82.4	98.9	91.5	94.7	90.5	89.6	93.0
13–14	86.3	91.9	88.2	87.2	88.0	84.1	90.8
15–16	88.0	95.3	92.4	88.3	93.5	95.3	90.1
17–18	97.0	96.7	97.8	93.4	99.0	97.4	98.0
19–20	91.0	100.2	98.1	90.5	100.8	99.7	96.7
21–22	103.0	104.6	107.1	90.0	111.8	102.8	110.4
23–24	116.3	109.0	115.1	95.9	121.8	109.9	119.5
25–26	137.7	127.1	137.8	111.8	146.4	132.5	141.4
27–28	134.5	147.2	140.3	115.7	150.5	150.8	130.0
29–30	162.6	148.3	155.8	123.8	170.6	161.3	150.8

SOURCE: Irwin, *9*, *13*, *14*.

TABLE 13. Earliest Ages at Which Sounds Were Correctly Produced, in Positions Indicated, by 75 Percent of 204 Children

Consonants	Initial	Medial	Final	Vowels and Dipthongs		Consonant Blends			
m	2	2	3	i	2	pr-	5		
n	2	2	3	ɪ	4	br-	5		
ŋ	–	3	nt[a]	ɛ	3	tr-	5		
p	2	2	4	æ	4	dr-	5	sl-	6
b	2	2	3	ʌ	2	kr	5	sw-	5
t	2	5	3	ə	2	gr-	5	tw-	5
d	2	3	4	ɑ	2	fr-	5	kw-	5
k	3	3	4	ɔ	3	θr-	6	-ŋk	4
g	3	3	4	ʊ	4	pl-	5	-ŋg	5
r	5	4	4	u	2	bl-	5	-mp	3
l	4	4	4	ɝ	2	kl-	5	-nt	4
f	3	3	3			gl-	5	-nd	6
v	5	5	4	ju	3	fl-	5	spr-	5
θ	5	nt	nt			-ld	6	spl-	5
ð	5	5	nt	oʊ	2	-lk	5	str-	5
s	5	5	5	aʊ	3	-lf	5	skr-	5
z	5	3	3	eɪ	4	-lv	5	skw-	5
ʃ	5	5	5	aɪ	3	-lz	5	-ns	5
ʒ	nt	5	nt	ɔɪ	3	sm-	5	-ps	5
h	2	nt	–			sn-	5	-ts	5
ʍ	5	nt	–			sp-	5	-mz	5
w	2	2	–			st-	5	-nz	5
j	4	4	–			-st	6	-ŋz	5
tʃ	5	5	4			sk-	5	-dz	5
dʒ	4	4	6			-ks	5	-gz	5

[a] nt: Not tested.
SOURCE: Wellman et al., 34.

TABLE 14. Earliest Age Levels at which 100 Percent of Children Tested by Davis Correctly Articulated Consonant Sounds Listed

Age Levels Yrs.	Consonants						
3.5	m	p	b	w	h		
4.5	n	t	d	ŋ	k	g	j
5.5	f	v	s	z[a]			
6.5	ʃ	ʒ	l	θ	ð		
8.0	r	ʍ	s	z[a]			

[a] [s] and [z] develop consistently in words at 4 or 5 years of age; then they often become distorted with loss of upper anterior deciduous teeth. This distortion is usually corrected automatically when anterior dentition is permanent at about 8 years.
SOURCE: Davis, 4.

TABLE 15. Earliest Age Levels at which 75 Percent of Children Tested by Templin Correctly Articulated Consonant Sounds Listed

Age Levels Yrs.	Consonants						
3.0	m	n	ŋ	p	f	h	w
3.5	j						
4.0	b	d	k	g	r		
4.5	s	ʃ	tʃ				
6.0	t	l	v	θ			
7.0	ð	z	ʒ	dʒ			

Sound tested but not articulated correctly by 75 percent of the subjects at the oldest age tested (8.0) : [ʍ].
SOURCE: Templin, 26.

TABLE 16. Ten Consonant Sounds (Tested as Singles) Most Frequently Misarticulated as Reported in Four Studies

	Sample Studied				
Rank	25 Elementary School Children Aged 7-2 to 13-5 Functional Articulation Problems (1)	1989 Children in Grades I Through VI[a] (2)	1998 Children in Grades VII Through XII[a] (3)	1661 University Students (4)	83 University Freshmen with Articulation Problems (5)
1	s	θ	z	s-z	s
2	z	s	v	hʍ-w	z
3	ʃ	t	tʃ	ʃ-ʒ	dʒ
4	tʃ	ð	ŋ	θ-ð	ʃ
5	dʒ	z	ð	tʃ-dʒ	tʃ
6	ʒ	dʒ	hʍ	t-d	hʍ
7	hʍ	tʃ	f	m-n-ŋ	ʒ
8	θ	r	s	r	ð
9	r	v	θ	l	ŋ
10	ð	k	g	f-v	θ

[a] Minor errors excluded.
SOURCE: (1) Hall, 7; (2) Roe and Milisen, 21; (3) Sayler, 22; (4) Barnes, 2; (5) Hall, 7.

TABLE 17. Mean Scores, with Standard Deviations, of Children
on 50-Item Screening Test

Age Yrs.	Girls (N=30)[a]		Boys (N=30)		Both Sexes (N=60)		Upper SE[b] (N=18)		Lower SE[c] (N=42)	
	Mean	SD	Mean	SD	Mean	SD	Mean	SD	Mean	SD
3	20.1	12.9	22.5	13.5	21.3	13.2	21.5	13.2	21.2	13.3
3½	30.5	13.1	25.1	15.2	27.8	14.2	28.8	13.6	27.4	14.8
4	34.2	10.6	34.7	11.2	34.4	10.9	37.3	7.3	33.2	11.9
4½	37.3	10.3	34.3	13.4	35.8	11.8	38.7	11.6	34.6	12.1
5	40.6	12.0	34.7	14.5	37.7	13.3	41.6	9.4	36.0	14.8
6	44.3	8.7	38.5	13.8	41.4	11.3	42.1	11.9	38.8	14.6
7	47.8	3.9	44.0	8.4	45.9	6.2	48.2	4.3	42.7	12.1
8	47.9	4.6	47.8	4.2	47.8	4.4	48.8	2.2	47.5	5.0

[a] N=number of subjects at each age level.
[b] Upper SE=subjects in classes I, II, and III of Minnesota Scale of Paternal Occupations.
[c] Lower SE=subjects in classes V, VI, and VII of Minnesota Scale of Paternal Occupations.
SOURCE: Templin, 27.

TABLE 18. Cut-off Score on Screening Test at Each Age Level

Age in years	3	3½	4	4½	5	6	7	8
Cut-off score	12	18	23	26	31	34	39	44

SOURCE: Templin, 27

TABLE 19. Mean Scores, with Standard Deviations, of Children
on 176-Item Diagnostic Test

Age Yrs.	Girls (N=30)[a]		Boys (N=30)		Both Sexes (N=60)		Upper SE[b] (N=18)		Lower SE[c] (N=42)	
	Mean	SD	Mean	SD	Mean	SD	Mean	SD	Mean	SD
3	88.2	31.8	98.3	35.0	93.3	33.8	97.6	33.1	91.5	34.0
3½	118.2	31.0	105.5	37.6	111.9	35.0	115.9	31.1	110.1	36.5
4	125.5	26.7	127.2	31.6	126.4	29.3	136.1	18.9	122.2	31.8
4½	131.2	29.5	127.2	32.2	129.2	31.0	141.7	29.8	123.8	29.9
5	141.8	33.9	128.8	38.1	135.3	36.7	146.0	26.8	130.3	39.1
6	156.9	21.8	143.7	33.8	150.3	29.2	154.5	28.6	140.4	42.7
7	166.4	10.8	157.3	21.7	161.9	17.7	167.8	11.4	151.4	38.9
8	166.6	13.2	167.6	8.6	167.1	11.1	169.7	7.3	166.0	12.3

[a] N=number of subjects at each age level.
[b] Upper SE=subjects in classes I, II, and III of Minnesota Scale of Paternal Occupations.
[c] Lower SE=subjects in classes V, VI, and VII of Minnesota Scale of Paternal Occupations.
SOURCE: Templin, 26.

A. RECORD SHEET

Key: Mark correct sound (√); substitutions with sound substituted; omitted sounds (—); distorted sounds (×); no response (nr).

	I	M	F

1. i____   19. m____ ____ ____   **r-blends**

2. ɪ____   20. n____ ____ ____   44. pr-____

3. ɛ____   21. ŋ   ____ ____   45. br-____

4. æ____   22. p____ ____ ____   46. tr-____

5. ʌ____   23. b____ ____ ____   47. dr-____

6. ə____   24. t____ ____ ____   48. kr-____

7. ɝ____   25. d____ ____ ____   49. gr-____

8. ɚ____   26. k____ ____ ____   50. fr-____

9. ɑ____   27. g____ ____ ____   51. θr-____

10. ɔ____   28. r____ ____   52. ʃr-____

11. ʊ____   29. l____ ____ ____

12. u____   30. f____ ____ ____

13. ju____ 31. v____ ____ ____

14. oʊ____ 32. θ____ ____ ____   **l-blends**

15. ɑʊ____ 33. ð____ ____ ____   76. pl-____

16. eɪ____ 34. s____ ____ ____   77. bl-____

17. ɑɪ____ 35. z____ ____ ____   78. kl-____

18. ɔɪ____ 36. ʃ____ ____ ____   79. gl-____

        37. ʒ   ____ ____   80. fl-____

        38. h____ ____

        39. ʍ____ ____

        40. w____ ____

        41. j____ ____   **s-blends**

        42. tʃ____ ____ ____   95. sm-____ -sm____

        43. dʒ____ ____ ____   96. sn-____

        97. sp-____ -sp____

        98. st-____ -st____

        99. sk-____ -sk____ -ks____

        100. sl-____

        101. sw-____

	æ			æ		Other 2-element Blends

æ Syllabic | æ Nonsyllabic | Other 2-element Blends

ʒ

Syllabic	Nonsyllabic	Other 2-element Blends
53. -mɚ_____	64. -ɚm_____	109. tw-_____
54. -nɚ_____	65. -ɚn_____	110. kw-_____
55. -pɚ_____	66. -ɚp_____	111. -zm_____
56. -bɚ_____	67. -ɚb_____	112. -ŋk_____
57. -tɚ_____	68. -ɚt_____	113. -d3d_____
58. -dɚ_____	69. -ɚd_____	114. -mp_____
59. -kɚ_____	70. -ɚk_____	115. -nt_____
60. -gɚ_____	71. -ɚg_____	116. -nd_____
61. -fɚ_____	72. -ɚf_____	117 -kt_____
62. -ðɚ_____	73. -ɚθ_____	118. -pt_____
63. -ʃɚ_____	74. -ɚtʃ_____	119. -ft_____
	75.-ɚd3_____	

Vowel 1 | 3-element Blends

Vowel 1		3-element Blends
81. -pl̩_____	88. -lp_____	120. spl-_____
82. -bl̩_____	89. -lb_____	121. spr-_____
83. -tl̩_____	90. -lt_____	122. str-_____
84. -kl̩_____	91. -lk_____	123. skr-_____
85. -gl̩_____	92. -lf_____	124. skw-_____
86. -fl̩_____	93. -lθ_____	125. -kst_____
87. -sl̩_____	94. -lz_____	126. -mpt_____
		127. -mps_____
		128. -ntθ_____

ɚ, ɝ and vowel 1 with blends

102. -stɚ_____	106. -nkl_____
103. -skɚ_____	107. -ngl_____
104. -mbɚ_____	108. -lfθ_____
105. -ɝst_____	

B. ANALYSIS SHEET

1. Comparison with norms:
   a. Of the 50 Screening Test items, how many did subject
      produce correctly?   _____
   b. According to the table of norms for the Screening Test,
      what is the mean number of items correctly produced by
      children of this age and sex?   _____
   c. According to Screening Test norms, what cut-off score
      separates adequate from inadequate performance at the
      age of this subject?   _____
   d. Of the 176 Diagnostic Test items, how many did subject
      produce correctly?   _____
   e. According to the table of norms for the Diagnostic Test,
      what is the mean number of items correctly produced by
      children of this age and sex?   _____
   f. How many singles (numbers 1-43) were defective in any
      position?   _____

2. Analysis of misarticulations: Analyze the subject's production of the phonemes
   listed as singles (numbers 1-43).
   a. List all error sounds, indicating position of error (I, M, F).

   Omissions   Substitutions   Distortions
   _____   _____   _____

   b. Which of these phonemes (1-43), incorrectly articulated as singles in the
      positions indicated above, were correctly articulated as singles in at least
      one position?

   c. Which of these phonemes (1-43), incorrectly articulated as singles in any
      position, were correctly produced in any of the blends in which they were
      further tested?

d. Which phonemes (1-43), not correctly produced as singles in any position or subsequently in blends, were correctly produced following stimulation as described below?

As a single			In a Blend
In Isolation	In a Syllable	In a Word	in a Word

e. The following phonemes were never articulated correctly anywhere in the test or following any type of stimulation:

3. Factors possibly related to patterns of misarticulation:

* Permission for the reproduction of the record sheet and analysis sheet portions of the Articulation Test Form developed for use with the Templin-Darley Screening and Diagnostic Tests of Articulation has been kindly given by the Bureau of Educational Research and Service, Extension Division, University of Iowa, Iowa City. The four-page articulation test form prepared originally for use with the Templin-Darley Tests of Articulation can be ordered from the publisher in limited numbers or in quantity.

The items followed by double lines constitute the 50-item Screening Test.

Additional copies of this form may also be obtained from the Interstate Printers and Publishers, 19-27 North Jackson Street, Danville, Illinois.

REFERENCES

1. Anderson, Patricia W., "The relationship of normal and defective articulation of the consonant [s] in various phonetic contexts to auditory discrimination between normal and defective [s] production among children from kindergarten through fourth grade," unpublished M.A. thesis, University of Iowa, 1949.

2. Barnes, H. G., "A diagnosis of the speech needs and abilities of students in a required course in speech training at the State University of Iowa," unpublished Ph.D. disseration, University of Iowa, 1932.

3. Buckingham, D. R., and E. W. Dolch, *A Combined Word List*, Chicago: Ginn, 1936.

4. Davis, Irene Poole, "The speech aspects of reading readiness," *17th Yearbook of the Department of Elementary School Principals*, NEA, 1938, *17* (7):282-289.

5. Gates, A. I., *A Reading Vocabulary for the Primary Grades* (revised and enlarged), New York: Teachers College, Columbia University, 1935.

6. Goodenough, Florence, *Mental Testing*, New York: Rinehart, 1949.

7. Hall, Margaret E., "Auditory factors in functional articulatory speech defects," *Journal of Experimental Education*, 1938, *7*:110-132.

8. Horn, Madeline D., *A Study of the Vocabulary of Children Before Entering the First Grade*, International Kindergarten Union, Child Study Committee, 1928.

9. Irwin, O. C., "Development of speech during infancy: curve of phonemic frequencies," *Journal of Experimental Psychology*, 1947, *37*:187-193.

10. Irwin, O. C., "Infant speech: variability and the problem of diagnosis," *Journal of Speech Disorders*, 1947, *12*:287-289.

11. Irwin, O. C., "Infant speech: consonantal sounds according to place of articulation," *Journal of Speech Disorders*, 1947, *12*:397-401.

12. Irwin, O. C., "Infant speech: development of vowel sounds," *Journal of Speech and Hearing Disorders*, 1948, *13*:31-34.

13. Irwin, O. C., "Infant speech: the effect of family occupational status and of age on use of sound types; on sound frequency," *Journal of Speech and Hearing Disorders*, 1948, *13*:224-226, 320-323.

14. Irwin, O. C., "Infant speech: speech sound development of sibling and only infants," *Journal of Experimental Psychology*, 1948, *38*:600-602.

15. Irwin, O. C., and H. P. Chen, "Development of speech during infancy: curve of phonemic types," *Journal of Experimental Psychology*, 1946, *36*:431-436.

16. Jordan, E. P., "Articulation test measures and listener rating of articulation defectiveness," *Journal of Speech and Hearing Research*, 1960, *3*:303-319.

17. Mase, D. J., *Etiology of Articulatory Defects*, New York: Teachers College, Columbia University, 1946.
18. "Public School Speech and Hearing Services," *Journal of Speech and Hearing Disorders*, 1961, Monogr. Suppl. 8, pp. 1-163.
19. Rinsland, H. D., *A Basic Vocabulary of Elementary School Children*, New York: Macmillan, 1945.
20. Rinsland, H. D., *The Vocabulary of Elementary School Children of the United States*, Norman, Okla.: University of Oklahoma Press, 1938.
21. Roe, Vivian, and R. Milisen, "The effect of maturation upon defective articulation in elementary grades," *Journal of Speech Disorders*, 1942, *7*:37-45.
22. Sayler, Helen K., "The effect of maturation upon defective articulation in grades seven through twelve," *Journal of Speech and Hearing Disorders*, 1949, *14*:202-207.
23. Snow, Katherine, and Robert Milisen, "The influence of oral versus pictorial presentation upon articulation testing results," *Journal of Speech and Hearing Disorders*, 1954, Monogr. Suppl. 4, pp. 30-36.
24. Spriestersbach, D. C., and J. F. Curtis, "Misarticulation and discrimination of speech sounds," *Quarterly Journal of Speech*, 1951, *37*:483-491.
25. Stetson, R. H., *Motor Phonetics*, Amsterdam: North-Holland Publ. Co., 1951.
26. Templin, Mildred C., *Certain Language Skills in Children* (*Institute of Child Welfare Monograph Series*, No. 26), Minneapolis: University of Minnesota Press, 1957.
27. Templin, Mildred C., "Norms on a screening test of articulation for ages three through eight," *Journal of Speech and Hearing Disorders*, 1953, *18*:323-331.
28. Templin, Mildred C., "Spontaneous versus imitated verbalization in testing articulation in preschool children," *Journal of Speech Disorders*, 1947, *12*:293-300.
29. Templin, Mildred C., and F. L. Darley, *The Templin-Darley Tests of Articulation*, Iowa City: University of Iowa Bureau of Educational Research and Service, 1960.
30. Terman, L. M., and Maud A. Merrill, *Stanford-Binet Intelligence Scale: Manual for the Third Revision, Form L-M*, New York: Houghton-Mifflin, 1960.
31. Thorndike, E. L., *The Teacher's Word Book*, New York: Teachers College, Columbia University, 1921.
32. Thorndike, E. L., *A Teacher's Word Book of Twenty Thousand Words*, New York: Teachers College, Columbia University, 1932.
33. Thorndike, E. L., and I. Lorge, *The Teacher's Work Book of 30,000 Words*, New York: Teachers College, Columbia University, 1944.
34. Wellman, Beth L., Ida Mae Case, Ida G. Mengert, and Dorothy E. Bradbury, "Speech Sounds of Young Children," *University of Iowa Studies in Child Welfare*, 1931, *5*, (2).

35. Whipple, G. M., *The Twenty-Fourth Yearbook of the National Society for the Study of Education*, Bloomington, Ill.: Public School Publ. Co., 1925, pp. 185-193.

36. Winitz, Harris, and O. C. Irwin, "Infant speech: consistency with age," *Journal of Speech and Hearing Research*, 1958, *1*:245-249.

5 *THE SPEECH MECHANISM*

In Chapter 1 we were reminded that oral expression involves, in addition to symbolic formulation, the processes of respiration, phonation, resonance, and articulation. The structures involved in these processes include the respiratory mechanism, larynx, tongue, hard and soft palates, teeth, lips, pharynx, and nasal cavities. To be sure, these structures are controlled during oral expression by the nervous system, but we shall not be concerned here with measurements and judgments dealing primarily with the nervous system. These lie fundamentally within the province of the neurologist; neurological considerations of particular importance to the speech pathologist are included mainly in the sections of this manual that deal with dysphasia and cerebral palsy.

You will note, too, that Form 4 (Speech Mechanism Examination) does not include an evaluation of the larynx. Laryngeal assessment is omitted from this examination because the larynx is the only speech structure that cannot be observed or evaluated rather directly. In our opinion, direct and indirect laryngoscopy is the proper province of the laryngologist rather than the speech pathologist. As speech clinicians we do, of course, make inferences about the condition and functioning

111

of the larynx from our observations of oral expression. In this manual we consider these inferences in Chapter 6, in relation to examination of voice quality.

Evaluation of the speech structures is difficult even for the experienced clinician, since many of the observations involve estimates or judgments rather than direct measurements. The range in motility, shape, and size of the structures is great. Since certain particulars of normative data on the shape, size, and motility of many of the structures are not available, you must as a clinician make your evaluations of them largely on the basis of your own experience. Furthermore, the relationships between the sizes of contiguous structures and spaces is the important consideration rather than the measures of size as such. Finally, the combined effect of several deviations of the speech mechanism tends to be cumulative and may prove to be disabling to the speaker even though the magnitude of the individual deviations may be of little clinical significance; yet it is extremely difficult to assign the weight to be given to each of the several deviations in evaluating their combined effects. For these reasons it is important that you make as many observations of oral structures as you possibly can so that you will acquire a firsthand knowledge of the usual and the exceptional and a practical sense regarding the significance of the effect of any given structural condition on speech.

We do not usually find dramatic deviations of the oral structures which can be conclusively related to specific deviations in speech. While unusual size and shape of these structures may contribute to a speech problem, most individuals show very considerable ability to compensate for structural irregularities. Many individuals who have poorly aligned or missing teeth, short and immobile upper lips—indeed, some who have unrepaired cleft palates—may speak quite satisfactorily, at least in certain contexts and for specific purposes. We must be careful, therefore, in relating findings from examination of the speech mechanism to the speech imperfections that we observe. As a general rule, if the speaker can produce a sound correctly in some contexts, particularly those involving connected speech, any structural deviations he may have, even in apparently marked degrees, cannot be extremely significant in relation to his misarticulations of that sound.

It is important that we understand clearly why we examine the oral structures. Almost always we are chiefly interested in their functional adequacy. If, in our judgment, the structures are not adequate for speech, we must decide whether the speaker can be helped to obtain more effective function from the deviant structures or whether physical changes must be made in them before we attempt to change their function. Only rarely are we interested in explaining why the deviation exists. To be sure, some speech pathologists, working in certain kinds of specialized settings, may make observations of the motility of the speech structures which will have significance to workers in other disciplines, such as neurologists who are attempting to arrive at a diagnosis concerning possible pathology of the nervous system. However, even in these instances, the speech pathologist limits his reporting to the observations and evaluations concerning function. As a consequence, the Speech Mechanism Examination calls for a rating of the adequacy for speech of each of the oral structures in terms which are suggestive of the possible practical clinical decisions to be made. The ratings to be made are as follows:

1 Normal.
2 Slight deviation—probably no adverse effect on speech.
3 Moderate deviation—possible adverse effect on speech; remedial services may be required, particularly if other structures of the speech mechanism are also deviant.
4 Extreme deviation—sufficient to prevent normal production of speech; modification of structure required, either with or without clinical speech services.

When as a clinician you give a structure a rating of 4 you are indicating that, in your judgment, the speaker will not be able to produce certain sounds or qualities of voice until some changes are made in the function or potential for function of the affected structures of his speech mechanism. If you feel that physical changes must be effected before function can be changed, your retraining program will likely not include efforts to change the speech behavior until the indicated changes have been made. It follows, of course, that you should be prepared to recommend that the speaker secure the services of the appropriate professional person who can effect the desired physical changes.

When you give a structure a rating of 3 you are indicating that you may be able to provide a retraining program which will enable the speaker to make the necessary compensations required by the deviant structure. Structural changes may not be required in this case unless several related structures are involved. In any event a rating of 3 implies that you feel that a program of experimental speech therapy is justified. You would use a rating of 2 to indicate that a structure does not fall clearly within the normal range but that the deviation has no practical clinical significance so far as speech is concerned.

The specific observations called for in the Speech Mechanism Examination may best be considered against a background of essential information about the functional contribution made by each of the various structures to the speech act.

THE LIPS

Normally the lips serve to modify the breath stream in the production of the labial sounds. In general, however, a highly precise modification of the breath stream is not essential in producing the labial sounds. Furthermore, since the lips are highly mobile, it is quite possible, for example, for the lower lip to make contact with even an unusually short upper lip. As a consequence, deviations of the lips will rarely be rated as *Extreme*. Such a point of view is consistent with the findings of Fairbanks and Green (5). It is consistent also with data reported by Spriestersbach, Moll, and Morris (21), who concluded that deviations of the lip structure do not play a significant part in accounting for the articulation problems of speakers with cleft lips and palates. In fact, they reported that persons with clefts only of the lip had essentially normal articulation.

Nevertheless, we must evaluate the lips and make judgments of their contribution to the articulation problems of the speakers we observe because, if for no other reason, professional workers from other fields frequently relate structural deviations of the lips to articulation errors. We must be prepared, therefore, to explain the lack of a relationship when such a judgment is consistent with our observations. It should also be appreciated that lip structures, particularly in the case of any speaker with a repaired cleft lip, need to be evaluated because of the important role they play in the appearance of the individual. The psychological impact of a badly scarred lip may sometimes be great enough to cause a speaker to react negatively to speaking situations.

The motility of the lips can be evaluated by observing labial movements involving both speech and nonspeech acts. However, the Speech Mechanism Examination requires observations of speech acts only. Sprague (20) found that normal 8-year-old boys articulate, on the average, 4.39 [pʌ] sounds per second. Bloomquist (2) found that normal 9-, 10-, and 11-year-old boys and girls could produce the same sound, on the average, 4.9 times per second. In both studies the standard deviation was approximpately 0.60. Thus, conservatively using Sprague's mean as the reference point and allowing a range of variation of two standard deviations, you would consider speeds of less than 3.0 [pʌ] sounds per second below average and speeds above 5.50 per second above average.

THE TEETH

Normally the teeth play an important role in the production of labiodental, linguadental and postdental fricatives. However, as in the case of the lips, ample clinical and research evidence exists to support the view that speakers are able to make major compensations for dental deviations, particularly if they are not accompanied by other relevant deviations of the speech mechanism. Fymbo (8), for example, found that 38 percent of his speakers who had severe malocclusions and 24 percent of his speakers with facial deformities resulting from malocclusions had satisfactory speech. Fairbanks and Lentner (6) found that 10 out of 30 young adults who had been rated as superior speakers had one or more marked dental deviations. Snow (19) observed that a group of children with missing or grossly defective incisors were able to produce from 63 to 94 percent of the dental sounds correctly. Again, as in the case of the lips, dental deviations are easily observed and inexperienced examiners frequently attempt to account for articulation difficulties on the basis of these deviations. In contrast to the situation with the lips, however, dental conditions may frequently be considered extreme in relation to the production of consonant sounds, particularly the sibilants, if there is severe openbite or mesioclusion.

Eruption of Teeth

Because of the possible importance of dental deviations in accounting for certain misarticulations, it is important to review basic information about dental development and dental relationships. Tables 20 and 21 provide information about dental development.

Dental Occlusion

Use Angle's categories, summarized briefly below, in describing dental occlusion. For a detailed description of the categories see Graber (9, pp. 166-189). However, before we consider definitions of the various categories, a word of explanation is in order concerning the definition of *mesial* and *distal* in this context. The usual dictionary definition of *mesial* is "toward the middle or center." *Distal,* on the other hand, is defined as "away from the middle or center." In this context, however, the reference point is *not the center of the body, as one might assume, but the midpoint of the dental arch,* that is, the point between the central incisors. Thus, when the lower arch is displaced in an *anterior* direction in relation to the upper arch, it is said to be in a mesial position. When it is displaced in a *posterior* direction in relation to the upper arch, it is said to be in a distal position.

Here, then, are the definitions essential in Angle's system of classification of dental occlusion patterns:

Normal Occlusion: The teeth are well aligned and the upper and lower arches are in correct anteroposterior and laterial relationship to each other and to the rest of the skull anatomy. An important aspect of this relationship involves the occlusion of the upper and lower first permanent molars. See Bloomer's discussion and diagrams (*23*, pp. 625-629) for a clear presentation of the nature of this relationship. As used here "normal" does not mean "average." Several studies have shown that only about one-third of the population have normal occlusion as here defined.

Neutroclusion (Angle's Class I): The upper and lower dental arches are in correct front-to-back (anteroposterior) and side-to-side (lateral) relationship to each other and to the skull but there is malalignment of individual teeth, for example, rotated, or jumbled teeth, or teeth displaced toward the lips or cheeks or tongue from their normal positions.

Distoclusion (Angle's Class II): The lower jaw with its superimposed dental arch is too far back (posterior) in relation to the upper arch and to the rest of the skull.

Mesioclusion (Angle's Class III): The lower jaw with its superimposed dental arch is too far forward (anterior) in relation to the upper dental arch and the rest of the skull.

The following terms are defined to assist you in describing conditions of the anterior teeth:

Openbite—absence of contact between the upper and lower anterior teeth resulting in open spaces between them when the posterior teeth are in occlusion.

Closebite—the upper anterior teeth overlap the lower front teeth excessively when the posterior teeth are in occlusion.

Crossbite—dental arches of upper and lower teeth cross over each other from side to side instead of maintaining a parallel relationship; the lower jaw may be swung to one side of the midline.

Edentulous spaces—spaces resulting from the absence or loss of teeth.

Lack of proximal contact—lack of contact between any two adjacent teeth—that is, space between the teeth.

Misalignment or malalignment—an abnormal position of a tooth in the dental arch.

Jumbling—a piling-up or crossing-over of several teeth.

Supernumerary teeth—teeth in excess of the normal number.

Linguoversion—deflection of a tooth toward the tongue from its normal position.

Labioversion—deflection of a tooth toward the lips from its normal position.

Buccalversion—deflection of a tooth toward the cheeks from its normal position.

THE TONGUE

Normally the tongue is a very mobile structure. It can be moved rapidly and precisely. When it functions in conjunction with the other oral articulators, it participates in the production of speech sounds by channeling, impeding, and obstructing the breath stream as it passes through the mouth. It also assists in modifying the resonance cavities used in speech. Its strength and motility may be impaired as the result of poor muscular development, paresis due to pathology of the nervous system, or disease or accident resulting in the removal of portions of the tongue. While there are reports of individuals who have developed satisfactory speech without tongues, under usual conditions the tongue is one of the most important structures of the oral mechanism.

Tongues vary in size and shape. So do the oral cavities in which they function. Sometimes the two do not seem to fit together very well. Unfortunately, there is no easy way to quantify the size of the tongue. Judgments concerning its size in relation to the dental arches are made largely on the basis of experience in viewing these structures.

The motility of the tongue is necessarily affected by pathologies which effect its innervation. However, individuals with articulation problems who do not have neural pathology affecting the tongue are able to manipulate the tongue as effectively, at least when tested on unlearned nonspeech tasks, as individuals with normal speech (7, 14).

On the basis of the findings of Fairbanks and Spriestersbach (7), the following scale might be used for judging the rate at which a person can touch the alveolar ridge with the tongue without speech: below average, less than 3.5 contacts per second; average, from 3.5 to 6.0 contacts per second; above average, more than 6.0 contacts per second. On the basis of the work of Sprague (20), the following scale might be used in judging the rate at which a speaker can articulate [tʌ]: below average, less than 3 sounds per second; average, from 3.0 to 5.5 sounds per second; above average, more than 5.5 sounds per second. There are no available data to indicate the rate at which speakers can touch the corners of the mouth. However, clinical experience indicates that the rate of performing complete cycles of contacts, touching both corners of the mouth with the tongue, is of the same order of magnitude as the rates quoted above.

It is possible that the lingual frenum may restrict the activity of the anterior portion of the tongue. When this condition is severe the speaker will have difficulty touching the alveolar ridge with the tip of his tongue and the blade of the tongue will look like the top of a heart when he attempts to protrude it between his teeth. However, restriction by the frenum will typically not be marked enough to impair the functioning of the tongue for speech. As Curtis points out (*12*, p. 102), "If the child has been able to nurse, can extend his tongue between the teeth, and can touch the upper gum ridge with the tip of his tongue, the judgment that he is 'tongue-tied' is probably irrelevant so far as his ability to speak is concerned."

THE HARD PALATE

Comprehensive evaluation of the hard palate includes consideration of the molar and cuspid width and length, the nature of the palatal vault, etc. However, you may appropriately limit your observations of this structure to those aspects which, in your judgment, are most apt to influence speech. Specialized examinations conducted for research purposes, or to evaluate specific problems such as those of cleft palate, may require more detailed observations.

The two deviations of palatal contour which tend to be of most significance in speech production are flat palatal vaults and very high and narrow palatal vaults, particularly if the sizes of the tongues which function within the oral cavities which have these types of palatal contours are inappropriate for the available space. There are no objective techniques for making routine clinical measurements of these aspects, however. This is another instance in which you as the clinician must make use of your background of experience in making the required evaluations.

THE VELOPHARYNGEAL PORT MECHANISM

As in the case of the hard palate, so in that of the velopharyngeal port, the descriptive observations called for in the Speech Mechanism Examination are gross and based on norms derived from clinical experience rather than from measurements which can be made objectively.

Calnan (*4*) has observed a close relationship between the bifid or divided uvula and submucous cleft of the hard palate. In view of his evidence, you should be alert to the need for a medical examination to consider the possible existence of a submucous cleft if the speaker has a bifid uvula and exhibits speech which suggests the existence of an incompetent velopharyngeal mechanism. In such cases the soft palate does not function properly, even though it appears to be normal, because maldevelopment and malfunction of the palatal muscles are generally found with submucous cleft of the hard palate.

Evaluation of the function of the velopharyngeal port mechanism on the basis of a peroral examination (examination made by looking directly into the mouth rather than by radiographic or other indirect means) is complicated by several factors. First, the crucial area to be observed—the area where the port is most constricted during speech—cannot be directly observed in a peroral examination because the inferior borders of the soft palate and the uvula block its view. Secondly, the views you can obtain of the functioning of the mechanism are limited to those that you can make during the sustained phonation of low vowels or of actions resulting from eliciting the gag reflex. It has been well documented that the action of the velopharyngeal mechanism involved in both of these tasks may not be representative of its actions during connected speech. You can infer from such investigations as those of Calnan (*3*), Bloomer (*1*), and Moll (*17*) that you will generally observe less action of the port mechanism during the sustaining of low vowels and more action during the gag reflex than would exist during connected speech. To complicate the evaluation problem still further, there is considerable evidence to indicate that given individuals may differ markedly from these generalizations. In fact, there is considerable variability even in the reflex activity of the velopharyngeal port mechanism. The neurology staff at the Mayo Clinic (*15*, p. 193) has noted that "The pharyngeal reflex may be absent in apparently healthy people." Furthermore, some speakers who have normal gag reflexes do not necessarily exhibit normal function of the velopharyngeal port mechanism during speech.

The Speech Mechanism Examination calls for observations of the symmetry of velar elevation while the person is prolonging the vowel [ɑ] or when the gag reflex is induced. Lack of symmetry of this movement may be an indicator of a palatal neuromotor problem.

The observations of the soft palate and oropharynx included in the Speech Mechanism Examination serve to emphasize the fact that the velopharyngeal mechanism is complex; that it involves, at least in some individuals, mesial movement of the lateral walls of the oropharynx as well as elevation and posterior retraction of the soft palate; and that the functioning of the involved structures may vary from one type of activity to another.

Radiographic information can, of course, tell us a good deal about the dynamic functioning of the velopharyngeal port mechanism. It helps us to understand not only how the various structures which make up the mechanism work together in an integrated fashion but also how their movements are related to each other in time (*16*). However, such information is not readily available to most clinicians nor is it required in many instances. Certainly it is possible for you to make observations of activities which involve the velopharyngeal port mechanism and from which you can make at least some gross assessments of its function. Thus, you can observe the individual as he blows out a match and drinks through a straw; you know that he must achieve some degree of velopharyngeal closure in order to do these things. Again, in this instance, however, you should be careful not to assume that because a person can do these things his velopharyngeal mechanism is adequate for speech; if he cannot do them, however, you may properly consider the possibility that speech is affected accordingly.

Considerable recent research has been concerned with the ability of speakers to develop positive breath pressure in the oral cavity. We are interested in this measurement because we know that the production of stop-plosives and fricatives requires some minimal amount of pressure, as yet unspecified. We also know from the work of Spriestersbach and Powers (22) that velopharyngeal closure, as measured from lateral head X-ray films, is highly related to the ability to develop intra-oral breath pressure. Therefore, measurement of a speaker's ability to develop intra-oral breath pressure provides us with some indirect information about the functional efficiency of his velopharyngeal port mechanism.

Various types of instruments, including wet and dry spirometers and oral manometers, are available for the measurement of intra-oral breath pressure. Air flow through the oral and nasal cavities can be measured by an instrument called the pneumotachograph. For clinical purposes, however, we are more interested in the ratio obtained by comparing the amount of air pressure that an individual can develop with the nostrils open to the amount that he can develop with the nostrils occluded. Individuals vary greatly in their ability to impound air in the oral cavity although there is reason to believe that most persons with normal breathing mechanisms are capable of developing far more pressure than the minimal amount required for the articulation of consonant sounds. Because of the individual variability in this regard, the measure we obtain of the individual's ability to impound air with the nostrils occluded is used as his personal norm against which we compare his ability to impound air in the oral cavity when he does his best to close the velopharyngeal port. Presumably, if he is able to close the velopharyngeal port for this task, he should be able to build up as much oral breath pressure with the nostrils open as when they are occluded. Consequently, the ratio of these two measures has more functional significance than do the absolute pressure values. It is best, incidentally, to use a device which allows the pressure to be measured while the air is flowing through the mouth rather than one which measures static intra-oral breath pressure. That is why some models of manometers currently in use employ a constant leak or bleed. Such a provision prevents the examinee from valving with the tongue and soft palate in order to impound air in the oral cavity. It is clear that when the subject does this the pressure ratio we obtain is irrelevant to the evaluation of the competence of the soft palate-pharyngeal wall valving mechanism.

Spriestersbach, Moll, and Morris (21) have shown that ratios of .89 or better are likely to reflect adequate functioning of the velopharyngeal port mechanism. A ratio of .89 means that the intra-oral breath pressure achieved with the nostrils open is 89 percent of that achieved with the nostrils occluded. Most speakers without any organic involvement of the speech mechanism should be able to achieve ratios of this order. However, we may infer from the work of Spriestersbach, Moll, and Morris and from that of Hardy (10) that incompetence of the velopharyngeal port mechanism of individuals with cleft palates, cerebral palsy, and other pathological conditions which may result in palatal paresis or inadequacy of palatal tissue is likely to be one of the major factors in accounting for the articulation difficulties of these speakers. As a consequence, you will be well advised to obtain substantial amounts of clinical experience in making intra-oral breath pressure measurements. Incidentally, we have found that the subject's nostrils can be closed best if the examiner holds his fingers gently against the nares rather than the alae. Speakers, especially children, do not like to have their noses pinched while being given intra-oral breath pressure tests.

In view of the importance which intra-oral breath pressure plays in the articulation of stop-plosives, the speed and manner of articulating [kʌ] and [pʌtəkʌ] are to be observed. Individuals who do have velopharyngeal incompetence may produce these syllables, if at all, at speeds that are slower than normal, not because of poor motor ability but because they have learned that they can produce the sounds involved in the syllables more acceptably if they articulate them at slower rates. On the basis of the work of Bloomquist (2) and Sprague (20) speakers without involvement of the velopharyngeal mechanism who produce less than 3.5 [kʌ] syllables per second are to considered to be below average; those producing from 3.5 to 5.5 syllables may be considered average; and those who can articulate more than 5.5 syllables per second are to be considered to be above average. On the basis of Sprague's work individuals who can produce less than 1.0 [pʌtəkʌ] per second may be considered to be below average; those producing from 1.0 to 1.75 per second are to be considered average; and those who can articulate more than 1.75 per second can be considered to be above average. For this series of syllables we have included in our examination the counts noted both when the nostrils are open and when they are closed. Our assumption is that if there is velopharyngeal incompetence, the speaker may be able to say the series at a faster rate with the nostrils closed. In any case you should interpret this ratio with some tentativeness since its validity has not been subjected to test.

THE FAUCES

We are interested in examining the area of the fauces because we are sometimes able to make inferences from these observations concerning the functioning of the velopharyngeal port mechanism and because, in some instances, the faucial isthmus may be restricted to a degree that makes the free movement of air from the oropharynx into the oral cavity difficult. In some instances the tonsils may be so much enlarged that they touch at the midline during phonation. Such a condition may result in a muffling of the laryngeal tone and in placing an unusual requirement on the velopharyngeal port mechanism to achieve a very tight closure if nasal escape of air is to be prevented. This reasoning is consistent with the observations of Kaltenborn (13) that in the production of non-nasal tones there is a higher degree of velopharyngeal closure when the opening into the oral cavity from the oropharynx is small than when the opening is large.

The muscles which underlie the mucous membranes of the faucial pillars are intermeshed with the muscles of the soft palate, pharynx, and tongue. On the basis of clinical observations it is assumed that mesial movement—movement toward the midline—of the posterior pillars during phonation and gagging is an indication that the muscles of the lateral walls of the pharynx are playing some part in velopharyngeal closure. It has also been assumed that such movements reflect a desirable type of possible compensatory activity in those instances in which adequate velopharyngeal closure is not achieved by action of the soft palate. On the other hand, some individuals have only remnants of pillars or none at all. Their absence should not be viewed with alarm since there is no evidence that such speakers have any unique problems in achieving velopharyngeal competence.

THE NASAL CAVITIES

We are interested in making observations of the nasal passageways because they must be relatively open for the production of nasal sounds. Furthermore, it has been our clinical experience that constriction of the nares during speech is a positive indicator of either some degree of velopharyngeal incompetence or a habit pattern which was developed at an earlier time when incompetence did exist.

THE BREATHING MECHANISM

Most authorities agree that sublaryngeal air pressure causes the vocal folds to vibrate when they are in the adducted position. The laryngeal tones which result from these vibrations are used in the production of speech sounds. The breathing mechanism provides us with the means for producing the necessary sublaryngeal air pressure. This pressure must be controlled in the sense that it must be present in adequate degrees to enable us to produce series of laryngeal tones which are long enough for the usual phrasal units of our language. The Speech Mechanism Examination does not include any evaluation of sublaryngeal pressure, however, because it is our clinical experience that speakers, except those whose breathing mechanisms are severely involved, appear to develop such pressures that are well within the range required for speech production.

It will also be noted that the Speech Mechanism Examination includes no observations or measurements of "breathing type" and vital capacity. We agree—with one qualification to be noted presently—with the conclusion of Van Riper and Irwin (24, p. 353) : "On the basis of evidence now available, then, it must be admitted that we cannot establish any predictable relationship between vital capacity and good voice. Moreover, with the exception of extreme upper clavicular breathing, good voice can be and is produced by any of the breathing types. Certainly so far as area of activity is concerned, there is no one best type of breathing. Whatever method gives us enough air pressure is good enough." We would modify this statement by Van Riper and Irwin by deleting the exception concerning upper clavicular breathing, for two reasons. First, we have serious doubts about the reliability of judgments made concerning the types of breathing, including clavicular breathing, used by speakers. Second, we feel that the term "clavicular breathing," and any other term purporting to describe breathing type, tends to carry the implication that other regions of the breathing mechanism are not involved in the breathing cycle. Such an implication, of course, is obviously incorrect. We have included in our examination, however, observations concerning the raising of the shoulders during the respiratory cycle, because we believe that this particular characteristic has clinical significance in alerting us to the possibility of poor breath control during phonation.

The observations of the breathing mechanism called for in the Speech Mechanism Examination are designed to help you make inferences about the control of the breathing mechanism for speech. We agree with Hardy (10, pp. 317-318) that breath control for speech should refer not only to the provision of adequate sublaryngeal pressures at the appropriate times but also to the speaker's "ability to accelerate or decelerate the volume flow of air from his lungs at will, expire or inspire at will, and otherwise regulate his breathing pattern." As a general rule, breath control is not an important factor in accounting for significant communicative problems unless there is a paresis of the breathing mechanism.

Unfortunately, there are no appropriate norms against which to evaluate observations of breath control. For the time being at least, you will have to develop your own standards of adequacy for judging the observations involved. However, in making these observations you focus your attention on this very important aspect of speech production, and gain thereby a more comprehensive appreciation of the speech function in any given case.

In order to acquaint yourself more fully with principles and procedures of examination of the speech mechanism you may want to view and study the film, "Examining the Speech Mechanism," produced in the Department of Speech Pathology and Audiology of the University of Iowa, and available on a rental basis from the Bureau of Audiovisual Education, Extension Division, University of Iowa, Iowa City.

SUMMARY

As we indicated in our introductory comments, it is frequently difficult to pin a particular type of misarticulation to a particular structural deviation in a given instance. A given structural deviation may be of significance only if it occurs as one of a constellation of deviations. In the summary section of the Speech Mechanism Examination we suggest that you view the deviations as constellations. We also, and most importantly, suggest that you interpret the results of the Speech Mechanism Examination in the light of the findings from the testing you have done of the person's speech. No big point is to be made of a space between the upper incisors, for example, when the speaker's only misarticulation is a [w] for [r] substitution.

ASSIGNMENTS

1. Select five speakers, at least two of whom present articulatory problems other than foreign dialect.
2. Examine each speaker with respect to the items listed on the Speech Mechanism Examination. In making your evaluations consider both of

the following factors: (a) the normal range of the population of persons of the same sex and age; (b) the relationships between the structures of the particular person being examined. For example, an individual's tongue might be small when compared to the average of other persons of the same age and sex, but in good proportion in relation to the size of his mandible and the various dimensions of his own oral cavity.

3. After completing this examination, rate the connected speech of each person using Form 2 (p. 78). Note particularly any consistently misarticulated speech sounds, voice characteristics, etc., which logically might be accounted for by some observed feature of the speech mechanism. Relate your findings from the General Speech Behavior Rating to your observations of the speech mechanism as suggested in Section 9, Form 4.

TABLE 20. Ages in Months of Eruption of Deciduous Teeth of 1962 Normal Boys and Girls

Tooth	Earliest Age Erupted	Median Age Erupted	Latest Age Not Yet Erupted
Mandibular central incisor	4	7.8	17
Maxillary central incisor	5	9.6	15
Maxillary lateral incisor	6	11.5	21
Mandibular lateral incisor	6	12.4	27
Maxillary first molar	8	15.1	28
Mandibular first molar	8	15.7	27
Mandibular cuspid tooth	8	18.2	29
Maxillary cuspid tooth	8	18.3	29
Mandibular second molar	8	26.0	34
Maxillary second molar	8	26.2	34

SOURCE: Sandler, *18*.

TABLE 21. Mean Ages of Eruption of Permanent Teeth of White Children Living in the Northern Temperate Zone (N=more than 93,000)

Order of Emergence	Tooth Maxilla	Tooth Mandible	Mean Age of Emergence Boys yrs.	Mean Age of Emergence Girls yrs.	Sex Difference mos.
1		Molar 1	6.21	5.94	3.5
2	Molar 1		6.40	6.22	2.0
3		Incisor 1	6.54	6.26	3.5
4	Incisor 1		7.47	7.20	3.5
5		Incisor 2	7.70	7.34	4.5
6	Incisor 2		8.67	8.20	5.5
7 (Boys) 8 (Girls)	Premolar 1		10.40	10.03	4.5
8 (Boys) 7 (Girls)		Cuspid	10.79	9.86	11.1
9		Premolar 1	10.82	10.18	7.7
10	Premolar 2		11.18	10.88	3.6
11		Premolar 2	11.47	10.89	7.0
12	Cuspid		11.69	10.98	8.5
13		Molar 2	12.12	11.66	5.5
14	Molar 2		12.68	12.27	4.9

SOURCE: Compiled from 24 published reports, after Hurme, *11*.

FORM 4. SPEECH MECHANISM EXAMINATION*

Name _____ Age _____ Sex _____

Examiner _____ Date _____

upper alveolar ridge asymmetrical
right tonsil enlarged
high palatal arch
enlarged papiloma

1. Lips
   a. Structure:
      Touch when upper and lower teeth in contact: yes _____ no __X__
      Upper lip length: normal __X__ somewhat short _____ markedly short _____
   b. Function:
      Can protrude: yes _____ no _____
      Can retract unilaterally, left: yes __X__ no _____; right: yes __X__ no _____
      Equal retraction bilaterally: yes _____ no _____
      Number of times can say [pʌ] in 5 seconds:
         Trial 1 _____ Trial 2 _____ Trial 3 _____
         above average _____ average _____ below average _____
   c. Adequacy for speech: 1 _____ 2 _____ 3 _____ 4 _____

2. Teeth
   a. Structure: *overbite*
      Occlusion normal: _____ neutroclusion _____ distoclusion _____ mesioclusion _____
      Anteroposterior relationship of incisors: normal _____; mixed—some in labioversion, some in linguoversion but all upper and lower teeth in contact _____; all upper incisors lingual to lower incisors but in contact _____; not in contact _____
      Vertical relationship of incisors: normal _____ openbite _____ closebite _____
      Continuity of cutting edge of incisors and cuspids: normal _____; rotated, jumbled _____; missing teeth _____; supernumerary teeth _____
      If lack of continuity, identify teeth involved and describe nature of deviation.
   b. Adequacy for speech: 1_____ 2 _____ 3 _____ 4 _____

* The ratings 1, 2, 3, and 4 are defined as follows:
  1 Normal
  2 Slight deviation—probably no adverse effect on speech
  3 Moderate deviation—possible adverse effect on speech; remedial services may be required particularly if other structures of the speech mechanism are also deviant
  4 Extreme deviation—sufficient to prevent normal production of speech; modification of structure required, either with or without clinical speech services

3. Tongue
   a. Structure:
      Size in relation to dental arches:
         too large _____ appropriate _____ too small _____
      Symmetrical _____ asymmetrical _____
   b. Function:
      Can curl tongue up and back: yes _____ no _____
      Number of times can touch anterior alveolar ridge with tongue tip without
      sound in 5 seconds:
         Trial 1 _____ Trial 2 _____ Trial 3 _____
         above average _____ average _____ below average _____
      Number of times can touch the corners of mouth with tongue tip in 5
      seconds:
         Trial 1 _____ Trial 2 _____ Trial 3 _____
         above average _____ average _____ below average _____
      Number of times can say [tʌ] in 5 seconds:
         Trial 1 _____ Trial 2 _____ Trial 3 _____
         above average _____ average _____ below average _____
      Restrictiveness of lingual frenum:
         not restrictive _____ somewhat restrictive _____ markedly restric-
         tive _____
   c. Adequacy for speech: 1 _____ 2 _____ 3 _____ 4 _____

4. Hard Palate
   a. Structure:
      Intactness: normal _____ cleft, repaired _____ cleft, unrepaired _____
      Palatal contour: normal configuration _____ flat contour _____ deep and
      narrow contour _____
   b. Adequacy for speech: 1 _____ 2 _____ 3 _____ 4 _____

5. Velopharyngeal Port Mechanism
   a. Structure:
      Soft palate:
         Intactness: normal _____ cleft, repaired _____ cleft, unrepaired _____
         Symmetrical _____ asymmetrical _____
         Length: satisfactory _____ short _____ very short _____
      Uvula:
         Normal _____ bifid _____ deviated from midline to right _____ to
         left _____ absent _____
      Oropharynx:
         Depth: shallow _____ normal _____ deep _____
         Width: narrow _____ normal _____ wide _____
   b. Function:
      Soft palate:
         Movement during prolonged phonation of [ɑ]: none _____ some _____
         marked _____

128

Movement during short, repeated phonations of [ɑ]: none _____
some _____ marked _____

Movement during gag reflex: none _____ some _____ marked _____

If some movement, is amount:
    same for both halves _____ more for right half _____ more for
    left half _____

Oropharynx:
    Mesial movement of lateral pharyngeal walls during phonation of [ɑ]:
    none _____ some _____ marked _____

    Mesial movement of lateral pharyngeal walls during gag reflex:
    none _____ some _____ marked _____

Velopharyngeal closure:
    Can blow out a match: yes __X__ no _____
    Can drink through a straw: yes __X__ no _____
    Pressure ratio (instrument_____):
        Trial 1: nostrils open _____, nostrils closed _____; ratio _____
        Trial 2: nostrils open _____, nostrils closed _____; ratio _____
        Trial 3: nostrils open _____, nostrils closed _____; ratio _____

    Number of times can say [kʌ] in 5 seconds:
        Trial 1 _____ Trial 2 _____ Trial 3 _____
        above average _____ average _____ below average _____

    Number of times can say [pʌtəkʌ] in 5 seconds with the nostrils open:
        Trial 1 _____ Trial 2 _____ Trial 3 _____
        above average _____ average _____ below average _____

    Number of times can say [pʌtəkʌ] in 5 seconds with the nostrils closed:
        Trial 1 _____ Trial 2 _____ Trial 3 _____
        above average _____ average _____ below average _____

    Mean speed per second in saying [pʌtəkʌ]:
        nostrils open _____, nostrils closed _____; ratio _____

c. Adequacy for speech: 1 _____ 2 _____ 3 _____ 4 _____

6. Fauces
  a. Structure:
    Tonsils: normal _____ enlarged _____ atrophied _____ absent _____
    Pillars: normal _____ scarred _____ inflamed _____ absent _____
    Area of faucial isthmus: above average _____ average _____
        below average _____

  b. Function:
    Posterior movement during phonation of [ɑ]:
        none _____ some _____ marked _____
    Mesial movement during phonation of [ɑ]:
        none _____ some _____ marked _____
    Restriction of velar activity by pillars:
        none _____ some _____ marked _____

Degree to which faucial isthmus is closed during phonation of [ɑ]:

    none _____ some _____ marked _____

c. Adequacy for speech: 1 _____ 2 _____ 3 _____ 4 _____

7. Nasal Cavities
    a. Structure:

        Septum: normal _____ deviated right _____ deviated left _____

        Nasal obstruction:

            Right: none _____ some _____ marked _____

            Left: none _____ some _____ marked _____

    b. Function:

        Nares constriction during speech:

            none _____ some _____ marked _____

    c. Adequacy for speech: 1 _____ 2 _____ 3 _____ 4 _____

8. Breathing Mechanism
    a. Function:

        Inhalation:

            deep and inaudible _____ deep and audible _____ shallow _____

        Breathing movements: rhythmical _____ jerky _____

        Heaving of the shoulders during speaking:

            none _____ some _____ marked _____

        Can pant rapidly for 5 seconds: yes _____ no _____

        Can shout: yes __X__ no _____

        Number of seconds can prolong [ɑ] following deep inhalation:

            Trial 1 _____ Trial 2 _____ Trial 3 _____

            above average __X__ average _____ below average _____

        Number of times can say [pʌ] in 10 seconds on one exhalation:

            Trial 1 _____ Trial 2 _____ Trial 3 __X__

            above average _____ average __X__ below average _____

    b. Adequacy for speech: 1 _____ 2 _____ 3 _____ 4 _____

9. Summary and Evaluation
    a. Specify the deviations which you have rated as significant:

        Rating of 4: _____

        Rating of 3: _____

        Rating of 2: _____

    b. Relate these deviations to your findings from testing the speech of the examinee. Comment on account to be taken of these deviations in planning a program of remedial speech services for the examinee.

Additional copies of this form may be obtained from the Interstate Printers and Publishers, 19-27 North Jackson Street, Danville, Illinois.

REFERENCES

1. Bloomer, H. H., "Observations on palatopharyngeal movements in speech and deglutition," *Journal of Speech and Hearing Disorders*, 1953, *18*:230-246.
2. Bloomquist, Betty L., "Diadochokinetic movements of nine-, ten-, and eleven-year-old children," *Journal of Speech and Hearing Disorders*, 1950, *15*:159-164.
3. Calnan, J., "Movements of the soft palate," *British Journal of Plastic Surgery*, 1953, *5*:286-296.
4. Calnan, J., "Submucous cleft palate," *British Journal of Plastic Surgery*, 1954, *6*:264-282.
5. Fairbanks, G., and Evelyn Green, "A study of minor organic deviations in 'functional' disorders of articulation: 2. Dimensions and relationships of the lips," *Journal of Speech and Hearing Disorders*, 1950, *15*:165-168.
6. Fairbanks, G., and Mary Lentner, "A study of minor organic deviations of 'functional' disorders of articulation: 4. The teeth and hard palate," *Journal of Speech and Hearing Disorders*, 1951, *16*:273-279.
7. Fairbanks, G., and D. C. Spriestersbach, "A study of minor organic deviations in 'functional' disorders of articulation: 1. Rate of movement of oral structures," *Journal of Speech and Hearing Disorders*, 1950, *15*:60-69.
8. Fymbo, L. H., "The relation of malocclusion of the teeth to defects of speech," *Archives of Speech*, 1936, *1*:204-216.
9. Graber, T. M., *Orthodontics, Principles and Practice*, Philadelphia: Saunders, 1961.
10. Hardy, J. C., "Intraoral breath pressure in cerebral palsy," *Journal of Speech and Hearing Disorders*, 1961, *26*:309-319.
11. Hurme, V. O., "Ranges of normalcy in the eruption of permanent teeth," *Journal of Dentistry for Children*, 1949, *16*:11-15.
12. Johnson, W., S. Brown, J. Curtis, D. Edney, and J. Keaster, *Speech Handicapped School Children*, rev. ed., New York: Harper, 1956.
13. Kaltenborn, A. L., "An x-ray study of velopharyngeal closure in nasal and non-nasal speakers," unpublished M.A. thesis, Northwestern University, 1948.
14. Matthew, J., and Margaret Byrne, "An experimental study of tongue flexibility in children with cleft palates," *Journal of Speech and Hearing Disorders*, 1953, *18*:43-47.
15. Mayo Clinic and Mayo Clinic Foundation for Medical Education and Research, *Clinical Examinations in Neurology*, Philadelphia: Saunders, 1956.
16. Moll, K. L., "Cinefluorographic techniques in speech research," *Journal of Speech and Hearing Research*, 1960, *3*:227-241.
17. Moll, K. L., "Velopharyngeal closure on vowels," *Journal of Speech and Hearing Research*, 1962, *5*:30-37.

18. Sandler, H. C., "The eruption of deciduous teeth," *Journal of Pediatrics*, 1944, *25*:140-147.
19. Snow, Katherine, "Articulation proficiency in relation to certain dental abnormalities," *Journal of Speeech and Hearing Disorders*, 1961, *26*:209-212.
20. Sprague, Ann L., "The relationship between selected measures of expressive language and motor skill in eight-year-old boys," unpublished Ph.D. thesis, University of Iowa, 1961.
21. Spriestersbach, D. C., K. L. Moll, and H. L. Morris, "Subject classification and articulation of speakers with cleft palates," *Journal of Speech and Hearing Research*, 1961, *4*:362-372.
22. Spriestersbach, D. C., and G. R. Powers, "Articulation skills, velopharyngeal closure, and oral breath pressure of children with cleft palates," *Journal of Speech and Hearing Research*, 1959, *2*:318-325.
23. Travis, L. E. (Ed.), *Handbook of Speech Pathology*, New York: Appleton-Century-Crofts, 1957.
24. Van Riper, C., and J. V. Irwin, *Voice and Articulation*, Englewood Cliffs, N. J.: Prentice-Hall, 1958.

6 EXAMINATION OF VOICE QUALITY DISORDERS

In Chapter 3 we gave attention to certain general procedures for noting various deviations of voice. We considered ways of describing and recording what we hear while observing samples of connected speech. While it is true that by such means we may gain numerous cues for use in planning therapy, we usually need to make more extensive and systematic observations of voice problems before we can proceed effectively with retraining. Voice problems are typically complex, because there are so many factors which may be associated, singly or in combination, with a given voice deviation. They are complex, too, because they may be significantly related to the speaker's personal adjustment patterns. The clinician needs to be sensitive to the significance of deviant behavior in areas other than voice, particularly that of language, in order to evaluate effectively the relationship, if any, of a given form of unusual behavior to a specific characteristic of voice. Finally, voice problems seem complex to the average clinician because they are relatively rare. Most of us have so little experience with cases of breathiness, for example, that we lack the insight which comes from frequent clinical study of such a problem.

For these reasons the examinations of voice quality disorders presented here are fairly detailed. It is, perhaps, impractical to follow them in their entirety in the field; they are designed to be training devices which require the student to get into the habit of looking at the many details that may possibly be significant in a given instance.

Note that we confine our examinations of voice quality deviations to those of nasality, breathiness, and harshness. While many other terms purporting to describe deviations of voice quality are mentioned in the literature, we prefer to follow the criterion established by Fairbanks that "the test of the existence of a voice quality disorder is whether or not the quality that is heard is independent of phonemes, or, in other words, whether or not the phenomenon heard can be superimposed upon a good example of a voiced sound" (1, p. 202). Research data indicate that there are, according to this criterion, fewer voice quality disorders than some authors indicate.

In the General Speech Behavior Rating blank (Form 2, p. 78) hoarseness is also listed as a type of voice quality. Here again we accept Fairbanks' statement (2, p. 182) that hoarseness combines the acoustical features of breathiness and harshness and is rare as a functional disorder. This does not mean that there is no such thing as hoarseness; it means simply that hoarseness can be understood as combining the characteristics of breathiness and harshness. Moreover, while it is rare as a functional disorder it is, of course, relatively common in cases of laryngitis, and it is also found in association with other laryngeal pathologies. For this reason, it is to be emphasized that any case of hoarseness should be referred to a physician before any therapeutic procedures are undertaken. After having received medical clearance on such cases, of course, we will need to do the same careful and detailed diagnostic evaluations of them that we would do of any other type of voice problem. The essential observations, however, are those described here in the sections dealing with breathy and harsh voices. In view of these considerations, we do not include examination procedures for hoarseness, per se.

It will also be noted that we do not include techniques for investigating the attributes of pitch, loudness, and time. With respect to loudness and time there are few deviations which cannot be handled adequately by making use of the descriptive information obtained from the General Speech Behavior Rating. Significant loudness deviations are most frequently related to hearing loss or severe psychogenic conditions. These relationships should be reported if suspected. A further diagnostic work-up in such instances, however, lies beyond the scope of the training covered by this manual. So far as pitch is concerned the General Speech Behavior Rating can be used to note whether or not the pitch is too low or too high to be effective, or whether there is a distracting pitch pattern or too little pitch variation. Frequently, however, it is desirable to go beyond these judgments and determine whether or not the pitch range which the speaker is using is appropriate for his vocal mechanism. If it is not, some sort of voice quality deviation may develop.

The terms "habitual" and "natural," which are commonly used in speaking of pitch levels, need to be clearly understood. In defining these terms Fairbanks refers to habitual pitch level as the "central tendency of the pitches used by the individual" (2, p. 123); and of natural pitch level he says, "It is proposed that each speaker has an individual level, determined by such characteristics of his vocal mechanism as size, manipulability, etc. at which his voice is most efficient for speech . . ." (2, p. 122). He defines "pitch level" as the mode of the distribution of the fundamental frequencies in a speech sample of adequate length. When used in these contexts, then, "level" represents a statistic derived from a frequency distribution of the pitches observed in a given sample of vocal tones. Many clinicians tend to forget the definitions of these terms and behave as though habitual and natural pitch levels were specific pitches. Van Riper and Irwin (15, p. 451) remind us of the proper definition of these terms when they say: "It is our belief that the appropriate pitch of the larynx is indeed a function of its range, and that the most appropriate or optimum pitch is in itself a range rather than a specific tone or frequency. . . . Finally, we believe that the optimum range may vary with the actual intensity of the voice; in general, the optimum range will become higher as the fundamental of the voice increases in intensity." Thus, whenever you use "pitch level" in speaking of voice you should keep in mind that you are referring to a range of pitches.

Several techniques have been used to determine natural pitch level. One involves having the speaker vary the general pitch level at which he phonates and noting whether his voice becomes louder or swells in a given range of pitches. This technique is based on the assumption that there is a band of vocal tone frequencies for each speaker within which the tones are assumed to become louder, fuller, more resonant, and that his vocal mechanism functions most efficiently within this frequency range. Thurman (13), however, was not able to demonstrate the validity of this assumption in a study of normal speakers. In other words, the voices of his speakers, on the whole, simply did not swell observably within a frequency range which could logically be judged as most effective for speech. In fact, the "swells" that were observed did not even occur for a given speaker at the same place on the frequency scale when he sang or hummed the scale more than once.

While Thurman's findings certainly suggest that we should not expect to establish an individual's natural pitch level by a simple singing technique, clinical experience has amply demonstrated that cues for the establishment of an appropriate pitch level can frequently be obtained by having the individual speak on a variety of pitch levels and observing the effects on his voice.

Another method of determining the speaker's natural pitch level is based on the assumption that a superior speaker is superior partly because he uses a level at which his vocal mechanism functions most effectively and that this level has a definite relationship to his total pitch range. Fairbanks (2, pp. 123-126) has outlined a method which can be used to determine the natural pitch level on this basis. You will be wise to use both of the methods referred to in examining persons with voice problems.

Other possible observations include those which can be made by means of examination procedures used to evaluate the condition of the laryngeal structures or the more obscure regions of the nasal cavities. While we do not wish to minimize in any way the importance to voice of these anatomical regions, it is our opinion that the examination of them is properly reserved for the physician. We assume, however, that the speech pathologist should include in his examination the observations of structural deviations that can be readily made by persons without specialized medical training. On the basis of these observations, and of inferences which can be drawn from the characteristics of the voice as heard, most significant organic deviations can be detected or suspected. Any speaker in whom such organic factors are noted or suspected should be promptly referred to a physician.

In examining a person with a voice problem, you might use the indicated procedures in the following order. First, administer the General Speech Behavior Rating (Form 2, p. 78) in order to get an overview of his problem. Then complete your evaluation of the speech mechanism (Form 4, p. 127). Finally, administer the General Voice Quality Examination (Form 5) and such supplementary examinations of voice quality (Forms 6, 7, and 8) as are indicated on the basis of the general examination. The information obtained from some sections of the General Voice Quality Examination will not be equally relevant to all types of quality deviations, but since you can best learn about the shortcuts in diagnosis through experience, you should complete all sections of the General Voice Quality Examination for all types of quality deviations in order to increase your awareness of those circumstances under which certain observations can be omitted.

For many of the observations included in the voice quality examinations the rationale is presumably sufficiently clear that explanatory comments are unnecessary. Comprehensive discussions of the various techniques would fill many books; indeed, they have. We assume that you have read some of the available books before you attempt to make the voice examinations described below. In the following sections, we shall, therefore, make comments about specified items of the various examinations only to provide essential clarification or to make our relevant personal biases a matter of record.

THE GENERAL VOICE QUALITY EXAMINATION

1. Complaint

Record the actual words used by the individual in telling about the problem as he sees it and in explaining how he happened to come to you about it. See Van Riper and Irwin's discussion of the initial interview in the clinical study of voice problems (15, pp. 277-280).

2. Primary Voice Quality Problem

On the basis of your observations in completing the General Speech Behavior Rating (Form 2, p. 78), indicate here your tentative classification of the problem in order to provide direction for your observations during this examination.

3. Pertinent History

It is important that you understand the rationale for including the items under "General physical development and health." It should be emphasized that this section is located in the general section concerning history. These items are not intended to suggest that as a speech pathologist you should, or would have need to, make physical diagnoses. The fact is that if the conditions listed have played a part in causing and maintaining the voice problem, it is likely that they are quite obvious and have been identified already by competent medical authority. It is not within the scope of this manual to discuss the relationships which each of the listed conditions might have to specific voice quality deviations. Moore (in Travis, 14, ch. 22) presents a systematic discussion of the possible relationships. The basic point is that you should be aware of the factors in question and consider their possible relevance to your own professional responsibilities. If they are among the factors maintaining the voice problem you must take them into account in making prognostic and remedial judgments. Moreover, with due awareness of them you are able to ask more meaningful questions in making referrals to the laryngologist. For example, in making a referral you might say "The patient gives a history of hypothyroidism which he says is still present. The patient has a hoarse voice. It would be helpful to know if he does have hypothyroidism or any other medically significant condition and if so whether it might be related to the voice problem. If it is present and related, will you kindly advise me concerning your prognosis for changing the condition and the time involved in the medical treatment so that I might plan a program of voice therapy accordingly?"

4. Examination of Pertinent Physical Mechanisms

Since you will have completed a Speech Mechanism Examination (Form 4, p. 127), the items included here are meant to suggest additional observations which might further illuminate the voice problems.

Larynx: By "pinched throat" is meant that condition in which the thyroid cartilage is drawn up toward the hyoid bone and tilted from its normal plane so that the thyroid notch is not exposed to palpation as it normally is.

The item concerning similarity of the muscular contractions exhibited during phonation and swallowing is included because some speakers exhibit marked and abnormal contraction of the extrinsic laryngeal musculature during phonation. Van Riper and Irwin (*15*, p. 187) suggest that you can evaluate this phenomenon by using the following procedure: "The finger is placed in the angle of the jaw and the individual is asked to swallow, the muscular contraction being carefully noted. The person is then asked to phonate loudly. If he can produce voice only by a muscular contraction similar to (though less pronounced than) that of swallowing, he is obviously using the swallowing muscles in phonation. This will have an adverse effect upon voice production."

"Two-toned" voice, or diplophonia, refers to a condition in which there are two sources of tone of different pitches. Usually it is assumed that the sources of the tones are the vocal folds and the ventricular bands. It is possible, however, that a supplementary source other than the ventricular bands may be operating. In any event, the presence of two tones is an indication of unusual tensions in the larynx and the laryngopharynx.

In interpreting the significance of the percentage of tones that are in the total pitch range between the lowest tone and the habitual pitch level, you should use Fairbanks' method of determining natural pitch level (*2*, p. 122).

Articulatory Mechanism: The extent of mouth opening during speech is related to degree of restriction of egress of the breath stream and of sound waves from the oral cavity. Unnecessary or unusual restrictions placed upon the breath stream by action of the tongue, teeth, and lips may result in tones which are muffled and lacking in clarity.

If the quality of the vowels is changed when the nostrils are occluded, you may assume that a portion of the acoustic energy resulting from the phonation is being channeled through the nasal cavity. From the data of Spriestersbach and Powers (11), we can infer that velopharyngeal competence and nasality are related. Thus, if you obtain marked changes in the vowel quality when the nostrils are occluded, you may wish to investigate the possibility that some degree of velopharyngeal incompetence exists, at least while the speaker is performing tasks of this sort. The use of pressure ratios in evaluating velopharyngeal competence is discussed on pp. 120–121.

We define the velopharyngeal space, for the purposes of judging its depth and width from peroral examinations, as that space which can be seen between the posterior and inferior edge of the soft palate and the posterior and lateral pharyngeal walls when the speaker is not phonating. It must be remembered, of course, that the closure effected by contact of the palate and pharyngeal walls does not occur on the plane from which you are able to make your observations and judgments. Even so, there is such a considerable degree of variation in this space among speakers that you can make gross estimates of the adequacy of the size of the palate within the pharyngeal space by the means of these observations, and you can obtain from them some feeling for the importance of the concept of "degree of critical closure" (5).

Posture: We have consistently tried to organize the observations to be made of the speech-producing mechanism around the four main processes of oral expression. We have done this in the hope that the significance of these observations may be more apparent in considering those aspects of speech behavior that need to be changed in order to effect improvement in speech. However, there are a few observations which we have rather arbitrarily placed under the heading of "Posture" for want of a better term. In the absence of relevant research findings, clinical experience and current knowledge concerning the speech-producing mechanism suggest that the articulators and resonators function most effectively when they are held in positions that are not markedly deviant in relation to the long axis of the body.

5. Associated Variables

We agree with the statement of Van Riper and Irwin (15, p. 273) that "Seldom does the abnormal variation exist along one dimension of voice alone." Fairbanks (2, p. 171) makes the same point when he says, "The prominence of any of the types of deviations varies significantly in relation to changes in other variables of speech. For example, the relationship between pitch, intensity, and voice quality is powerful in most voices, as would be expected from the involvement of the vocal folds in all three. . . ." It is imperative, then, that we observe the changes that take place in one dimension of voice when we manipulate another dimension which may be related to it. We are interested in determining how we can change the speaker's vocal behavior. We develop the nucleus for a plan of attack when we observe, for example, that the harshness is diminished by raising the pitch level, or that the breathiness decreases when the speaker uses more effort and speaks more loudly.

Frequently in dealing with both functional and organic cases it is not enough to have determined that the low pitch, or chronic inflammation, or poor breath control is the cause of the voice quality problem. These manifestations may simply be symptomatic of some more basic psychological problem. Certainly we cannot predict from a harsh or breathy voice that the speaker has personal adjustment problems, or vice versa, but we should be alert to the possibility of such relationships. It goes without saying that we can modify the vocal quality much more effectively if we can improve the individual's general adjustment to speaking situations, or if we are able to provide for him the counseling he needs in order to deal with his feelings of inadequacy. By such means we may be able to get the speaker to relax generally and become the type of person who can produce vocal tones easily with a physical mechanism free from excessive tensions.

SUPPLEMENTARY VOICE QUALITY EXAMINATIONS

The supplementary voice quality examinations provide for additional investigation of breathiness, harshness, and nasality. All three of these examinations are organized in a similar fashion. In each examination the speaker is asked to say a series of test words selected to reveal any relationships that may exist between his voice quality problem and the phonetic context of his speech, and to indicate the conditions under which changes can be effected through the manipulation of other attributes of voice. It is assumed that when you have completed the appropriate supplementary examinations you will attempt to relate the findings from them and from the General Speech Behavior Rating, the General Voice Quality Examination, and the appropriate sections of the Speech Mechanism Examination.

The supplementary examinations for both breathiness and harshness include observations of the influence of *arresting* and *releasing* consonants on the voice quality of adjacent vowels. These terms are here used as they were employed by Stetson in defining the *syllable:* "The smallest indivisible phonetic unit. Basically, the syllable is a puff of air forced upward through the vocal canal by a compression stroke of the intercostal muscles. It is usually modulated by the actions of the vocal folds. It is accompanied by accessory movements (syllable factors) which characterize it. These are the *release* (by the action of either the chest muscles or the releasing consonant), the *vowel shaping* movements of the vocal canal, and the *arrest* (by the action of either the chest muscles or the arresting consonant)" (*12*, p. 200). He defines *arresting consonants* and *releasing consonants* as follows: "Arresting consonant—The syllable factor which brings the syllable pulse to a close. Releasing consonant—The syllable factor which initiates the syllable pulse" (*12*, pp. 193, 198). In these terms, then, [t] serves as a *releasing* consonant in such words as *too, ten,* and *top*. It serves as an *arresting* consonant in such words as *cot, rat* and *suit*.

Breathiness: Breathiness results from improper coordination of the breath supply with the degree of closure and tension of the vocal folds. It is possible for an individual to have satisfactory breath control for speech and still have a breathy voice if he does not control the vocal folds in such a way as to use the available air supply effectively. On the other hand, some speakers may have apparently faulty breath control without having breathy voices.

In evaluating your findings from the supplementary examination for breathiness you will want to consider them in relation to information obtained from your observations of the breathing mechanism during the Speech Mechanism Examination. However, as we indicated when discussing that examination, you will probably find that most speakers have the requisite degree of breath control. In that event, the relationship of the breathiness to phonetic context and the other dimensions of voice will probably provide the main basis for your remedial program.

Harshness: While you look mainly at the level of the larynx for the conditions responsible for harshness, you are interested in any particular case in attempting to determine whether the causes are mainly functional or organic. If you suspect that the causes are primarily organic, you will, of course, refer the speaker to a physician for a laryngeal examination. Serious injury can be caused by vocal drills when there is chronic laryngeal pathology. Most clinicians agree that tension is commonly associated with harsh voices, and so in any given case you will want to determine whether the harshness is due primarily to the improper use of the laryngeal mechanism or a combination of improper laryngeal function and generalized tension. See Sherman and Linke (*10*), Rees (*8, 9*) and Fairbanks (*2*, pp. 175-179) for additional information and suggested types of observation concerning variations in harshness as a function of phonetic context, and for related material useful in planning a remedial program.

Nasality: There are two types of nasality, hyponasality (less than ordinary amount) and hypernasality (more than ordinary amount). However, because hypernasality is one of the most commonly observed impairments of voice quality, "nasality" is frequently used to mean an excess amount of nasality. It is so used here. It will be noted that in this manual we provide for no specific observations of hyponasality beyond those included in the General Speech Behavior Rating. According to our experience, hyponasality is commonly related to such organic conditions as enlarged adenoidal pads or nasal obstructions. When these are removed the hyponasality nearly always disappears without voice retraining. Therefore, we have not included observation of hyponasality in our supplementary examination for nasality.

The relevant data strongly indicate that nasality is a complex phenomenon and does not have a simple etiology. Lintz and Sherman (4) support this point of view: "It is apparent that perceived nasality varies with a number of parameters. Examination of data on velopharyngeal closure related to those parameters suggests that relatively inadequate closure may be the most important cause of functional nasality. There is some indication that lack of precision of articulation of consonants may be associated with this voice quality. A consideration of the obtained results leads also to the conclusion that degree of perceived nasality varies with fundamental frequency, duration and intensity of vowels." The paired words in the supplementary examination for nasality have been selected to point up some of the possible parameters which may make a difference in the perception of nasality. Fairbanks (2, pp. 172-175) presents material specifically designed to demonstrate variation in the degree of perceived nasality as a function of phonetic context.

Nasalization characteristic of the nasal consonants that is carried over into adjacent vowels and diphthongs is called assimilated nasality. If the carry-over affects a vowel or diphthong that precedes the nasal consonant, the assimilation is said to be anticipatory; if it affects a vowel or diphthong that follows the nasal consonant, the assimilation is classified as retentive. McIntosh (6) and, more recently, Moll (7) have reported that anticipatory assimilation is observed more frequently than retentive assimilation. These comments are not meant to imply that any degree of assimilation is abnormal. However, if assimilated nasality is observed, it may be possible to reduce the degree of perceived nasality through exercises designed to reduce the relative contribution which assimilation makes to it.

Complete diagnostic work-ups on three speakers who are breathy, three who are harsh, and three who are nasal. These work-ups should include the following sets of observations: General Speech Behavior Rating (Form 2, p. 78), Speech Mechanism Examination (Form 4, p. 127), General Voice Quality Examination (Form 5), and the appropriate supplementary voice quality examinations (Forms 6, 7, and 8). Discuss your findings in each case in the space following section 3 of the supplementary examination form.

FORM 5. GENERAL VOICE QUALITY EXAMINATION

Name _____ Age _____ Sex _____

Examiner _____ Date _____

1. Complaint

2. Primary voice quality problem as revealed by General Speech Behavior Rating: breathiness _____ harshness _____ hoarseness _____ nasality _____

3. Pertinent History
   a. History of the problem:
      Nature of onset:

      Duration of the problem:

      History of vocal misuse (talking in a noisy environment, excessive speaking, shouting, screaming): yes _____ no _____. If Yes, describe circumstances:

      History of total loss of voice: yes _____ no _____. If Yes, describe the circumstances:

      Description of how voice is used in daily work:

      Variations in the severity of the problem noted by the speaker and circumstances when variations occur:

      Has speaker had voice therapy: yes _____ no _____. If Yes, what was the nature of the therapy:

What were the results of therapy:

b. Family history of voice and speech problems:
   Other members of the family with voice or speech problems: yes _____
   no _____. If Yes, describe the nature of the problem and relation of person to the speaker in each case:

c. General physical development and health:
   Is there a history of:

	Yes	No		Yes	No
allergies	_____	_____	hormone therapy	_____	_____
anemia	_____	_____	diptheria	_____	_____
glandular imbal-			influenza	_____	_____
ance	_____	_____	typhoid fever	_____	_____
hyperthyroidism	_____	_____	rheumatic fever	_____	_____
hypothyroidism	_____	_____	scarlet fever	_____	_____
chronic colds	_____	_____	poliomyelitis	_____	_____
chronic rhinitis	_____	_____	mumps	_____	_____
sinus infection	_____	_____	excessive		
chronic laryn-			smoking	_____	_____
gitis	_____	_____	broken nose	_____	_____
ear disease	_____	_____	mouth-breathing	_____	_____
incoordination of			retarded sexual		
face or tongue			development	_____	_____
muscles	_____	_____	other _____	_____	_____
gait peculiarities	_____	_____	other _____	_____	_____
random purpose-			other _____	_____	_____
less movements	_____	_____			

If the answer to any of the items above is Yes, give the relevant details:

4. Examination of Pertinent Physical Mechanisms
   a. Respiratory Mechanism:
      Breath supply and control appear to be adequate: yes _____ no _____
      (See Form 4 for suggestions of pertinent observations.)
      Any apparent muscular tensions of the chest and neck which appear to
      be related to faulty breath supply and control: yes _____ no_____

Describe and discuss any such deviations:

b. Larynx:

	Yes	No
History of laryngeal pathology (growths, inflammations, chronic pain or tickling)	____	____
Complaint of "tired throat"	____	____
Evidence of "pinched throat" during phonation	____	____
Muscular contractions exhibited during phonation which are similar to those exhibited during swallowing	____	____

If the answer to any of the items above is Yes, give the relevant details:

Does the speaker exhibit any of the following during phonation: hard glottal attack _____ two-toned voice _____ infrequent pitch breaks _____ frequent pitch breaks _____ phonation interspersed with whispering _____ tremulous voice _____. Give the relevant details concerning any of the items that have been checked above:

Has speaker done any formal singing: yes _____ no _____. If Yes, what part has he sung?

Can the speaker sing up and down the musical scale: yes _____ no _____

Can speaker imitate inflectional patterns: yes _____ no_____

Number of tones in total pitch range including falsetto: _____

Number of tones habitual pitch level is above lowest tone: _____

Percentage of tones in total pitch range that are between lowest tone and habitual pitch level: _____

c. Articulatory Mechanism:

Activity of lips and jaws (extent of mouth opening) while speaking: immobile and clenched _____ slight movement _____ average movement _____ above average movement _____

Quality when nostrils occluded during sustained phonation of vowels: changed _____ unchanged _____

Pressure ratio: nostrils open _____ nostrils occluded _____; ratio _____

Discuss the significance of any deviations noted above:

d. Resonators:

   Size of velopharyngeal space:

       depth: shallow _____ normal _____ deep _____

       width: narrow _____ normal _____ wide _____

   Tonsils: none _____ small _____ moderately large _____ very large _____

   Nasal obstruction:

       right nostril: none _____ some _____ complete _____

       left nostril: none _____ some _____ complete _____

   Discuss the significance of any deviations noted above:

e. Posture:

   Overall posture of the body generally adequate: yes _____ no _____

   Head held in reasonably upright position during speaking: yes _____
   no _____

   Is the position of the larynx in the neck symmetrical: yes _____ no _____

   If the answer to any of the items above is No, describe the deviation
   and discuss any possible relationships it may have to the voice problem:

5. Associated Variables

   a. Pitch and loudness:

      Quality changed under any of the following conditions:

      sustained vowels:

          lower than habitual pitch level: yes _____ no _____

          higher than habitual pitch level: yes _____ no _____

          softer than habitual loudness level: yes _____ no _____

          louder than habitual loudness level: yes _____ no _____

      oral reading:

          softer than habitual loudness level: yes _____ no _____

          louder than habitual loudness level: yes _____ no _____

   b. Personal and social adjustment:

      What is the degree of obvious concern that the speaker has about his
      voice problem:

      none _____ some _____ marked _____

      Does the language which the speaker uses tend to be well-qualified,
      normally cautious, specific, or does it tend to be rigidly either-orish, ab-
      solute, inappropriate to the situation, etc.? (See Johnson, 3, Chapters
      11 and 12, for a relevant account of normal and abnormal varieties of
      language behavior.)

Does the speaker's interpretation of objective events tend to be competent, impersonal, factual, or does it tend to be exaggerated, self-defensive, vague, etc.?

Does the speaker tend to have a relaxed appearance, a smooth, rhythmical gait, firm handshake, direct gaze, or does he tend to appear physically tense, move jerkily, remain quietly at ease only with difficulty, refuse to look directly at the examiner, etc?

Does the speaker tend to appear hostile (curt, cryptic, indifferent), extremely dependent, generally insecure, or does he tend to appear cooperative, pleasant, helpful, interested, etc.?

In talking about the voice problem itself is the speaker reticent, apologetic, embarrassed, depressed, and self-defensive, or does he discuss it freely in a forthright manner, with an interested, objective, problem-solving attitude?

Specify and discuss any other aspects of the speaker's behavior which appear to be indices of his adjustment:

Do the speaker's maladjustments, if any, appear to be related largely to specific problems and situations or do they appear to be characteristic of his behavior generally? List any situations to which the speaker appears to adjust poorly.

How would you rate the speaker's over-all adjustment:
above average _____ average _____ below average _____

6. Relationship of the voice quality problem to other variables, if any, not discussed above:

7. Summary of the relationship of findings recorded under "Associated variables" to the voice quality problems revealed by the General Speech Behavior Rating:

FORM 6. SUPPLEMENTARY EXAMINATION FOR BREATHINESS

Name _____ Age _____ Sex _____

Examiner _____ Date _____

1. Detailed Speech Examination
   a. Rating of breathiness of vowels and diphthongs in specified contexts:
      Place a check mark in the space before the one of each of the following
      pairs of words that is the more breathy. If there is no difference leave
      both spaces blank.

_____pup	_____up	_____coop	_____cap
_____hold	_____old	_____sham	_____am
_____heat	_____deed	_____gauze	_____fought
_____set	_____suit	_____heat	_____eat
_____bathe	_____hate	_____cake	_____coke
_____ease	_____seize	_____pot	_____gob
_____am	_____ham	_____ode	_____sawed
_____put	_____pet	_____groove	_____grave
_____ate	_____mate	_____air	_____hair
_____it	_____hit	_____rude	_____spoof

Discuss any patterning that you observe with reference to voiced, aspirated
consonants vs. unvoiced, nonaspirated consonants adjacent to the vowels;
high, back vs. low, front vowels; releasing consonants preceding the vowels
vs. the absence of releasing consonants preceding the vowels; aspirated
sounds preceding the vowels vs. the absence of aspirated sounds preceding
the vowels:

b. Evaluation of changes in degree of breathiness (check the appropriate blanks):

	More Breathy	Less Breathy	Unchanged
Reading at a louder than habitual loudness level	_____	_____	_____
Reading at a softer than habitual loudness level	_____	_____	_____
Reading with a pitch level above the the habitual level	_____	_____	_____
Reading with a pitch level below the habitual level	_____	_____	_____
Spontaneous conversation while expending physical effort	_____	_____	_____
Prolonging vowels at pitch levels higher than habitual pitch level	_____	_____	_____
Prolonging vowels at pitch levels lower than habitual pitch level	_____	_____	_____
Prolonging vowels at louder than habitual loudness levels	_____	_____	_____
Prolonging vowels at softer than habitual loudness levels	_____	_____	_____
Prolonging vowels while expending physical effort	_____	_____	_____
Staccato phonation of vowel vs. prolonged vowels	_____	_____	_____
Phonations at beginning of expiratory cycle vs. end of expiratory cycle	_____	_____	_____
Imitation of nonbreathy, prolonged vowels of examiner	_____	_____	_____

Discuss the significance of any changes observed in indicating possible etiological factors and their implications concerning the possibility and desirability of changes in breathiness:

2. Discuss the relationships of the findings of this examination, the General Voice Quality Examination, and the Speech Mechanism Examination to the voice problems revealed by the General Speech Behavior Rating, and indicate the implications of these findings concerning procedures to be employed in attempting to change voice quality:

Additional copies of this form may be obtained from the Interstate Printers and Publishers, 19-27 North Jackson Street, Danville, Illinois.

FORM 7. SUPPLEMENTARY EXAMINATION FOR HARSHNESS

Name _____   Age _____ Sex _____

Examiner _____   Date _____

1. Detailed Speech Examination:
   a. Rating of harshness of vowels and diphthongs in specified contexts:
      Place a check mark in the space before the one of each of the following pairs of words or sounds that is the more harsh. If there is no difference leave both spaces blank.

____leaf	____leap	____hat	____at
____of	____dove	____[i]	____[ɔ]
____[æ]	____[i]	____fool	____cool
____vale	____sale	____bed	____fez
____as	____has	____[ɔ]	____[u]
____ton	____sun	____tan	____fan
____feel	____eel	____his	____is
____[u]	____[æ]	____pit	____it
____eel	____heel	____[ɛ]	____[I]
____fall	____bawl	____loop	____lose
____roof	____rude	____bowl	____toll
____at	____cat	____ease	____seize
		____it	____hit

Discuss any patterning that you observe with reference to stop-plosives vs. fricatives, high vowels vs. low vowels, syllables released by consonants vs. syllables not released by consonants, voiced vs. voiceless consonant environments:

b. Evaluation of changes in the degree of harshness (check the appropriate blanks):

	More Harsh	Less Harsh	Unchanged
Reading at a louder than habitual loudness level	____	____	____
Reading at a softer than habitual loudness level	____	____	____
Reading with more than habitual activity of the lips and jaws	____	____	____
Reading with less than habitual activity of the lips and jaws	____	____	____
Reading at a pitch level above the habitual pitch level	____	____	____
Reading at a pitch level below the habitual pitch level	____	____	____
Reading at a faster than habitual rate	____	____	____
Reading at a slower than habitual rate	____	____	____
Reading vs. spontaneous conversation	____	____	____
Spontaneous conversation while expending physical effort	____	____	____
Spontaneous conversation vs. prolonged vowels	____	____	____
Spontaneous conversation vs. humming at habitual pitch	____	____	____
Prolonging vowels at pitch levels higher than habitual pitch level	____	____	____
Prolonging vowels at pitch levels lower than habitual pitch level	____	____	____
Prolonging vowels at louder than habitual loudness levels	____	____	____
Prolonging vowels at softer than habitual loudness levels	____	____	____
Prolonging vowels while expending physical effort	____	____	____
Prolonged vowels vs. vocalized yawns	____	____	____
Imitation of nonharsh, prolonged vowels of examiner	____	____	____

Discuss significance of any changes observed in indicating possible etiological factors and their implications concerning the possibility and desirability of changes in harshness:

2. Discuss the relationships of the findings of this examination, the General Voice
   Quality Examination, and the Speech Mechanism Examination to the voice
   problems revealed by the General Speech Behavior Rating, and indicate the
   implications of these findings concerning procedures to be employed in attempting to change voice quality:

Additional copies of this form may be obtained from the Interstate Printers an l
Publishers, 19-27 North Jackson Street, Danville, Illinois.

FORM 8. SUPPLEMENTARY EXAMINATION FOR NASALITY

Name _____ Age _____ Sex _____

Examiner _____ Date _____

1. Detailed Speech Examination:
    a. Rating of nasality of vowels and diphthongs in specified contexts:
        Place a check mark in the space before the one of each of the following pairs of words that is the more nasal. If there is no difference leave both spaces blank.

_____teen	_____tea	_____vat	_____cat
_____peep	_____poop	_____rude	_____red
_____doom	_____mood	_____pop	_____peep
_____toot	_____tot	_____do	_____doom
_____make	_____came	_____boot	_____bet
_____head	_____hood	_____dude	_____dead
_____odd	_____nod	_____ton	_____nut
_____zoo	_____too	_____heat	_____hat
_____bat	_____beat	_____dad	_____dude
_____tile	_____vile	_____meat	_____eat
_____dean	_____need	_____rave	_____rake
_____veal	_____teal	_____tam	_____mat
_____may	_____bay		

Discuss any patterning that you observe with reference to front vs. back vowels, high vs. low vowels, voiceless vs. voiced consonants adjacent to the vowels, words with the nasal consonants preceding the vowels vs. words with the nasal consonants following the vowels; words with the nasal consonants adjacent to the vowels vs. words without the nasal consonants adjacent to the vowels:

156

b. Production of nasal consonants:

Evaluate the production of [m] in the following series and check the appropriate blank following the series: made, came, almost, famous, map, dime

_____satisfactory _____slighted _____substitution

Evaluate the production of [n] in the following series and check the appropriate blank following the series: night, down, another, train, only, now

_____satisfactory _____slighted _____substitution

Evaluate the production of [ŋ] in the following series and check the appropriate blank following the series: bring, ring, single, wing, longer, banker

_____satisfactory _____slighted _____substitution

c. Evaluation of changes in degree of nasality (check the appropriate blanks):

	More Nasal	Less Nasal	Unchanged
Nostrils open vs. occluded during the production of [a]	_____	_____	_____
Closing vs. opening the nostrils during the humming of [m]	_____	_____	_____
Reading at a louder than habitual level	_____	_____	_____
Reading at a softer than habitual level	_____	_____	_____
Reading with more than habitual activity of the lips and jaws	_____	_____	_____
Reading with less than habitual activity of the lips and jaws	_____	_____	_____
Reading at a pitch level above the habitual level	_____	_____	_____
Reading at a pitch level below the habitual level	_____	_____	_____
Imitation of non-nasal, prolonged vowels of examiner	_____	_____	_____

Discuss the significance of any changes observed in indicating possible etiological factors and their implications concerning the possibility and desirability of changes in nasality:

d. In general, is the precision of articulation of speech sounds:
less than average_____ average_____ more than average_____
e. Does the severity of the nasality vary from one type of speaking situation to another? yes_____ no_____. If yes, describe:

2. Physical condition of the nasal cavities
Recent removal of tonsils, adenoids, or other nasal obstructions: yes_____ no_____
History of chronic inflammation of the nasal mucosa due to hay fever, asthma, etc. yes_____ no_____
Does the speaker have a cold: yes_____ no_____
If yes is checked on any of these items, discuss the possible implications in accounting for the problem:

3. Discuss the relationships of the findings from this examination, the General Voice Quality Examination, and the Speech Mechanism Examination to the voice problems revealed by the General Speech Behavior Rating, and indicate the implications of these findings concerning procedures to be employed in attempting to change voice quality:

Additional copies of this form may be obtained from the Interstate Printers and Publishers, 19-27 North Jackson Street, Danville, Illinois.

REFERENCES

1. Fairbanks, G., *Voice and Articulation Drillbook*, New York: Harper, 1940.
2. Fairbanks, G., *Voice and Articulation Drillbook*, rev. ed., New York: Harper, 1960.
3. Johnson, W., *People in Quandaries: The Semantics of Personal Adjustment*, New York: Harper, 1946.
4. Lintz, Lois B., and Dorothy Sherman, "Phonetic elements and perception of nasality," *Journal of Speech and Hearing Research*, 1961, *4*:381-396.
5. McDonald, E. T., and H. K. Baker, "Cleft palate speech: an integration of research and clinical observation," *Journal of Speech and Hearing Disorders*, 1951, *16*:9-21.
6. McIntosh, C. W., "An auditory study of nasality," unpublished M.A. thesis, University of Iowa, 1937.
7. Moll, K. L., "Velopharyngeal closure on vowels," *Journal of Speech and Hearing Research*, 1962, *5*:30-37.
8. Rees, Maryjane, "Harshness and glottal attack," *Journal of Speech and Hearing Research*, 1958, *1*:344-349.
9. Rees, Maryjane, "Some variables affecting perceived harshness," *Journal of Speech and Hearing Research*, 1958, *1*:155-168.
10. Sherman, Dorothy, and E. Linke, "The influence of certain vowel types on degree of harsh voice quality," *Journal of Speech and Hearing Disorders*, 1952, *17*:401-408.
11. Spriestersbach, D. C., and G. R. Powers, "Nasality in isolated vowels and connected speech of cleft palate speakers," *Journal of Speech and Hearing Research*, 1959, *2*:40-45.
12. Stetson, R. H., *Motor Phonetics*, Amsterdam: North-Holland Publ. Co., 1951.
13. Thurman, W. L., "An experimental investigation of certain vocal frequency-intensity relationships concerning natural pitch level," unpublished M.A. thesis, University of Iowa, 1949.
14. Travis, L. E. (Ed.), *Handbook of Speech Pathology*, New York: Appleton-Century-Crofts, 1957.
15. Van Riper, C., and J. V. Irwin, *Voice and Articulation*, Englewood Cliffs, New Jersey: Prentice-Hall, 1958.

7 APPRAISAL OF LANGUAGE DEVELOPMENT AND LANGUAGE DISORDERS

THE PROBLEM OF LANGUAGE

Professional workers in speech pathology and audiology are concerned not only with the mechanics of speech production and reception, but also with language itself—the symbolization process and the symbolic systems that distinguish man uniquely from all other creatures. As a speech pathologist you will become increasingly intrigued with the meaning of meaning, with what can be meant by the word "word" and such other words as "phrase," "sentence," "proposition," "abstracting" and, indeed, "speaking." You will, of necessity, become interested in problems of language structure (17), in relationships between words and things (17) and between speaking and behaving (17, 39), in the still relatively unexplored and even largely unimagined interaction of language and feeling and thought (17) and in laws governing the development of language and other symbolic forms and their purposeful uses.

You will be interested in these matters because as your clinical experience expands you will deal with more and more persons whose

160

crucial handicap is one of language comprehension and formulation—
the mentally retarded individual, the brain-injured child, the dysphasic
adult, the psychotic patient. You will become increasingly aware of the
content and the *structure* of what is spoken and you will puzzle over
how language patterns are learned, how some are lost and others retained, and how lost ones are regained. The farther you go, the clearer
it will become that to understand Henry as a speaker (see Chapter 1)
you must listen to what he says as well as to how he says it. You must
listen especially with an informed ear to the talking he does. It would
be naive and indeed careless to study a speaker's production and reception of language symbols apart from the symbols he uses and the
meanings they hold for him—or, more precisely, the meanings he pro-
jects into them, for the meanings of a word are not to be found in the
word, nor indeed in the dictionary, but in the persons who respond to
the word and by means of it.

There has been much speculation about, and some study of, the
origin and growth of language as a human achievement and the development of language skills by the individual. In this chapter we skirt
the larger issue of the origin of language in the misty dawn of human
history and focus instead upon a set of techniques—developed largely
as research procedures and recently adapted to clinical purposes—by
means of which the language usage of a given person can be sampled
and analyzed. We also briefly examine the procedures we may follow
and certain specific instruments we may use in appraising the nature and degree of language impairment in persons who, once having
acquired normal language skills, lose them through damage to the
brain, whether induced by trauma, infection, neoplasm, or cerebrovascular accident. The speech pathologist has batteries of tests suitable for
evaluating the level of language achieved by children and the degree
of language impairment of persons appropriately called aphasic or
dysphasic.

The procedures we suggest for children provide results that can be
compared with normative data based upon well-selected samples of
respectable size and known composition. (See Tables 22-33). Out of
your use of these procedures and the normative data related to them
can emerge a new appreciation of what a staggeringly difficult set of
skills a child must master before he is old enough even to know what
he is up against. The processes of language comprehension, formulation, and expression, which at first thought may appear simple, automatic, and obvious because they are so commonplace, soon impress one
who works with them as being intricate, obscure, unstable, and even
hazardous. Consider the child's bewilderment and challenge when
confronted by the "blooming, buzzing confusion" of his environment.
As Delacroix (*8*) put it:

To analyze the sonorous continuity of heard speech, to take the sentence apart, to deduce the logical relationships of inflections and endings, to retain in one simultaneous grasp that fleeting melody which builds itself up in proportion as it fades away, to construct a whole, an ensemble from elements which proportionately disappear, to make a synthesis at the same time as one makes an analysis, to expect something even while knowing what it is he is expecting, to imagine, to foresee, to interpret, to work from knowledge of the whole to knowledge of its elements and vice versa—such is the game of very complex operations which at least to a certain degree and in a certain form the comprehension of language inevitably involves.

Before he has had a chance to master the rules of *this* game, the child is expected to begin playing another: to talk back to the talkers who are relentlessly bombarding him with sound. And, strangely enough, most children by the age of one and a half have so mastered the technique that they are successfully exercising a degree of control over some of those other talkers, their parents, demonstrating to them that two can play at *that* game!

Certainly it behooves you as a student of communication problems to delve into the process of language and find out all you can about how it develops and sometimes goes awry. As a speech clinician you have a need to learn not to focus your attention in a given case too narrowly on the traditional dimensions of articulation and fluency, for example, and thus overlook other crucial speech and language behavior. It is essential, certainly, to distinguish general language retardation from a functional articulatory problem, or impaired voice or articulation associated with a hearing loss or with mental deficiency. Children who are retarded only in speech-sound articulation present a kind of problem that is manifestly different from the problems of children who are retarded in several dimensions of language. The diagnosis of speech retardation or delayed language development is best reserved for children who show significant deviations from the average in several dimensions. The problem limited to articulation is best identified simply as a problem of impaired articulation or articulation disorder.

There are several dimensions of language development to be considered. Perhaps the best review of these dimensions and the various measures that have been applied to them is that of McCarthy (*18*). A reading of this review and scrutiny of some of the research studies quoted in it reveal that investigators who have tried to describe how children grow in language behavior have used many frames of reference and diverse measures. Whereas one has concentrated on the age at which words are first spoken, another has been more interested in the order and rate of appearance of speech sounds, the over-all intelligibility of speech, or the amount and rate of talking. Whereas one investigator has studied the length of children's responses, others have been interested in the egocentricity of the responses, their grammatical construction, or the number of different words used.

What measures should speech pathologists employ? The decision rests largely upon the clinical usefulness of the various measures. Some that have been reported to be of considerable value will be found too time-consuming or technical or difficult to apply. The phoneme type and phoneme frequency measures used by Irwin (see references 9-15, Chapter 4) in his research on children from birth to 30 months of age, though highly reliable and of demonstrated use for appraisal, give their best results only with repeated observations over extended periods. Moreover, they require special skill in phonetic transcription of fleeting bits of babbling or speech, a kind and degree of skill which demand unusually intensive specialized training. Johnson's several type-token ratios, as well as the ratio of actional words to qualitative words, the percentages of self-reference terms, "allness" terms, and quantifying terms, and measures of total verbal output (17, pp. 500-518)—all of these and others require much time, relatively elaborate recording techniques, and detailed analysis of speech samples obtained. The same is true in considerable degree for highly accurate analysis of speech in terms of sentence structure, grammatical form, and the use of different parts of speech.

Another factor that may help some day to determine which measures to use is the degree of intercorrelation among the various measures. Only a beginning has been made toward determining the relative importance of the various dimensions (see Williams, 40, and Schneiderman, 25).

PROCUREMENT OF STANDARD LANGUAGE SAMPLE

In order to evaluate the language development and status of a child you need to obtain a sample of his speech that will lend itself to rather comprehensive analysis. This sample can be supplemented by other kinds of special samples which will enable you to answer specific questions about the child's language status. The procedure for securing the primary sample was devised by McCarthy (19) and further developed and used by Day (7) Davis (6), Templin (36), Winitz (41), Spriestersbach, Darley, and Morris (35), Morris (22), Miller (20), and others.

1. General

You are to elicit and record verbatim for analysis as indicated below at least 50 utterances (not necessarily consecutive) from each person tested. Researchers have found that with increase in age children present in conversation increasingly long and structurally more complicated responses; the functions served by language also appear to change with increasing age, as noted by Piaget (24) and others. The 50-utterance sample of the child's connected speech will allow you to compare him with his peers of like age and sex with respect to at least three dimensions of language—length of response, structural complexity, and size of use vocabulary.

The choice of 50 utterances to comprise the language sample is a matter of some interest and concern because of the amount of time required to record and analyze this much of a person's speech. The question arises as to whether equally reliable information can be obtained from an analysis of fewer than 50 responses. Nice (23), an early advocate of this procedure for studying children's language development, and the person who apparently first suggested the use of mean length of response as a measure of linguistic achievement, offered the following comment concerning the size of speech sample: "Although as few as 30 such sentences ought to show clearly a child's stage of speech development, for any comparative or detailed study there should be at least 100 sentences and preferably more."

McCarthy (19) explained her choice of the speech sample of 50 responses thus: "This number was decided upon because it would give a fairly representative sample of a child's linguistic development in a relatively short period of time, without tiring the child with a prolonged observation." In his research Williams (40) used only 40 expression units and considered these to constitute "a fairly representative sample of a child's expressive control over the language." Schneiderman (25), in a study of the relationship between articulatory ability and language ability, used for her measure of sentence length the mean length of 15 sentences (oral definitions of 15 common nouns after a practice session defining five other nouns).

Darley and Moll (4) studied speech samples of seven different sizes (5, 10, 15, 20, 25, 35, and 50 responses) collected from each of 150 five-year-old kindergarten children. They found that for a group of subjects the means of two language measures (mean length of response and structural complexity score) remain essentially the same regardless of the number of responses on which the scores are based. But they also found that the fewer the number of responses obtained, the greater the variability of the scores. They evaluated the reliabilities of the two language measures in relation to size of language sample. They concluded that 50 responses will yield mean length of response scores of adequate reliability for most research purposes but that the reliability of structural complexity score values based on 50 responses may be less than is desired in some situations. Their data suggest that a sample of 50 responses is the smallest sample affording adequate reliability.

2. Materials and Their Use

Under usual circumstances you will elicit the speech sample while alone with the child, no parent being present. If the child refuses to co-operate in the absence of a parent, take the parent along but ask him to be as quiet and unobtrusive as possible.

Materials: In order to overcome the child's self-consciousness, to establish rapport, and to stimulate spontaneous speech, use pictures, picture books, and toys. McCarthy found that with younger children an animal picture book having one central object in each picture was particularly suitable. For older children she used a book containing group or situation pictures illustrating Mother Goose rhymes. Davis (6) used ship pictures, a book showing simple school situations, and several colored animal books.

For toys McCarthy used "a little red auto, a cat that squeaked, a telephone with a bell, a little tin mouse, and a small ball." Davis chose objects of special interest to boys (assuming that girls would enjoy them too), "a motley collection of little covered wagons with detach-able oxen, lassoing cowboys, buffalo hunters, scouts, Indians in atti-tudes of hostility, flight, or pursuit, and various animals or trees." Templin sought to avoid a "boy" bias in the language-stimulating materials and used toys similar to McCarthy's.

McCarthy and Templin used toys and pictures interchangeably. Davis preferred the toys and resorted to pictures only when toys failed to stimulate spontaneous speech.

How to Proceed: The materials need not be presented in the same way to all children; their use should be adapted to each child. You may allow the child to express a preference for toys or pictures first. If no preference is expressed, you can present the toy or picture you think might be most interesting to the child. Davis framed her opening remarks in such a way as to stimulate conversation, saying, for ex-ample, "I wonder what you play with at home," or "Here are some animals that not many children know," or "Now I'm going to show you something funny," or "Now we're going to look at some books. I want you to tell me about the pictures." You might say, "Tell me what they're doing here. What happened before? How will it all turn out?"

If the first picture or toy fails to bring forth any verbal response, try another. You may get your quota of utterances by presenting only one or two items; with other children you will need to go through the whole repertory of materials, perhaps more than once.

The purpose is to secure responses that are as spontaneous as possible. Therefore you should keep your own remarks to a minimum after your initial rapport-building introduction; if it is necessary to stimulate a response, avoid questions that can be answered by a single word. If older children are invited to play with toys, they may do it in silence unless they are instructed, as by Davis: "I want you to take these toys out of the boxes and play with them any way you like, just as you would if you were at home by yourself. But you must tell me what you are doing while you play so I will know."

Recording the Remarks: Do not record the first ten utterances secured in response to the stimulation materials. McCarthy found that the first ten responses were on the average shorter than the succeeding groups of ten responses, indicating "an overcoming of shyness during the observation." Record the next 50 utterances as they are spoken, using the best shorthand system you can develop. If you lose part of a remark, omit that remark and use the next one you can record in full. The 50 remarks need not be consecutive. Present 50 separate remarks that you have been able to record fully and accurately; they should represent all that the child said those 50 times.

After you have used your materials several times, you will have a fair estimate of the range of vocabulary you can expect. Formulate your own abbreviations: *h* for "horse," *t* for "truck," *cb* for "cowboy," *ll* for "looks like," etc. If an individual word in a response is unintelligible, record phonetically what you hear. If you make remarks or ask questions to stimulate a response, record what you say whenever possible; if you do not have time to do this, use some symbol to indicate that the child's next remark was elicited or followed a remark of the examiner.

An alternative procedure is to use a tape recorder and make a record of all that is said during the testing situation. This procedure, which was first used and reported by Winitz (*41*), has the advantage of reducing the burden on the examiner, who in the traditional procedure must make extremely rapid judgments concerning fleeting verbalizations. In the traditional procedure the tendency may be for the examiner to record some of the shorter responses that he can remember easily in their entirety and to skip some of the longer responses; the result of such a practice is to reduce the estimate of the amount of the child's verbal output. The tape recording procedure also permits the replaying of responses several times in order to make certain of what the child says; in this way a more accurate count of the words used and a more accurate analysis of the sentence structure are possible. A disadvantage arises from the extra time required to transcribe the responses from tape onto paper.

If you adopt the tape recording technique, you probably will find it useful to identify each response by recording on paper the first and last words of each as it is spoken, so as to know when 50 responses have been obtained.

Definitions. The following definitions are to be used in the determination of what constitutes an utterance (remark, response):

A response is considered a separate unit if it is marked off from the preceding and succeeding remarks by pauses (*19*).

A remark is considered finished if a child comes to a full stop, either letting the voice fall, giving interrogatory or exclamatory inflection, or indicating clearly that he does not intend to complete the sentence (*6*).

When one simple sentence is followed immediately by another simple sentence with no pause for breath, the two are considered to comprise one sentence if the second statement is clearly subordinate to the first (*6*). Examples: "I have a sister, she's in fourth grade." "There was buffaloes—no there wasn't buffaloes, there was maneaters." "I used to have—my brother used to have, a tricycle."

Remarks connected by interjections and conjunctions, such as "and," "um," "er," "uh," etc., are considered as separate remarks if the remarks appear to be clearly enumerative. Examples: "The girl, er . . . the boy, um . . . and the monkey." Each example is to be considered a single remark (*41*).

MEASURES OF VERBAL OUTPUT

A number of useful measures of verbal output can be calculated from the basic language sample. These are the mean length of response (MLR), the mean of the five longest responses (M5L), and the number of one-word responses (N1W).

1. Mean Length of Response

McCarthy (*19*) used mean length of response as her primary measure of children's linguistic achievement. This measure was earlier suggested by Nice (*23*) and used by Smith (*31*) in her analysis of hour-long samples of spontaneous speech recorded by hand in a group free-play situation. Nice suggested that "this average sentence length may well prove to be the most important single criterion for judging a child's progress in the attainment of adult language." McCarthy originally called MLR "the simplest and most objective measure of the degree to which children combine words at the various ages" (*19*, p. 50). More recently she has stated that no measure "seems to have superseded the mean length of sentence for a reliable, easily determined, objective, quantitative, and easily understood measure of linguistic maturity" (*18*, pp. 550-551). Information about the reliability of this measure and others to be introduced in this chapter has been reported by McCarthy (*19*) and Minifie (*21*).

The procedure consists of counting the number of words in each response, totaling these numbers, and dividing by 50 (or by the total number of responses if fewer than 50 were secured). The result can be compared with the norms for mean length of response given in Table 22.

The following standards, developed by McCarthy (*19*) and amplified by Davis (*6*) and Winitz (*41*), are used in determining how words should be counted.

a. Contractions of the subject and predicate like "it's" and "you're" are counted as two words.

b. Contractions of the verb and the negative like "can't" are counted as one word.

c. Hyphenated words and compound nouns, particularly proper nouns that are not hyphenated but function as single words and as names of single objects, are counted as single words. Examples: "merry-go-round," "Mother Goose," "Betty Lou."

d. Each part of a verbal combination is counted as a separate word. Example: "have been playing" would be counted as three words.

e. "Lookit" is counted as one word if it occurs alone and functions simply as "look"; if followed by an object, it is counted as the two words "look at."

f. Each of the following is to be counted as one word: oh boy, my gosh, darn it, doggone it, all right, maybe, giddy-up, someone, lighthouse, birdhouse, high school, ain't.

g. Each of the following is to be counted as two words: oh yes, oh no, oh gee, let's see, on to, Christmas tree, kinda, oughta, hafta.

h. Since repetitions can add substantially to the length of the uttered response, they should be excluded according to the following rules:

(1) *Word repetition.* When the same word is repeated several times consecutively it should be counted only once: "He *he he* went home." "The boy ran *ran* he ran away." The italicized words should not be counted.

(2) *Phrase repetition.* When a phrase is repeated it should be counted only once: "He was—*he was* hurt." "And he hit—*and he hit* him." You would not count the italicized words. However, if at least one different word is added when a phrase is repeated, all the words in the repetition should be included in the total count: "And he hit—and he spanked him." "They were going, they were having fun." Word

repetition within a phrase repetition does not nullify a phrase repetition; "And he's *he's, he's—and he's* home." The italicized words should not be counted. Contractions should be separated for purposes of this analysis and not be considered to nullify a repetition: "He's eating, *he is eating* the mouse." The italicized words should not be counted. This procedure should be followed for word repetition also.

(3) *Repetitions not excluded.* When a child repeats a word for enumerative purposes and for starting a new thought unit, he should not be penalized for repetition. "That's a bear there, that's a bear there, that's a bear there." (Child is pointing as he speaks). "I think that that is a bear." "That's what they are, they're bears." Both "that" and "they're" are to be judged as part of a new subordinate or independent clause and are to be counted. Where it cannot be determined whether a repetition is used for emphasis or constitutes a disfluency, the repetition should be excluded.

i. Words not completed by the child should be recorded as though they were completed. Examples: "I th- (think)—I know he's going home." "He might ma- (make)—build a fire." It is especially important to follow this procedure with regard to the analysis of repetition. In many instances a child repeats phrases but does not complete words within the phrase. Example: "I th- (think) he—*I think* he went home." This sentence should be judged to include a phrase repetition, since it could hardly be interpreted as "I he, I think he went home." The italicized words would, therefore, not be counted in determining the number of words in the speech sample.

j. Noises should be counted only when they are considered to be an integral part of the sentence. "*Ahhh grrr,* the lion is eating the monkey," "The lion is going to *grrr* the monkey." In the first instance the *Ahhh grrr* can be considered unessential and should be excluded as not indicative of the child's linguistic maturity. In the second instance the *grrr* takes the part of the verb and should be included.

k. Interjections not considered dictionary items and functioning solely to connect words or phrases should not be counted: "er," "um," etc. However, like utterances which serve as words should be counted: "Uh-huh," "hmmm"—the first of these serves as a substitute for the affirmative word "yes" and the second as the negative word "no."

l. All colloquialisms and neologisms should be counted: "wham," "whoops," "yike," "ya," "yippee," "teensy-weensy," "naw," "yeah," etc.

2. Mean of Five Longest Responses

Davis (*6*) first suggested that the mean of the five longest responses produced by the child might serve as a good indicator of what can be thought of as the child's maximum linguistic skill, the best he can do in a given situation. This measure can be calculated by totaling the words in the five longest responses and dividing by five. The result of this calculation can be compared with the norms compiled by Templin (*36*) which are presented in Table 23.

3. Number of One-Word Responses

Davis (*6*), Templin (*36*), and others have been interested in the number of one-word responses among the total of 50 produced by the child. A decreasing number of one-word responses may be taken as a good indication of increasing language maturity in children. The number of one-word responses made by a given child can be compared with Templin's norms in Table 24, which represent the median number of one-word remarks made by children in her normative sample.

MEASURES OF LANGUAGE STRUCTURE

McCarthy was interested in the complexity of the utterances she obtained from the children in her sample because she wanted to learn "the stage of grammatical complexity that the child has reached, or in other words, how closely his sentence structure approximates adult conversation, his sole criterion upon which to model his speech" (*19*, p. 42). She reported high agreement among four judges in classifying responses with regard to structural complexity and considered the method reliable enough for use with groups. Day (*7*) used McCarthy's procedures and classification system in a study of the language of twins, and Davis (*6*) followed similar procedures with minor modifications. The classification system presented here is essentially that of McCarthy with some amplification of definitions and rules by Davis.

Use the following system for classifying children's remarks with regard to their structural (grammatical) complexity:

1. Complete Responses

a. Functionally Complete but Structurally Incomplete Response. McCarthy has pointed out that much of adult conversation is composed of phrases and other groups of words that are not strictly sentences. The sentence is not expressed in its full form but is merely implied or understood. "If a response is adequate in the situation, and is what an adult would say in such circumstances, the child is using the most complete form he has had the opportunity to learn," and his response should be classified as functionally complete though structurally incomplete. Examples of responses belonging in this category:

> Practically all single-word sentences
> Most responses to questions, where omitted words are implied
> Names
> Expletives
> Other remarks, incomplete in themselves, which are clearly continuations of preceding remarks

b. Simple Sentence Without Phrase. Example: "He has a dog."
c. Simple Sentence With Phrase, or with Compound Subject, Object, or Predicate. Examples:
"He has a puppy with black spots."
"The boy and the girl have sleds."
"He has a dog and a cat."
"He comes up here and slides down."
d. Complex and Compound Sentence. Examples:
"When he pushes her, she slides down."
"He has a sled, and he likes to slide."
e. Elaborated Sentence. This category includes the following types of more involved sentences:
   (1) Simple sentence with two or more phrases, or with compound subject or predicate and a phrase.
   (2) Complex sentence with more than one subordinate clause, or with a phrase or phrases.
   (3) Compound sentence with more than two independent clauses, or with a subordinate clause or phrases.

2. Incomplete Responses

This category, not formally subdivided, includes fragmentary or incomprehensible responses:
> "Well—not this—but—"

Responses without:
> Verb, subject, introductory "there," pronoun, preposition. conjunction.

Responses interrupted by changes in form:
> "We have—my brother has a motorcycle."

Sentences left dangling:
> "He wants to. . . ."
> "She said that she. . . ."

(McCarthy (19) pointed out that in recording children's speech it is often difficult to be sure whether one hears the articles. If a response is complete except for an article, consider it complete.)

Winitz (*41*) has suggested that otherwise complete sentences beginning with the words "but," "and," and "then" should be considered complete, and that sentences beginning with the conjunctions "because," " 'cause," and "for" should be considered incomplete.

3. Analysis

Classify each remark made by the child tested, placing it in one of the divisions and subdivisions listed above. Calculate the total number of remarks falling in each division and subdivision, and divide by the total number of responses elicited to determine the percentage in each category. The percentages can be compared with the norms presented in Table 25.

You will find such lists of percentages rather cumbersome in trying to evaluate the linguistic maturity of the child in question. Obviously a single numerical score that would indicate the relative maturity of the child's grammatical usage would be much more convenient, even though it would not reflect some details of the child's performance. Williams (*40*) was the first to develop a quantitative method for indicating the completeness and complexity of children's remarks. Templin (*36*) also has devised a quantitative method of representing sentence completeness and complexity. She has assigned weights as follows to the categories of the McCarthy-Davis outline in order to obtain a structural complexity score (SCS):

Classification of Remark	*Weight*
Incomplete responses, 1a and 2	0
Simple sentences as described in 1b and 1c	1
Simple sentences with two or more phrases, or with a compound subject or predicate and a phrase, 1e(1)	2
Compound sentences, 1d	3
Complex sentences, 1d, and elaborated sentences as described in 1e(2) and 1e(3)	4

Assign the appropriate weight to each of the remarks made by the child and total these values to obtain the SCS. This score can be compared with the norms reported by Templin and presented in Table 26. It should be noted that the SCS has the meaning here intended only when based upon 50 responses. It is not an average but rather the sum of the weights assigned to 50 remarks. Comparison with the norms, therefore, is not valid if the number of responses is different.

With 50 responses, the SCS can range from 0 to 200. Fifty incomplete responses would give a score of 0, and 50 complex or elaborated sentences would give a score of 200.

Templin (*36*) has indicated that "the quantitative complexity score is not quite so stable as other language measures used in her study. However, it has the advantage of being a quantitative measure and thus permits some comparisons of grammatical complexity of the obtained remarks with other language skills." Similarly Darley and Moll (*4*) reported that SCS values are less reliable than MLR scores when both are based on the same number of responses, possibly because the structural complexity of a child's speech is more variable from response to response than is length of response. They suggested that it is also possible that the arbitrary weights assigned in the Templin scheme to the different grammatical categories may not be entirely appropriate.

It may seem that a study of the child's use of the various parts of speech could yield another index of his skill in language structure. You may find it informative to test this possibility. Classify each word used by a child in his 50 responses as a noun, verb, adjective, adverb, pronoun, conjunction, preposition, article, or interjection. Total the words falling into each of these categories and divide each of the nine totals by the total number of words uttered in order to obtain a percentage for each of the parts of speech. These values can be compared with Templin's norms presented in Table 27.

These norms show that the relative incidence of the various parts of speech in children's responses does not constitute a very discriminating index, as there is not much change in the proportion of the various parts of speech with increase of age from 3 years to 8. As Templin has said,

By the time a child begins to use sentences, the formal structure of the sentence imposes restrictions which partially determine the relative proportions of the use of the various parts of speech. . . . Soon after the child begins to use sentences, considerable stability in the proportion of the various parts of speech has been reported by various investigators, particularly when all words used are considered. The youngest subjects in the present study (aged three years) are already beyond the age when extensive change in proportion of various parts of speech is observed. . . . After the age of three the parts of speech used in . . . the total number of words . . . uttered show little change. This . . . is an indication that the language of children is functioning similarly to the language of adults. At this age the structure of adult grammar has already imposed the pattern of word selection upon the children (*36*, pp. 100, 102, 104).

MEASURES OF VOCABULARY

Children's knowledge of words has long served as an index of their language maturity. Investigators have based their judgments concerning progress in language development upon the age at which children first begin speaking intelligible words, the number of words they appear to know at any given age, and their ability to define, use, or indicate understanding of selected samples of words at various levels of difficulty. Your problem as a clinician is to select procedures that will give the most reliable and useful information about a given child's stock of words.

1. Age of First Word

To learn the age at which a child first used words, we depend upon a statement from the parent or some other informant familiar with the child's early development. How reliable will the information be? Westlake (*38*) stated, "It has been said that most children begin to speak when their parents think they do. The point is that most parents go all out with their children, accepting as words sounds which may slightly resemble words and assuming meanings and ideas that are probably not there at all." McCarthy elaborated the point thus:

Although it might seem as though it would be very easy to determine the actual onset of speech by noting the child's first word, there are a number of difficulties surrounding the determinations of the exact age at which the child uses his first word. The first use of sound with meaning is usually considered to constitute the child's first word. This event is so eagerly anticipated by parents that they often read meaning into the child's early babblings which happen to coincide with the presence of certain persons, objects, or events in the environment. If the child habitually uses "da-da" in his babbling, and sometimes uses it in the presence of his father, when can it be said that "Daddy" is uttered to designate his father? If the criterion of using the word to mean only one person, and not using it in any other situation, is accepted, it is necessary to observe over a period of time, to note consistency of usage, and to see that the sounds are not used in other situations. This is rather a negative way of establishing the fact that the word is used with meaning, and it does not indicate positively the first time the word is used with meaning. . . . Some observers consider the child's first word to be his first spontaneous utterance of a word with meaning (meaningfulness being inferred by the adult with little or no objective evidence as to the correctness of the inference); others consider it to be the first word that the child gives evidence of understanding; and still others consider it to be the speaking of a word in imitation of an adult's speech. With such varying criteria it is necessary to employ caution in interpreting data which have been reported on the appearance of the first word (*18*, p. 523).

Darley and Winitz have reviewed the research having to do with the ages at which children speak their first word. A summary table in their report dramatizes the fact that many definitions have been assigned to the concept of "age of first word" and that the average ages reported for groups of children studied have varied greatly. They identified the problems involved in the use of this measure as follows:

In summary, it would seem that the use of operational definitions of the first word have been so consistently different from investigator to investigator as to be an important source of error in the reported age of appearance of the first word. Coupled with it are other sources of error: the inadequacy of parental records; the fallibility of parents' memory; parents' "wishful hearing," "optimism," and pride; and the infrequency and meagerness of sampling of infants' vocalizations by observers other than parents (5, p. 283).

As they indicated, about the best one can say is that it appears the average child begins to say his first word at approximately one year. Delay of appearance of the first word beyond 18 months *may* indicate a serious physical, mental, or hearing impairment. The measure is so highly subjective that it is useful mainly in pointing up gross retardation or acceleration in language development. The same is true of age at first two-word or three-word combinations (such expressions as "me too," "all gone," and "me through"), and of age at first sentences (longer, more nearly complete constructions, such as those involving subject-verb-object relationships—for example, "Car bumps baby").

2. Number of Different Words Used

All of us draw upon numerous general and special vocabularies to meet our everyday conversational needs. Generally, such word groups can be divided into recognition vocabulary and use vocabulary. Methods of appraising an individual's recognition vocabulary will be discussed in the following section. A procedure for assessing an individual's use vocabulary involves analysis of words used in the basic speech sample of 50 responses.

Obviously a sample of 50 responses will not include all the words a child can use. It can be highly illuminating, however, to compare the number of different words a child uses under the specific conditions created with the number used by other children under similar conditions.

Make a list of all the different words used in the 50 responses, and compare the total with Templin's norms reported in Table 28.

3. Estimates of Size of Recognition Vocabulary

A pioneer investigator into the manner of growth of vocabulary in young children was Smith (*31*), who constructed a 203-word test and administered it to a representative sample of 273 children ranging in age from 2 to 6 years. For children between the ages of 8 months and

2 years the number of words was reported by their mothers. Children were asked to name pictures, but if they failed to say the appropriate word in response to the picture and a question, the examiner then asked another type of question in which the test word was used in such a way that the child could not answer the question unless he understood the word. It appears, then, that credit was given sometimes for recalling and speaking the word and sometimes for simply understanding the word.

The results of Smith's investigation are reported in Table 29. It is clear that the number of words known by children increases as they increase in age. The data presented in the column entitled "number of words" may be misleading in that they seem to indicate the absolute magnitude of children's vocabularies. In actuality Smith selected for her tests every twentieth word from Thorndike's list of 10,000 most common words, eliminating all words not found in any one of 77 published vocabularies of children. The sample of 203 words, then, was drawn from a total of only 10,000 words. Had the test sample been selected from an unabridged dictionary in a similar way, one would be able to generalize to a much larger population of words and therefore the values reported would be much greater.

Builders of vocabulary tests must grapple with a number of knotty problems. The test builder must decide upon a reasonable definition of the word "word." For example, he must decide whether the words "know," "knew," and "known" are three separate words or are to be lumped together as a single word, to be counted as one in the total population of words. He must also decide what constitutes "knowing" a word, that is, whether the test response shall involve saying a word in response to a picture, pointing to a picture in response to the aural stimulus of the word, selecting the correct synonym in a multiple-choice situation, defining the word, using the word in a sentence, giving an illustration of the meaning of the word, etc. He must also select the basis of his sampling, including the size of the dictionary providing the population of words and the manner of choosing the words to include in the test, whether on the basis of their position on the page, or their appearance at given intervals in the total distribution of words, or their demonstrated known difficulty as determined through a pilot study.

From the large number of tests that might be used in order to derive an estimate of the extent of a child's vocabulary three will be selected for particular discussion.

Peabody Picture Vocabulary Test: This test (*10*) conveniently measures a subject's "hearing vocabulary," as the author calls it. It has been standardized so as to provide norms for ages 2 years 6 months through 18 years. The subject is not required to read and the responses required are nonoral, so the test is usable with nonreading and speech-impaired children.

Stimulus materials consist of 150 plates contained in a spiral-bound booklet, each plate containing four pictures. The examiner speaks a test word for each plate and the subject in response either points to the appropriate picture on the plate or calls out the number of the picture which he has selected. The subject is encouraged to guess if he is not sure of the answer. The examiner begins at an appropriate point in the series of plates (for example, plate 25 for subjects between the ages of 4 years 3 months and 5 years 5 months). He establishes a basal value (eight consecutive correct answers) and a ceiling (six errors made in any eight consecutive presentations). The number of correct responses is then totaled and the resulting raw score can be converted to a mental age score and an intelligence quotient through the use of tables provided in the test manual. When using this test simply as a measure of vocabulary development, some may prefer to convert the raw score into a percentile through the use of other tables provided. Two equivalent forms of the test, A and B, are available, each with a separate table of norms.

The Ammons Full-Range Picture Vocabulary Test: This test (1) also is useful with nonreaders and those who, because of speech or physical handicap, find it difficult to respond orally or in writing. The stimulus materials consist of 16 cards or plates, on each of which four drawings appear. The examiner uses an answer sheet on which are listed the words to be tested by each plate. There are separate answer sheets for two equivalent forms of the test, A and B. The number of words tested by the several plates is not the same, some plates testing as few as two words, others testing as many as 11.

The subject is told that when he hears a word he is to "point to the best picture on the page to show what the word means." After a few practice items the examiner proceeds with the presentation of the test words, making an entry on the test blank to indicate the correctness or incorrectness of the subject's answer. The subject is told that he is not to guess; if the examiner feels that he has guessed on any words, he later asks him to point to those words again.

A point-level is shown after each word on the answer sheet. A point-level represents "approximately the mental age at which 50 percent of a representative population would fail the word." Words on a plate are given until three point-levels (*not necessarily words*) are passed consecutively and three failed consecutively.

At the completion of the test, the examiner counts the items answered correctly on the plates and derives a total, which then can be converted to mental age, using a table on the back of the answer sheet, and ultimately into IQ-equivalents if one wishes. An alternative method for interpreting the results is to compare the raw score (number of items correct on the total test) with the norms presented in Table 30.

The Seashore-Eckerson English Recognition Vocabulary Test: This test (*28*) was designed for school-age persons and can be self-administered by those who read with at least moderate ease. The test booklet presents three sets of words: 173 "general terms" or "basic vocabulary"; a supplementary list of 40 proper names, geographical locations, and rare words; and 46 derived terms. As a speech clinician you probably will find the "general terms" section most useful for your clinical purposes. Each test word is followed by four alternative words or sets of words from which the subject tested is to select the one which is the test word's synonym or is related to the test word's most common meaning.

Procedures vary with the grade level or reading proficiency of the subject being tested. Smith (*34*), who compiled the norms for this test that are presented in Table 31, has described in some detail the procedure she followed with different grade levels. Pupils in grades 7 through 12 usually can take the test independently with minimal instructions. Pupils in grades 4 through 6 probably will need to have the instructions read aloud to them, and the examiner usually will work out the test items together with a child needing help. These children may be tested in groups if necessary, but children in the lower elementary grades (1 through 3) must be tested individually. The recommended procedure is to ask the child to define each test word; if he fails to reply at once or does not make his meaning clear, read him the choice words and, if necessary, repeat the test word with each alternative response.

The range of difficulty of the words in the test is so great that whole pages of words may be unknown to the younger children. Smith has recommended that the examiner "suggest to the children that they leave out any words on pages 3, 4, and 5 which they have never seen or heard before. In general, fourth and fifth graders should attempt at least 100 words, sixth, seventh, and eighth graders at least 110 words."

Smith has pointed out that sometimes a child, regardless of grade level, gives stereotyped answers to the alternative responses on the basis of position cues—for example, always choosing the last foil without regard to its meaning. In such a circumstance, or if a child fails to respond at all, you should ask him to describe the word in his own way or tell something about it or to use the word in a sentence and then to explain his sentence. If his reply to such questions is correct, disregard his earlier incorrect choice of answers and give him credit for the word. As a last resort, Smith has suggested that leading questions be asked and half credit be given for correct replies to such questions.

Regardless of the child's mode of response award him credit for giving any correct meaning of a word. Count the number of errors made and multiply this number by 1.33 to correct for guessing. Subtract the product from the number of words attempted. Multiply the resulting value by 505 (since this sample is 1/505 of all such words in the Funk and Wagnall's unabridged dictionary). The result is an estimate of the size of the subject's basic vocabulary. You can interpret this estimate by referring to the norms given in Table 31. This table presents for each grade, on the basis of Smith's standardizing sample, the lowest and highest scores made, the mean score, and the 25th and 75th percentile scores.

For example, if a given twelfth grader is estimated to have a basic vocabulary of 22,000 words, you could report that he has a basic vocabulary smaller than that of any of the 66 children tested by Smith in her standardizing sample of twelfth graders. Indeed, his score is close to the mean score of Smith's group of 40 second graders. He appears to be seriously retarded in this particular dimension of language.

FUNCTIONAL ANALYSIS

Jean Piaget (*24*), of the Jean Jacques Rousseau Institute at Geneva, originated the analysis of children's language according to the functions of their responses in relation to their environment. According to Piaget, sometimes language conveys information, sometimes it provokes action in others, sometimes it serves to "let off steam," etc. McCarthy (*10*) adopted Piaget's classification system and modified it to fit the circumstances under which she made her observations and to allow for a more detailed analysis. Davis (*6*) modified it further, making it essentially what is to be described here. This system can be used in analyzing the 50 responses that constitute the basic language sample.

1. Egocentric Speech

The audience is disregarded in egocentric speech. The child "talks either for himself or for the pleasure of associating anyone who happens to be there with the activity of the moment. . . . He makes no attempt to place himself at the point of view of his hearer." He may talk about himself or about persons or things other than himself, but he disregards the audience. There are two subclasses:

Repetition or Echolalia: The child repeats words or syllables for the pleasure of talking with no thought of talking to anyone or even of making sense. This includes repetition of rhymes or songs.

Monologue: Here the child talks to himself as though thinking aloud, without addressing the examiner. This category can include remarks seemingly addressed to the examiner but without apparent expectation that he will hear, understand, or respond. The remark "Let's see" without amplification would be classified here.

2. Socialized Speech

Here the child addresses the listener, considers his point of view, tries to influence him, or exchanges ideas with him. Six subdivisions are used:

Adapted Information: The child offers his thoughts to the examiner, telling him something to interest him or influence his actions or actually interchanging ideas. This subdivision includes:

Naming—"This is an Indian."
Quantitative discrimination—"Here's two"; "You've got a lot of 'em."
Discrimination, comparison, choice—"These two are just alike"; "I like this kind best"; "That one is bigger."
Definition—"A sleigh is a kind of sled, isn't it?"
Judgment, deduction, interpretation—"This has to go here"; "I don't know what this is"; "I'd like to keep 'em." Also remarks introduced by such expressions as "he has to," "I think," "I guess," "I wonder," "I bet," "It needs."
Criticism—"I don't like that"; "It won't work."
Remarks about the immediate situation (includes descriptions of actions or intentions of self, examiner, or toys): "Then this one comes galloping up"; "I'll take this one next"; "Here goes a sheep."
Remarks associated with the immediate situation (additional information volunteered by the child obviously in connection with the current situation or the immediately preceding remark and the situation): "I go downstairs that way sometimes"; "I used to have some like these."
Irrelevant remarks (those in which the examiner cannot notice any connection with previous remarks or actions).

Emotionally Toned Remarks: Exclamations such as "Gee!" "Lands sakes!" "Will you look at that!" Also "H'm!" if uttered with marked astonishment, and "There!" if uttered with clear satisfaction. In addition, all commands and threats are classified here.

Questions: Classified here are formally interrogative sentences and also declarative sentences with an interrogative function—that is, any remarks that definitely require an answer from the hearer. This category does not include declarative sentences with a question tacked on the end simply for approval of the statement and not really requiring a reply: "I made it go, didn't I?" However, a sentence begun as a question, left unfinished, and then completed in declarative form is classified as a question: "Is it—this is a real Indian."

Answers: This class includes all answers to real questions and to commands. All elicited responses are classified here.

Social Phrases: These are responses which the child makes only in social situations, saying them parrot-fashion. They probably function as single words: "Please," "Thank you," "You're welcome," "Bye-bye," "Excuse me."

Dramatic Imitation: Here are classified all talk in imitation of adult conversation, such as imaginary telephone conversations. Imitations of sounds of animals, horns, etc. are also classified here: "Meow," "Moo-moo," "Now he shoots *bang bang*," "Bow-wow."

3. Interpretation

After classifying each remark made by the child tested, calculate the total number of responses falling in each division and subdivision. Divide each sum by 50 (or by the total number of responses elicited) to determine the percentage in each category. Compare these percentages with the values in Table 32 reported by Piaget (*21*), based upon his observation of two subjects, or with the norms presented in Table 33, based upon data summarized by McCarthy (*18*).

Approximately 38 percent of the remarks made by Piaget's 6-year-old boys were egocentric (*24*). McCarthy (*18*, p. 563) summarizes other findings of Piaget as follows: "Piaget reported a higher percentage of egocentric remarks in ages from three to five than at age six and stated that there occurs a definite socialization in the child's speech at seven to eight years of age. He implied that adult conversation is highly socialized and that this egocentricism is a symptom of psychological immaturity, which is outgrown with age." You will note a considerable discrepancy between the percentages of egocentric speech reported by Piaget (*24*) and the percentages reported by McCarthy (*19*), Day (*7*), and Davis (*6*) in Table 33. The values reported by Smith fall somewhere between. In discussing her results Smith (*33*) noted that "A far higher proportion of sentences in the records used in this study were classified as egocentric . . . than in that by McCarthy but a considerably lower proportion than in that by Piaget. Perhaps we do not all agree as to just the meaning of this term."

A more likely cause of the noted discrepancies is the fact that the speech samples in these studies were collected in different ways. Piaget had a researcher follow each boy at the morning class for about a month and take down in minute detail and in context everything that was said by the child. The class situation was almost completely unstructured; the two subjects and their fellows had complete freedom of movement from room to room and formed their groups as they wished. Their remarks, then, were collected in an essentially free-play situation. In contrast, McCarthy, Day, and Davis collected the remarks from their subjects in a highly structured situation, each child being alone with the adult looking at pictures and playing with toys. Some of Smith's records were taken while the child was at play with other children, others while the child was observed with adults in his own home or in another home.

It might well be expected that when children are playing freely alongside each other, sometimes interacting and sometimes not, the subject might well, to use the words of Piaget, "not bother to know to whom he is speaking or whether he is being listened to. He talks either for himself or for the pleasure of associating anyone who happens to be there with the activity of the moment." In the more structured situation with an adult, the child does not have this freedom; and he is afforded little or no opportunity or encouragement to engage in egocentric speech. The very nature of the situation demands that his responses be socialized. As a result, you will find that typically the functional analysis of 50 responses elicited from a child in the manner prescribed in this chapter yields little or no egocentric speech. It is well, however, to know about this particular dimension of language proposed by Piaget and to keep it in mind when analyzing the language of children you may have occasion to study, particularly if you can observe them during free-play situations.

FORM FOR RECORDING MEASURES OF SPEECH AND LANGUAGE DEVELOPMENT

Form 9 (Measures of Speech and Language Development), presented on pages 196–197, provides a convenient way to record several kinds of information about a child's language development status. The various sections of the form will be described in turn.

1. Acquisition of Language

Record the information you have secured from the child's parents or some other appropriate informant concerning the ages at which the child first spoke words, word combinations, and sentences.

2. Articulation

Abstract the information recorded on the Articulation Test (Form 3, pp. 104–105). Indicate the number of items the child produced correctly on the 50-item screening test, and following it record the appropriate cut-off score selected from Table 18, p. 103. Similarly, indicate the total number of items correct on the 176-item diagnostic test, and following it record the mean number of items produced correctly by children of comparable age and sex as presented in Table 19, p. 103. On the next line, "Sounds Consistently Misarticulated," list all sounds shown in section 2e of the analysis sheet of the Articulation Test. These are the sounds that the child never produced correctly during the test or following any kind of stimulation. On the next line, "Sounds Inconsistently Misarticulated," record all other sounds which the child produced incorrectly part of the time (all those listed after items 2b, 2c, and 2d of the analysis sheet). Finally make a judgment of the intelligibility of the child's conversational speech, using the four-point scale suggested.

3. Estimate of Vocabulary Size

If you have given a vocabulary test, name the test in the space provided and record the score obtained. In addition, enter after the space marked "Norm" any normative or other interpretative data which will indicate how the child's performance compares with that of others who have been given this test. If you gave no formal vocabulary test make a subjective judgment of the adequacy of the child's vocabulary. You may base this judgment on his ease or difficulty in responding to the picture articulation test and the variety and difficulty of words he has used in conversation, as well as his parents' judgment of his vocabulary size.

Then record the index of the child's use vocabulary that you obtained when you counted up the total number of different words he used in the 50 responses you obtained. Enter this number and also the corresponding normative value extracted from Table 28.

4. Measures of Verbal Output

The first entries concerned with amount of verbal output are your subjective ratings of the child's verbalization, made by using a five-point scale to compare the child with other children. Make the first three ratings—(a) amount of babbling; (b) amount of talking when child first began to speak, according to parent; and (c) amount of talking at present, according to parent—on the basis of answers supplied by the parent or some other informant. Make the other two ratings—(d) amount of talking at present, according to examiner; and (e) rate of speech—on the basis of the speech sample you elicit. In addition, characterize the child's conversation by checking one of the entries shown after "Description of conversation."

The remaining items in this section are based upon the basic sample of 50 responses. Indicate the actual number of responses you elicited. Then enter the mean length of response which you have calculated, together with the appropriate normative value indicating the mean length of response of children of similar age and sex as reported in Table 22. Also record the mean length of the child's five longest responses and the corresponding normative value extracted from Table 23. Finally, record the number of one-word responses in the total of 50, and with it the appropriate normative value selected from Table 24.

5. Structural Analysis

Having classified each of the 50 responses with regard to completeness and complexity according to the classification system presented on pp. 170–171, enter the number of sentences falling in each of the six categories, the corresponding percentage of the total number of responses represented by each of these entries, and the appropriate normative percentage values extracted from Table 25 of this chapter. Just after this enter the structural complexity score calculated according to the system described (warning: remember that this score can be computed only if a total of 50 responses has been elicited), and enter the appropriate normative value selected from Table 26 of this chapter.

In the portion immediately following, you will have an opportunity to record your impression of the child's use of various tenses and of other grammatical forms. The more advanced a child is in language use, the more refined will be his sense of time relationships and his mastery of verb forms that express them. Check the various tenses you hear the child use correctly in conversation—past, future, present perfect, and past perfect. Further, the skill with which he manipulates pronouns and the irregular verbs is partially indicative of his level of language development. Does he use "me" for all cases— nominative, objective, and possessive—or does he discriminate correctly between "I," "me," and "my"? When he should use a past participle or the past tense of an irregular verb, does he use the correct form or does he say "have did," "have saw," "I fighted him," or "I comed"? Check the blanks if you have observed correct use of pronouns and irregular verbs.

Finally, determine the total number of each of the various parts of speech (nouns, verbs, etc.) the child used. Use the category "miscellaneous" for proper names and unintelligible words. Divide each of the values obtained by the total number of words used by the child to secure the percentages of occurrences of the various parts of speech.

Following each of these percentage values enter the appropriate normative percentage value extracted from Table 27 of this chapter.

6. Functional Analysis

Enter the numbers of the child's egocentric and socialized responses, respectively, as well as the percentage of the total number of responses represented by each of these values. In addition, indicate for each an appropriate normative percentage extracted from Table 33.

7. Description of Testing Situation

Finally, describe how you elicited the speech sample on which many of the above judgments are based: the testing situation—degree of rapport, interference of distractions, fatigue, etc; the physical environment; any other aspects that may have served somehow to affect the reliability of the judgments. It is plain that an eager outpouring of whole paragraphs of bubbling conversation by a lonely child in a hospital ward, who has been yearning to talk to someone and finds you a pleasant audience, is a speech sample hardly comparable to the reluctant monosyllabic grunts and mumbles of the shy and weepy child clinging to her mother's skirt in a noisy clinic room—and neither sample should be considered "typical" for the child concerned.

APPRAISAL OF LANGUAGE IMPAIRMENT IN DYSPHASIA

The speech pathologist is concerned not only with children's problems in language acquisition but also with the problems of individuals, young or old, who as a result of any of several misfortunes involving damage to the brain, suffer a loss or impairment of their facility with language. The speech pathologist's importance as a member of the rehabilitation team concerned with any person so affected arises largely from the fact that he is properly charged with responsibility for ascertaining and describing the person's impairment of function in the various modalities of language and providing a systematic program of language retraining which will facilitate his recovery of language comprehension and expression.

Tests developed for appraising aphasic or dysphasic language impairment typically sample a patient's performance in the input modes of listening and reading and the output modes of speaking, writing, and calculation. Some tests sample certain nonlanguage behavior as well to detect agnosias (failures to recognize and comprehend the import of sensory information although sensation is intact) and apraxias (inabilities to perform purposeful skilled acts even though there is no paralysis) which are sometimes found in association with the problems of understanding, formulating, and using language which we commonly call aphasia. (As we stated previously, this disability is usually more correctly designated as dysphasia, a term which denotes a degree of impairment less than the total absence of language denoted by the term aphasia.)

Two widely used tests for degree of dysphasia, including aphasia. are Eisenson's *Examining for Aphasia (11)* and the *Halstead-Wepman Screening Test for Aphasia (14)*. Both of these tests are fairly brief and provide a sampling of the subject's performance in the language modalities mentioned above. Because each of the component batteries of these tests is relatively restricted and is not designed to provide opportunity for detailed examination of the many possible combinations of input and output channels, these tests are best used as screening instruments. They are not intended to detect minimal or subtle forms of impairment and they do not always lend themselves well to the charting of a patient's progress during language retraining.

The *Minnesota Test for Differential Diagnosis of Aphasia (26)*, developed by Schuell at the Minneapolis Veterans Administration Hospital, provides for relatively exhaustive testing of each language modality and for the use of several combinations of input and output channels. The test has not yet been published commercially but has been made available by the author in limited quantities in a series of research editions. Schuell has used the test on sufficient numbers of patients, whose language recovery she has followed for substantial periods of time, to derive an empirical five-fold classification of dysphasic disorders which the clinician may find useful. The classifications are based upon patterns of test performance and are related to prognosis for language recovery.

Responding to requests for a less lengthy test which would yield comparable (though necessarily somewhat less reliable) information about patterns of disability and prognosis, Schuell developed "A Short Examination for Aphasia" *(27)*. This test, which takes between 30 and 45 minutes to administer, consists of a selection of those items and batteries from the *Minnesota Test for Differential Diagnosis of Aphasia* judged to be of greatest diagnostic and prognostic value. Materials required for administration of the test are few in number and easily manipulated.

The latest newcomer in the field of aphasia testing is the *Language Modalities Test for Aphasia* developed by Wepman and Jones *(37)*. This test has been standardized and provides a useful clinical and research tool. Stimuli are presented to the subject through the medium of filmstrips and five different response categories are used. The test is available in two equivalent forms, the initial items of both constituting a "Screening Section." The time required for administering one complete form is usually about one hour. A manual provides detailed instructions for administration and scoring, and booklets for the examiner's record and the subject's responses are provided.

ASSIGNMENTS

1. In connection with Assignment 1, Chapter 4, complete Form 9 for the five children tested. In your report on each child include answers to the following questions:
    a. Along which dimensions, if any, does the child appear to be retarded?
    b. Along which one dimension is there the greatest degree of retardation?
    c. Are there marked discrepancies between any of the measures, which you feel suggest the need for further investigation?
    d. How adequate do you consider the sample of speech elicited?
    e. How reliable and valid do you consider the various ratings to be?
2. On the basis of your reading and experience, compile a list of all the possible measures of developmental status in speech that you can think of. Evaluate each one briefly with regard to its reliability, clinical usefulness, usefulness as a research tool, and relevance in the diagnosis of language retardation.
3. In view of the difficulty in eliciting responses longer than "yes" and "no" from some young children who offer little spontaneous conversation, prepare a list of questions for a clinician's use which you think would most surely elicit samples of connected speech. (It is obvious that the "mean length of response" can be no more than one word if all questions asked demand only one-word answers.)
4. Why are the measures "use of different parts of speech" and "percentage of egocentric speech" less useful clinically than other measures presented in this chapter?
5. Study the data presented in Table 22 derived from the researches of Templin, McCarthy, and Davis. Note that the values for mean length of response reported by Templin are consistently larger than those reported by McCarthy and Davis. How might such discrepancies be accounted for? What are the most reasonable explanations for these differences? (Templin, 36, has discussed the matter briefly.)

TABLE 22. Mean Length (in Words) of Oral Responses of White Boys and Girls (Results of Nine Investigations)

Type of Children Sampled

Age yrs.	Representative[a] N=480 (1)	Representative[a] N=140 (2)	Only[a] N=97 (3)	Singletons[a,b] N=173 (4)	Twins[a] N=166 (5)	All[a] N=436 (6)	Twins[a] N=160 (7)	Longitudinal[a] N=23 (8)	Gifted[c] N=72 (9)	Bilingual[d] N=1000 (10)	First Grade[a] N=300 (11)	First Grade[e] N=116 (12)	First Grade[f] N=116 (13)
1.5		1.2							3.7				
2.0		1.8					1.5	1.7	4.8	1.9			
2.5		3.1						2.7	4.7				
3.0	4.1	3.4					2.5	4.2	5.6	3.0			
3.5	4.7	4.3						4.5	6.9				
4.0	5.4	4.4					3.0		7.2	3.4			
4.5	5.5	4.6							9.5				
5.0	5.7						3.2			3.6			
5.5			5.1	4.4	4.4	4.6							
6.0	6.6		5.4	5.0	5.4	5.3				3.7			
6.5											5.4	6.9	10.4
7.0	7.3												
8.0	7.6												
9.5			7.3	6.5	6.2	6.5							

[a] Speech sample=50 utterances with adult.
[b] Singletons with siblings
[c] Speech sample=three 3-hour samples in play situations.
[d] Speech sample=50 utterances at play with children.
[e] Short speech samples with adult; 80 percent upper and middle class.
[f] Short speech samples from "share and tell" hours; 80 percent upper and middle class.

SOURCE: (1) Templin, 36; (2) McCarthy, 19; (3), (4), (5), (6) Davis, 6; (7) Day, 7; (8) Shirley, 30; (9) Fisher, 12; (10) Smith, 32; (11) Shire, 29; (12), (13) Hahn, 13. (This table was adapted from McCarthy, 18, Table 5, pp. 546-549.)

TABLE 23. Number of Words in Five Longest Oral Responses (M5L)
of Boys and Girls, Upper (USES) and Lower (LSES)
Socioeconomic Status in Templin's Normative Group

Age, Yrs.	Boys (N=30)		Girls (N=30)		USES (N=18)		LSES (N=42)		Total (N=60)	
	Mean	SD	Mean	SD	Mean	SD	Mean	SD	Mean	SD
3	7.95	2.63	7.82	1.83	8.75	2.72	7.52	1.93	7.89	2.27
3.5	8.66	2.08	9.46	3.05	9.99	2.19	8.67	2.00	9.06	2.14
4	10.35	3.05	10.66	3.43	10.64	2.34	10.45	2.89	10.51	2.74
4.5	10.73	3.03	10.78	2.23	11.84	2.26	10.28	2.68	10.76	2.66
5	10.82	2.98	12.63	3.61	12.57	3.73	11.36	3.23	11.73	3.43
6	12.42	2.78	12.11	1.90	13.09	2.23	11.91	2.37	12.27	2.39
7	13.76	1.81	13.37	2.45	13.80	1.71	13.47	2.32	13.57	2.16
8	13.55	2.87	14.75	2.69	14.30	2.70	14.09	2.90	14.15	2.85

SOURCE: Templin, *36*.

TABLE 24. Median Number (together with Semi-Interquartile Range) of
One-Word Oral Responses (N1W) of Boys and Girls, Upper (USES) and
Lower (LSES) Socioeconomic Status in Templin's Normative Group

Age Yrs.	Boys (N−30)		Girls (N=30)		USES (N=18)		LSES (N=42)		Total (N=60)	
	Median	Q	Median	Q	Median	Q	Median	Q	Median	Q
3	3.5	3.0	5.5	3.9	3.5	2.7	5.7	3.8	4.8	3.3
3.5	3.5	4.3	3.0	2.2	2.0	1.5	5.1	3.5	3.3	2.7
4	3.0	2.5	2.0	3.0	2.3	3.2	2.5	3.1	2.5	2.3
4.5	2.5	1.1	2.5	1.8	2.3	1.1	2.6	1.4	2.5	1.5
5	2.6	1.8	2.0	1.9	2.5	1.8	2.2	1.5	2.4	1.7
6	2.7	0.4	0.8	0.7	1.0	1.0	0.7	0.6	0.7	0.6
7	0.6	0.3	0.6	0.4	0.6	0.4	0.6	0.3	0.6	0.3
8	0.6	0.3	0.6	0.3	0.6	0.4	0.6	0.3	0.6	0.3

SOURCE: Templin, *36*.

TABLE 25: Mean Percentages of 50 Oral Responses Falling Within Each Category of Sentence Construction (Results of Four Investigations with White Boys and Girls)

Age, Yrs.	Source	Type of Sentence					
		Functionally Complete but Structurally Incomplete	Simple Sentence without Phrase	Simple Sentence with Phrase	Compound and Complex Sentences	Elaborated Sentences	Incomplete Responses
1.5	McCarthy	78.4	9.6	0.0	0.0	0.0	11.9
2.0	McCarthy	53.8	17.3	1.4	0.9	0.6	25.1
	Day[a]	70.0	7.5	2.0	0.2	0.0	19.7
2.5	McCarthy	35.3	38.7	5.3	1.5	1.2	18.1
3.0	McCarthy	27.2	45.1	8.7	1.5	1.3	16.2
	Templin	28.2	32.0	13.7	2.9	3.1	16.8
	Day[a]	48.0	23.0	4.0	0.5	0.3	24.6
3.5	McCarthy	30.6	35.3	11.4	6.5	2.3	13.9
	Templin	23.8	39.5	16.4	3.3	3.4	13.1
4.0	McCarthy	32.0	39.4	10.9	6.1	4.5	6.8
	Templin	19.7	37.2	18.5	6.9	6.5	11.2
	Day[a]	48.0	28.0	7.5	1.5	0.9	13.3
4.5	McCarthy	31.2	36.5	10.4	7.0	5.9	8.8
	Templin	19.5	37.6	16.2	6.8	7.5	12.1
5.0	Templin	17.2	35.8	16.8	8.7	8.1	12.6
	Day[a]	49.0	24.0	7.0	3.6	1.0	15.4
5.5	Davis	39.4	29.4	7.8	4.6	3.6	15.0
	Davis[a]	38.0	31.4	7.8	4.6	2.8	15.4
6.0	Templin	9.8	38.2	20.7	10.8	11.9	8.6
6.5	Davis	32.0	30.8	9.8	5.4	5.6	16.4
	Davis[a]	28.6	32.2	10.8	7.4	5.8	15.2
7.0	Templin	9.0	34.1	22.8	11.1	13.4	10.5
8.0	Templin	9.4	31.5	21.3	15.0	13.2	9.5
9.5	Davis	33.6	18.8	11.4	6.8	10.0	19.4
	Davis[a]	34.8	22.2	10.8	5.4	10.2	16.6

[a] Twin subjects.

SOURCE: McCarthy, *19*; Davis, *6*; Templin, *36*; Day, *7*. (This table was adapted from McCarthy, *18*, Table 7, p. 553.)

TABLE 26. Mean Structural Complexity Score (SCS) from 50 Oral Responses of Boys and Girls, Upper (USES) and Lower Socioeconomic Status (LSES), by Age in Templin's Normative Group

Age Yrs.	Boys (N=30) Mean	SD	Girls (N=30) Mean	SD	USES (N=18) Mean	SD	LSES (N=42) Mean	SD	Total (N=60) Mean	SD
3	36.4	19.7	32.2	16.5	40.6	20.4	31.4	16.6	34.3	18.3
3.5	38.1	17.3	43.2	18.2	49.2	19.1	36.9	16.1	40.6	17.9
4	48.0	18.8	54.9	20.7	50.6	14.2	51.8	22.1	51.6	20.1
4.5	50.9	24.0	52.9	16.6	61.8	16.3	47.7	20.9	50.4	24.1
5	50.6	18.8	63.2	23.5	55.6	19.4	57.4	22.3	56.9	21.5
6	71.5	22.1	68.7	17.4	70.5	16.0	69.9	21.4	70.1	22.7
7	69.7	20.0	73.9	16.6	70.0	16.5	72.6	19.2	71.8	18.5
8	74.4	18.7	79.2	28.7	91.0	23.5	71.9	21.3	77.7	33.8

SOURCE: Templin, *36*.

TABLE 27. Mean Percentages of Parts of Speech Used by Children in 50 Oral Responses

Age, Yrs.[a]	Noun	Verb	Adjective	Adverb	Pronoun	Conjunction	Preposition	Article	Interjection	Miscellaneous
3	17.7	22.6	6.3	10.0	19.4	1.5	6.5	6.8	2.1	7.1
3.5	17.1	23.0	6.9	9.9	19.2	2.3	6.9	6.5	1.8	6.5
4	16.3	23.1	6.7	10.1	20.3	2.8	6.9	6.8	1.3	5.7
4.5	16.5	23.6	7.7	10.0	18.9	2.5	6.8	7.3	1.2	5.6
5	16.1	23.5	7.5	10.6	20.0	2.6	6.7	6.7	0.8	5.4
6	17.1	25.0	7.6	10.0	19.3	2.6	7.6	7.0	1.0	3.1
7	17.0	24.0	7.3	10.4	18.0	3.3	8.0	7.9	1.4	2.8
8	17.0	24.3	7.4	9.1	17.8	3.7	7.9	8.1	1.2	2.9

[a] N=60 in each age group.
SOURCE: Templin, *36*.

TABLE 28. Mean Number of Different Words Used in 50 Oral Responses by Boys and Girls of Upper (USES) and Lower (LSES) Socioeconomic Status in Templin's Normative Group

Age Yrs.	Boys (N=30)		Girls (N=30)		USES (N=18)		LSES (N=42)		Total (N=60)	
	Mean	SD	Mean	SD	Mean	SD	Mean	SD	Mean	SD
3	94.3	29.9	90.7	21.4	102.4	26.7	88.3	24.6	92.5	26.1
3.5	100.6	20.5	109.0	19.4	115.0	17.9	100.4	19.8	104.8	20.4
4	115.7	28.9	125.2	25.3	127.8	27.1	117.3	27.2	120.4	27.6
4.5	128.6	28.3	125.4	16.5	136.2	17.4	123.0	28.1	127.0	23.9
5	125.8	26.5	139.1	26.1	141.3	25.6	128.6	26.9	132.4	27.2
6	155.2	25.8	138.8	27.0	151.0	23.9	138.6	42.2	147.0	27.6
7	156.0	29.1	159.4	24.9	164.1	22.6	145.8	42.3	157.7	27.2
8	164.7	28.1	168.4	30.6	173.8	30.1	163.4	28.4	166.5	29.5

Source: Templin, *36*.

TABLE 29. Increase in Size of Vocabulary with Age

Age Years-Months	N	Average IQ	Number of Words	Words Gained
8	13		0	
10	17		1	1
1–0	52		3	2
1–3	19		19	16
1–6	14		22	3
1–9	14		118	96
2–0	25		272	154
2–6	14		446	174
3–0	20	109	896	450
3–6	26	106	1222	326
4–0	26	109	1540	318
4–6	32	109	1870	330
5–0	20	108	2072	202
5–6	27	110	2289	217
6–0	9	108	2562	273

Source: Smith, *31*.

TABLE 30. Mean Raw Scores (Words Correct) and Standard Deviations on the Ammons Full-Range Picture Vocabulary Test (as Reported in Three Investigations)

Age Yrs.	Source	Male		Female	
		Mean	SD	Mean	SD
2	(1)	6.1	3.2	6.7	3.0
3	(1)	11.6	4.6	12.1	2.3
	(2)	13.4	3.4	12.3	2.9
3.5	(2)	15.5	2.8	14.6	2.7
4	(1)	17.4	3.6	15.7	4.1
	(2)	16.8	3.0	17.0	3.0
4.5	(2)	18.4	3.6	18.6	2.8
5	(1)	20.9	4.0	21.0	4.8
	(2)	19.4	3.3	21.5	3.2
6	(3)	24.7	4.2	25.3	5.0
7	(3)	28.5	4.4	29.3	4.8
8	(3)	33.2	5.2	29.9	4.3
9	(3)	36.2	6.3	34.9	6.5
10	(3)	42.9	5.3	41.7	4.9
11	(3)	52.8	6.8	43.2	6.6
12	(3)	53.5	5.5	47.8	5.7
13	(3)	55.7	5.5	50.3	6.0
14	(3)	58.4	5.5	57.8	5.2
15	(3)	63.7	6.3	59.3	4.4
16	(3)	63.7	6.1	62.5	5.8

SOURCE: (1) Ammons and Holmes, *3*; (2) Templin, *36*; (3) Ammons, Arnold, and Hermann, *2*.

TABLE 31. Distributions of Scores on the Seashore-Eckerson English Recognition Vocabulary Test Made by Subjects Tested in Each of 12 Grades

School Grade	N	Lowest Score	25th Percentile	Mean Score	75th Percentile	Highest Score
1	44	5,500	12,500	16,900	20,000	32,800
2	40	11,600	17,800	21,900	25,400	30,800
3	59	7,500	20,800	25,600	28,900	42,400
4	74	11,100	23,600	28,400	32,300	41,400
5	61	6,000	17,900	25,600	31,200	51,000
6	66	16,600	29,000	34,000	38,800	50,500
7	69	4,500	27,700	33,800	40,800	55,000
8	72	8,500	31,600	37,100	42,200	58,000
9	116	16,600	32,100	37,900	44,900	59,600
10	113	22,200	39,100	43,100	47,900	57,000
11	98	21,700	39,100	44,900	51,000	65,600
12	66	28,200	40,400	47,300	52,900	66,600

SOURCE: Smith, *34*.

TABLE 32. Percentages of Egocentric and Socialized Oral Responses Observed by Piaget in Speech of Two 6-Year-Old Boys

	Subject	
Classification of Remarks	A	B
Egocentric		
Repetition	2	1
Monologue	5	15
Collective monologue	30	23
Socialized		
Adapted information	14	13
Criticism	7	3
Commands, requests, threats	15	10
Questions	13	17
Answers	14	18
Totals		
Egocentric	37	39
Spontaneous socialized	49	43
Total socialized	63	61

SOURCE: Piaget, *24*.

TABLE 33. Mean Percentages of White Boys' and Girls' Oral Responses Falling in Each Main Functional Category
(Results of Four Investigations)

| | Egocentric Speech | | | | Adapted Information | | | | Socialized Speech | | | | | | | | | | | |
| | | | | | | | | | Emotionally Toned | | | | Questions | | | | Answers | | | |
Age Yrs.	(1)	(2)[a]	(3)[b]	(4)	(1)	(2)[a]	(3)[b]	(4)	(1)	(2)[a]	(3)[b]	(4)	(1)	(2)[a]	(3)[b]	(4)	(1)	(2)[a]	(3)[b]	(4)
1.5	3.1				60.5				14.6				10.8				0.3			
2.0	6.5	16		40	40.8	37		17	18.3	30		32	13.9	2		5	16.6	13		3
2.5	4.0				57.7				14.2				3.5				14.6			
3.0	3.6	1		33	50.9	52		20	9.4	18		30	13.2	7		8	19.1	19		6
3.5	4.7				53.2				9.4				9.7				20.4			
4.0	1.3	1		26	45.2	51		23	6.5	15		28	12.1	8		12	31.0	22		9
4.5	2.2				54.6				6.4				8.2				26.0			
5.0		2		26		50		25		14		22		9		16		21		7
5.5			.4				59.7				3.8				10.6				25.5	
6.5			.2				66.8				3.3				9.4				22.7	
9.5			.7				60.7				1.4				3.8				37.1	

[a] Twins.
[b] Singletons with siblings.
SOURCE: (1) McCarthy, 19; (2) Day, 7; (3) Davis, 6; (4) Smith, 33. (This table was adapted from McCarthy, 18, Table 9.)

FORM 9. MEASURES OF SPEECH AND LANGUAGE DEVELOPMENT

Name _____ Age _____ Sex _____

Examiner _____ Date _____

1. Acquisition of Language
   a. Age when first words were spoken:_____
   b. Age when first 2-word and 3-word combinations were spoken:_____
   3. Age when first sentences were spoken:_____

2. Articulation (information from Form 3)
   a. Screening Test: Number correct:_____ Cut-off score:_____
   b. Diagnostic Test: Number correct:_____ Norm:_____
   c. Sounds consistently misarticulated:_____
   d. Sounds inconsistently misarticulated:_____
   e. Intelligibility:
        Readily intelligible_____
        Intelligible if listener knows topic_____
        Words intelligible now and then_____
        Completely unintelligible_____
3. Estimate of Vocabulary Size
        Test used:_____
        Score:_____ Norm:_____
        Number of different words used_____ Norm:_____

4. Measures of Verbal Output
   a. Subjective ratings:

	Much More Than Average	Somewhat More Than Average	About Average	Somewhat Less Than Average	Much Less Than Average
Amount of babbling:	_____	_____	_____	_____	_____
Amount of talking when first began:	_____	_____	_____	_____	_____
At present, according to parent:	_____	_____	_____	_____	_____
At present, according to examiner:	_____	_____	_____	_____	_____
Rate of speech (more means fast; less, slow)	_____	_____	_____	_____	_____

b. Description of conversation:
    Voluble   _____
    Verbalizes easily   _____
    Brief responses   _____
    None   _____

c. Number of responses elicited:_____

d. Mean length of responses:_____ Norm:_____

e. Mean of five longest responses:_____ Norm:_____

f. Number of one-word responses:_____ Norm:_____

5. Structural Analysis

a. Sentence construction categories:

	Number	Percent	Norm Percent
Functionally complete but structurally incomplete	_____	_____	_____
Simple sentences without phrase	_____	_____	_____
Simple sentences with phrase or with compound subject, object, or predicate	_____	_____	_____
Compound and complex sentences	_____	_____	_____
Elaborated sentences	_____	_____	_____
Incomplete responses	_____	_____	_____

b. Structural complexity score:_____ Norm:_____

c. Correct use of the following forms was noted:
    Past tense   _____
    Future tense   _____
    Present perfect tense _____
    Past perfect tense   _____
    Irregular verbs
    Case of pronouns   _____

d. Parts of speech (based on total words uttered):

	Number	Percent	Norm Percent
Noun:	_____	_____	_____
Verb:	_____	_____	_____
Adjective:	_____	_____	_____
Adverb:	_____	_____	_____
Pronoun:	_____	_____	_____
Conjunction:	_____	_____	_____
Preposition:	_____	_____	_____
Article:	_____	_____	_____
Interjection:	_____	_____	_____
Miscellaneous:	_____	_____	_____

6. Functional Analysis

	Number	Percent	Norm Percent
Egocentric responses:	_____	_____	_____
Socialized responses:	_____	_____	_____

7. Description of Testing Situation

Additional copies of this form may be obtained from the Interstate Printers and Publishers, 19-27 North Jackson Street, Danville, Illinois.

REFERENCES

1. Ammons, R. B., and H. S. Ammons, *The Full-Range Picture Vocabulary Test,* Missoula, Mon.: Psychological Test Specialists, 1948.
2. Ammons, R. B., P. R. Arnold, and R. S. Hermann, "The Full-Range Picture Vocabulary Test. IV. Results for a white school population," *Journal of Clinical Psychology,* 1950, *6*:164-169.
3. Ammons, R. B., and J. C. Holmes, "The Full-Range Picture Vocabulary Test. III. Results for preschool-age population," *Child Development,* 1949, *20*:5-14.
4. Darley, F. L., and K. L. Moll, "Reliability of language measures and size of language sample," *Journal of Speech and Hearing Research,* 1960, *3*:166-173.
5. Darley, F. L., and Harris Winitz, "Age of first word: review of research," *Journal of Speech and Hearing Disorders,* 1961, *26*:272-290.
6. Davis, Edith A., "The development of linguistic skill in twins, singletons with siblings, and only children from age five to ten years," *Child Welfare Monographs,* No. 14, Minneapolis: University of Minnesota Press, 1937.
7. Day, Ella J., "The Development of Language in Twins. I. A Comparison of Twins and Single Children," *Child Development,* 1932, *3*:179-199.
8. Delacroix, H., *Le Langage et la Pensée,* Paris: Alcan, 1930.
9. Doll, E. A., *The Vineland Social Maturity Scale,* Philadelphia: Educational Test Bureau, 1946.
10. Dunn, L. M., *Peabody Picture Vocabulary Test.* Nashville: American Guidance Service, 1959.
11. Eisenson, J., *Examining for Aphasia,* rev. ed., New York: Psychological Corporation, 1954.
12. Fisher, Mary S., "Language patterns of preschool children," *Child Development Monographs,* No. 15, New York: Teachers College, Columbia University, 1934.
13. Hahn, Elise, "Analyses of the content and form of the speech of first grade children," *Quarterly Journal of Speech,* 1948, *34*:361-366.
14. Halstead, W. C., and J. M. Wepman, *The Halstead-Wepman Screening Test for Aphasia,* Chicago: University of Chicago Clinics, 1949.
15. Irwin, O. C., "Development of speech during infancy: curve of phonemic frequencies," *Journal of Experimental Psychology,* 1947, *37*:187-193.
16. Irwin, O. C., and H. P. Chen, "Development of speech during infancy: curve of phonemic types," *Journal of Experimental Psychology,* 1946, *36*:431-436.
17. Johnson, W., *People in Quandries: The Semantics of Personal Adjustment,* New York: Harper, 1946.
18. McCarthy, Dorothea, "Language development in children," in Leonard Carmichael, *Manual of Child Psychology,* New York: Wiley, 1954, Ch. 9.
19. McCarthy, Dorothea, "The language development of the preschool child,"

Child Welfare Monographs, No. 4, Minneapolis: University of Minnesota Press, 1930.

20. Miller, Judith C., "Linguistic skills of physically handicapped children," unpublished M.A. thesis, University of Iowa, 1961.

21. Minifie, F. D., "Temporal reliability of seven language measures," unpublished M.A. thesis, University of Iowa, 1961.

22. Morris, H. L., "Communication skills of children with cleft lips and palates," *Journal of Speech and Hearing Research*, 1962, 5:79-90.

23. Nice, Margaret M., "Length of sentences as a criterion of a child's progress in speech," *Journal of Educational Psychology*, 1925, 16:370-379.

24. Piaget, Jean, *The Language and Thought of the Child*, New York: Harcourt, Brace, 1926.

25. Schneiderman, Norma, "A study of the relationship between articulatory ability and language ability," *Journal of Speech and Hearing Disorders*, 1955, 20:359-364.

26. Schuell, Hildred, *The Minnesota Test for Differential Diagnosis of Aphasia* (Res. ed.), Minneapolis: Minneapolis Veterans Administration Hospital.

27. Schuell, Hildred, "A short examination for aphasia," *Neurology*, 1957, 7:625-634.

28. Seashore, R. K., and L. D. Eckerson, *English Recognition Vocabulary Test*, Evanston, Ill.: The authors, 1938.

29. Shire, Sister Mary L., "The relation of certain linguistic factors to reading achievement in first-grade children," unpublished Ph.D. thesis, Fordham University, 1945.

30. Shirley, Mary M., "The first two years: A study of twenty-five babies. Vol. II. Intellectual development," *Child Welfare Monographs*, No. 7, Minneapolis: University of Minnesota Press, 1933.

31. Smith, Madorah E., "An investigation of the development of the sentence and the extent of vocabulary in young children," *University of Iowa Studies in Child Welfare*, 1926, 3 (5).

32. Smith, Madorah E., "Some light on the problem of bilingualism as found from a study of the progress in mastery of English among pre-school children of non-American ancestry in Hawaii," *Genetic Psychology Monographs*, 1939, 21:121-284.

33. Smith, Madorah E., "A study of some factors influencing the development of the sentence in preschool children," *Pedagogical Seminary and Journal of Genetic Psychology*, 1935, 46:182-211.

34. Smith, Mary K., "Measurement of the size of general English vocabulary through the elementary grades and high school," *Genetic Psychology Monographs*, 1941, 24:311-345.

35. Spriestersbach, D. C., F. L. Darley, and H. L. Morris, "Language skills in children with cleft palates," *Journal of Speech and Hearing Research*, 1958, 1:279-285.

36. Templin, Mildred C., "Certain language skills in children: Their Development and interrelationships," *Child Welfare Monographs*, No. 26, Minneapolis: University of Minnesota Press, 1957.

37. Wepman, J. M., and L. V. Jones, *Studies in Aphasia: An Approach to*

Testing: The Language Modalities Test for Aphasia, Chicago: Education Industry Service, 1961.

38. Westlake, H., "A system for developing speech with cerebral palsied children," *The Crippled Child,* 1951, *29*:10-11.

39. Whorf, B. L., in John B. Carroll (Ed.), *Language, Thought, and Reality,* New York: Wiley, 1956.

40. Williams, H. M., "An analytical study of language achievement in pre-school children," Part I. of "Development of language and vocabulary in young children," *University of Iowa Studies in Child Welfare,* 1937, *13*:9-18.

41. Winitz, H., "Language skills of male and female kindergarten children," *Journal of Speech and Hearing Research,* 1959, *2*:377-386.

8

MEASUREMENT OF AMOUNT OF SPEAKING AND OF THE RATE AND DISFLUENCY OF SPEAKING AND ORAL READING

Among the basic dimensions of communicative behavior are those of amount of speaking and of rate and fluency, or disfluency, of speaking and oral reading. In the absence of findings from the substantial amount of relevant research to be done, surely, in the years ahead, available knowledge and general observations strongly indicate that amount or frequency of disfluency in its various forms, the amount of social speaking or verbal output, and the rate of speaking and of oral reading tend to change in relation to common variations in health and disease, shifts in emotional and psychological states, aging, certain neuropathologies, and such forms of psychopathology as manic agitation, depression, catatonia, or disorientation.

Johnson,[1] in a report of the investigation of a sampling of the tape-recorded public addresses and extemporaneous speaking of one person over a period of years, has quantitatively described increase in disfluency and reduction in rate of speaking and oral reading not only following but also preceding clinically significant cardiovascular and

[1] W. Johnson, unpublished research, University of Iowa.

201

cerebrovascular changes. He has also made informal observations of cases in which reduced speaking rate, increased disfluency, and errors in verbal formulation have provided the first noted indications of cerebrovascular malfunction (a brain tumor in one case and a blocked carotid artery in another, as examples).

Pertinent research designed to clarify the indicated functional interrelationships is much needed. Meanwhile speech clinicians are well advised to secure routinely a tape-recorded sample of the speaking and oral reading of each person served. Such a recorded sample may provide at some future time an essential base of reference against which to evaluate the rate and disfluency and other characteristics of utterance following a stroke, a laryngectomy, a head injury, brain tumor, or other event of medical or clinical significance. Moreover, such a recorded sample constitutes a base against which to make certain evaluations of some effects of speech therapy. For most stutterers, for example, improvement tends to be reflected in greater speech spontaneity—as represented by an increase in the rate of utterance—along with greater variability in pitch and loudness, as well as a decrease in the frequency of disfluency and associated strain and tension. Although, again, definitive research is needed to clarify the matter, it is likely that improvement in cases of functional articulatory disorder, certain voice problems, dysphasia, speech problems associated with cerebral palsy, and other kinds of language and speech impairment as well is to be observed in varying degrees in changes in the basic dimensions of amount, fluency or disfluency, and rate of speech.

In this chapter we present procedures for measuring or observing the rate, fluency or disfluency, and amount of oral reading and speaking, together with relevant normative data.

MEASURES OF RATE OF SPEAKING AND ORAL READING

Rate of utterance is a basic dimension of speech and of oral reading. As has been suggested above, measures of rate are of general interest in the examination of persons with speech and language problems. They have a particular relevance to the study of stuttering and dysphasia. In evaluating the problem sometimes referred to as "cluttering" the measurement of rate is of fundamental importance.

Measurements of rate of utterance may be expressed as words, or as syllables, per minute, or in other ways. In a study of rate of oral reading Darley (5) had each of 200 college students, 80 male and 120 female, read aloud three passages, each of which was 300 words in length. The passages differed in mean number of syllables per word. One passage contained only one-syllable words. One was made up of words which averaged 1.5 syllables in length, a word-length found by Lumley (*10*), Cotton (*4*), and Skalbeck (*13*) to be average for representative language samples. The mean word length of the third passage was 2.2 syllables. Darley reported that he perceived a slower rate of reading as the passages increased in word length and as less commonly used words, according to the word count of Thorndike (*14*), were added to the passages. Darley stated, "This progressively slower perceived rate corresponds directly to the measures of reading rate in words per minute, but bears an inverse relationship to the measures of reading rate in syllables per minute" (*5*). He concluded that, in this specific sense, a value representing words per minute provides a more valid measure of reading rate than one expressed as syllables per minute.[1]

Franke (*6*) obtained judgments of "slow," "normal," or "fast" made by seven observers listening to recorded samples of the oral reading of 42 subjects. These ratings correlated highly ($r-.93$) with measurements of rate in words per minute. Rate as measured in words per minute appears, thus, to correspond rather closely with rate as perceived by listeners, at least so far as oral reading is concerned under the conditions of Franke's study. However, Kelly and Steer (*9*) found that for extempore speaking, listeners' judgments of rate correlated .47 with over-all measurements of words per minute and .62 with measurements of words per minute within sentences.

The measure of words per minute is to be used with due regard to the findings of Kelly and Steer (*9*). Observing 2-minute samples of the extempore speech of 24 college speakers, they measured rate in words per minute for each sentence and computed a mean sentence rate as well as an over-all rate for each speaker. The average over-all rate of their subjects was 159 words per minute and the average sentence rate was 209 words per minute. Since the sentences contained all the words uttered, it may fairly be said that the mean sentence rate represented more closely than did the over-all rate the actual execution of the movements involved in the utterance of words, exclusive of pauses or nonspeaking intervals. Kelly and Steer reported a mean duration of syllables of .154 seconds and a correlation of $-.47$ between mean syllable duration and mean sentence rate in words per minute; the faster the mean sentence rate the shorter the mean syllable duration,

---

[1] It has been pointed out by Fred Minifie, Research Associate in the stuttering research program at the University of Iowa, that for adult stutterers rate in syllables per minute may be more closely related to severity of stuttering as rated than rate in words per minute. Pending the completion of additional relevant research, such a measure has not been included in this handbook. Its use would involve the transcription and inclusion in the syllable count of all 'extra" or "stuttered" syllables. A measure of this type was used by Donna Hedrick in an M.A. thesis directed by Dean Williams at the University of Iowa in 1961.

although the correlation coefficient of − .47, while significantly greater than a chance value, indicates that mean sentence rate is by no means to be accounted for wholly on the basis of mean syllable duration. Important also is the proportion of time during which voice is produced. Kelly and Steer found that in producing the average sentence their speakers phonated 71 percent of the total time.

The measure of mean sentence rate is probably more useful in general in evaluating spontaneous or extempore speech than in measuring the rate of oral reading, and in any instance the purposes of your examination should govern your decision as to which rate measure to use. A practical consideration, of course, has to do with the greater time and labor required to make the mean sentence rate measurement. In deciding which of these measures to use at any given time, due consideration is to be given to the correlation of .77 between over-all rate in words per minute and the mean sentence rate in words per minute.

For many ordinary clinical purposes rate can be meaningfully measured as words per minute. On Form 10, provision is made for computing either or both of the measures of over-all rate or mean sentence rate in words per minute. You can make measurements of the rate of oral reading and speaking most adequately by using tape recorded samples of speech, although the overall rate of oral reading may be readily measured directly by timing the reading of a test passage. A procedure for obtaining tape-recorded samples of speaking and oral reading from adults, developed by Johnson (7) and his associates, is described below. The basic procedure may be adapted, as required, for use with children and adults for whom modified instructions and techniques are needed.

PROCEDURES FOR OBTAINING TAPE-RECORDED SAMPLES OF SPEAKING AND ORAL READING FROM ADULTS

The Job Task

Seat the speaker in full view of the recording equipment and ask his cooperation in speaking into the microphone and following instructions so that a good tape recording may be secured. After essential explanation, turn on the tape recorder and ask the speaker for identifying information such as name, age, level of education, and marital status. Have him tell briefly about any previous experience in having his speech recorded. Ask additional questions concerning school, family, home town, etc., if necessary in order to accustom the speaker to the recording situation. After two or three minutes of conversation turn off the recorder, and instruct the speaker to talk for three minutes or so about his preferred, or possible, future job or vocation. Suggest to the speaker that he briefly describe the vocation, tell why he has chosen it, and say anything else about it that he wishes. If he does not seem able or inclined to talk about a possible future vocation ask him to tell about jobs he has held in the past. Do not encourage a formal speaking performance—that is, a performance resembling a public speech is not what is wanted. The objective is to obtain a sample of the person's representative speaking. Tell the speaker to take a minute or so to think about what to say. When he is ready turn on the recorder and ask him to begin speaking. If he stops before the end of about three minutes encourage him by means of leading questions to continue speaking. Make a reasonable effort to obtain a 3-minute sample of speech.

When the speaking performance has been completed turn off the recorder and hand the speaker a copy of the 300-word "Oral Reading Test Passage No. 1" reproduced on page 232. Instruct him to read it aloud *as he ordinarily would*. It is important that you not give him any more detailed instruction than this, and if he asks questions about the rate or loudness level at which he should read, or what he should do about stuttering, or related matters, tell him simply to read *as he ordinarily would*. When he is ready to begin, turn on the recorder again and ask him to begin reading aloud. Record a reading of the complete passage.

The TAT Task

If desired, a second speaking task, the TAT Task (7), may be employed. Presumably, this task induces somewhat more emotional involvement in some speakers, but the difference between the Job Task and the TAT Task seems not to be very great for most persons. In administering the TAT Task, show the person Card No. 10 from the Thematic Apperception Test (11) and ask him to tell a story based on the picture. Ask him to talk for three minutes or so about what is happening at the moment in the pictured situation, what events have preceded those represented in the picture, and what the outcome of the story is to be. Allow him up to one minute, while he studies the picture, to prepare his story. At the end of this minute, turn on the recorder again and ask the subject to begin talking. If he stops talking before the end of three minutes stimulate him to continue speaking by asking questions. Every reasonable effort should be made to get a 3-minute sample of speaking.

No observers, other than you—the examiner, that is—are to be present when these tape recordings are made.

Modifications of Procedure for Children and Atypical Adults

The procedures described above may be adapted, as required, for obtaining samples of speaking and oral reading from children—or adults—who are unable to follow exactly the indicated instructions.

A phonetically edited reading passage that is widely used in speech clinics and that is suitable for a large proportion of readers at younger age levels, as well as adults, is "Arthur, the Young Rat" (reproduced on page 233). It contains 180 words, and this number is to be used, therefore, instead of 300, in computations based on data obtained by means of this reading passage.

In securing samples of speaking from children, two types of procedure have been most commonly used. In the one, the examiner engages the child in conversation of a sort designed to encourage the youngster to talk as freely as possible until he has produced 200 to 300 words or more of representative speech. In the other, the child is asked to respond to pictures by talking about what the people shown in the pictures are doing, what they have been doing, what they probably will do next, whether the child would like to be doing what they are doing, where and when and with whom he or she has done such things, and so on until a sample of some 200 to 300 words or more has been obtained. The pictures in the Children's Apperception Test (CAT) by Bellak (1) were used in securing the children's speech samples involved in the study reported in *The Onset of Stuttering* (8, ch. 8), and the tables of normative data presented there, as well as Tables 51-54 in this manual which are taken from *The Onset of Stuttering*, can best be used for comparative purposes in evaluating the speech of a specific child if the CAT pictures are used. However, other pictures, such as those in current magazines or children's books, may be employed.

It is particularly important in timing children's speech samples for purposes of measuring speaking rate to time only the actual speaking, omitting the intervals of unresponsiveness and the speaking done by the examiner in order to encourage the child to begin or to continue speaking.

Procedures for Measuring Rate of Speaking and Oral Reading

The reading passage (No. 1) on page 232 contains 300 words. When this passage is used, over-all oral reading rate in words per minute is computed by dividing the number of words, 300, by the number of seconds required to read the passage, and multiplying the result by 60. For example, if the subject reads the 300-word passage in 200 seconds, you would make the following computations: $300/200 = 1.5 \times 60 =$ 90 words per minute. Always take 300 to be the number of words read when this test passage is used, provided it is completed, even though one or more words may be added or left out in the reading. If the 180-word passage (No. 2) on page 233 is used, 180 is, obviously, to be substituted for 300 in making these computations.

In order to compute either the over-all or the mean sentence rate of speaking it is desirable to make a transcript of the tape-recorded speech sample. It is essential, whether or not a transcript is made, to count the words spoken and to time the speaking of them, preferably with a stop watch, or by means of a watch with a second hand. One reason why it is advantageous to use tape recordings in making rate measurements is that with some speakers it is necessary to do a certain amount of prompting in order to obtain sufficient samples. In timing such samples, the use of tape recordings makes it possible to stop the watch with the completion of the last word uttered prior to each prompting and to start it again with the beginning of the first word uttered following the prompting. In each case indicate on the form whether the speaker was prompted while producing the speech sample.

In counting words in speech samples, count only those words that would have been spoken had the speaker performed no disfluencies. That is, for example, "Uh, when I wuh-wuh-wuh-was ten years old, I went I I went I went to New York" is regarded for word-counting purposes as consisting of "When I was ten years old, I went to New York," a total of 11 words. Count only once each word repeated singly or in a phrase. For example, count "We we we went home" as three words rather than five. Do not count sounds or words such as "well," "uh uh uh," and the like, which are not integral parts of the meaningful context. In any instance of revision, count only the words in the final form. That is, for example, count "I started to—I went to town and bought some bread" as eight rather than eleven words, disregarding the false start "I started to."

The computations to be carried out in determining either over-all or mean sentence rate in words per minute are indicated on Form 10.

Rate data, with which you may compare your own rate measurements, are summarized in Tables 34-36.

ASSIGNMENTS

Use Form 10 and the procedures described above.

1. For an adult stutterer, one adult with some other speech problem, and one adult with normal speech measure the following:
   a. Over-all oral reading rate in words per minute (use Oral Reading Test Passage No. 1)
   b. Over-all speaking rate in words per minute (Job Task)
   c. Mean sentence rate in words per minute (Job Task)
   d. Over-all speaking rate in words per minute (TAT Task)
   Write a report of the information and impressions you obtain by interviewing each subject about the differences and similarities among these performances, and of your observations of the differences and similarities among the speakers. Evaluate your rate measurements by reference to Tables 34-36. Discuss the difference between the over-all and the mean sentence rate in words per minute, indicating what you consider its implications to be. Comment on the variation in rate from sentence to sentence.

2. For one young stutterer, one youngster with some other speech problem, and one young normal speaker measure the following:
   a. Over-all oral reading rate in words per minute (use Oral Reading Test Passage No. 2)
   b. Over-all speaking rate in words per minute (use CAT pictures, or other pictures, or conversation)
   Write a report of the information and impressions you obtain by interviewing each subject about the differences and similarities among these performances, and of your observations of the differences and similarities among the speakers.

3. With the cooperation of a classmate or friend, obtain measurements of your own:
   a. Over-all oral reading rate in words per minute (use Oral Reading Test Passage No. 1)
   b. Over-all speaking rate in words per minute (Job Task)
   c. Mean sentence rate in words per minute (Job Task)
   d. Over-all speaking rate in words per minute (TAT Task)
   Write a report of your observations and impressions of the differences and similarities among these performances. Evaluate your rate measurements by reference to Tables 34-36. Discuss the difference between the over-all and the mean sentence rate in words per minute, indicating what you consider its implications to be. Comment on the variation in rate from sentence to sentence.

MEASURES OF DISFLUENCY IN SPEAKING AND ORAL READING

Samples of speaking and oral reading are fluent or disfluent in some degree. There are important differences among speakers—and in any given speaker from time to time, or from one condition or situation to another—in fluency or disfluency. As a practical matter, it is easier to think in terms of measuring disfluency than fluency. A forthright approach consists in identifying instances of disfluency and counting them. We can tabulate all disfluencies without regard to type, or we can classify them into various kinds of disfluency and tabulate each kind separately. We can make various combinations of kinds, or we can count some kinds but not others. Also, we can simply tabulate the number of words that are associated with any kind, or with some specified kinds, of disfluency. Several methods of measuring disfluency have been developed in the course of laboratory and clinical work with the stuttering problem. We shall describe these methods here, but shall reserve detailed discussion of them for Chapter 9 where their role in the clinical study of the problem of stuttering will be considered.

A system of classification of disfluencies and procedures for computing five different measures of disfluency are presented in the following pages.

A System of Classification of Disfluencies

A relatively comprehensive classification of disfluencies is essential to the systematic investigation of the disfluent aspects of speech. Such a classification and some of the uses that have been made of it have been discussed elsewhere by Johnson (7) and again in this manual (pp. 246-253). The classification includes the following categories:

Interjections of Sounds, Syllables, Words, or Phrases: This category includes extraneous sounds such as "uh," "er," and "hmmm" and extraneous words such as "well" which are distinct from sounds and words associated with the fluent text or with phenomena included in other categories. An instance of interjection may include one or more units of repetition of the interjected material; for example, "uh" and "uh uh uh" are each counted as one instance of interjection. (The number of times the interjection is repeated—that is, the number of units of repetition—within each instance may also be noted; "uh uh" is an example of an interjection repeated once and "uh uh uh" is an example of an interjection repeated twice.)

Part-Word Repetitions: Repetitions of parts of words—that is, syllables and sounds—are placed in this category. (Within each instance of repetition the number of times the sound or syllable is repeated may be counted; "buh-boy" involves one unit of repetition and "guh-guh-girl" involves two units.) No attempt is made to draw a distinction between sound and syllable repetitions. "Ruh-ruh-run," "cuh-come," "ba-ba-baby," and "abou-bout" are examples of part-word repetitions.

Word Repetitions: Repetitions of whole words, including words of one syllable, are counted in this category. (The number of repetition units within each instance may be counted. "I-I-I," "was-was," and "going-going" are samples of instances of word repetition; the first involves two units of repetition and each of the other two involves one unit.) A word repeated for emphasis as in "very, very clean," is not counted as a disfluency. A part-word repetition, or an interjection, does not nullify a word repetition; for example, "going uh going" or "guh-going going" is classified as a word repetition. In any such case, the interjected or associated disfluency is also tabulated in the appropriate category.

Phrase Repetitions: Repetitions of two or more words are included in this category. "I was I was going" is an example of this type of disfluency. (Again, if desired, the number of units of repetition within each instance of repetition may be separately noted.)

Revisions: Instances in which the content of a phrase is modified, or in which there is grammatical modification, are classified as revisions. Change in the pronunciation of a word is also counted as a revision. "I was—I am going" is an example in this category.

Incomplete Phrases: An incomplete phrase is one in which the thought or content is not completed and which is not an instance of phrase repetition or of revision. "She was—and after she got there he came" contains an example of an incomplete phrase.

Broken Words: This category is typified by words which are not completely pronounced and which are not classifiable in any other category, or in which the normal rhythm of the word is broken in a way that definitely interferes with the smooth flow of speech. "I was g-(pause)-oing home" is an example of a broken word.

Prolonged Sounds: Sounds or parts of words that are judged to be unduly prolonged are included in this category. It is usually the initial sound of a word that is prolonged.

Instances of any of these types of disfluency may be performed with ordinary or unusual degrees of tension, effort, or strain.

Procedures for Measuring Disfluency

On the basis of clinical experience and the findings of relevant research to date (to be reviewed in Chapter 9), five methods of measuring disfluency are to be considered. The background information which is presented in Chapter 9 is to be consulted and kept in mind in making use of these methods. Regardless of the method you use in a given instance, you will follow the procedure described on pages 204-206 in obtaining the necessary tape-recorded samples of speaking and oral reading. In each case make a verbatim transcription of the tape and then proceed by listening to the tape as you follow along on the transcription, identifying disfluencies for later tabulation on Form 11. Listen to each tape as often as you like, or until you are satisfied that you have identified and properly classified all, or as many as possible, of the disfluencies in the sample.

Total Disfluency Index

The Total Disfluency Index is the total number of disfluencies, of all types, per 100 words read or spoken. This represents the most thorough type of disfluency analysis, in which you identify, classify, and tabulate all the disfluencies in a sample of speech or oral reading. For this purpose, use the entire classification system described on pages 209-210. Use Form 11 to record your findings and make your computation. Table 40 contains norms against which to evaluate the measures you obtain in analyzing individual samples.

Disfluency Type Index

Form 11 provides for the computation of the number of each of eight types of disfluency per 100 words. Each such number is the Index of Disfluency for the type of disfluency which it represents. Norms against which to compare these values are presented in Tables 37-39.

Repetition Index

The Repetition Index is the number of repetitions—syllable or word or phrase, or any two of these or all of them combined—per 100 words read or spoken. Table 41 contains norms for frequencies of repetitions —syllable, word, and phrase—in the speech and oral reading of stutterers and nonstutterers. Counts of one or more of these types of repetition can be made and evaluated against the appropriate norms.

Sander's Disfluent Word Index

See page 250 for an account of the method developed by Sander (*12*), which involves the identification and tabulation of disfluent words.

Sander defines a disfluent word as one that involves a prolonged sound or a broken utterance, is interrupted by an interjection, or is repeated in whole or in part. Sander's Disfluent Word Index is the number of disfluent words, as defined by Sander, per 100 words read or spoken. Ranges, means, and standard deviations for counts of Sander's disfluent words in the oral reading and speaking of 40 adult stutterers are contained in Table 45. Approximate norms, computed from Tables 37-39 for the indicated types of disfluency, combined, are presented in Tables 42-44.

Young's Disfluent Word Index

Young's Disfluent Word Index is the number of disfluent words, as defined by Young, per 100 words read or spoken. Young (15) derived a single category of disfluency by means of a multiple correlational analysis of several measures of the disfluencies in the speech of 100 male adult stutterers. Although he called the category "repetitions," we shall call it "Young's disfluent words" in order to avoid confusion with the repetition categories in the classification system described in this chapter. A Young disfluent word is quite similar to a Sander disfluent word. Young defines it as a word "in relation to which a part-word repetition, a sound prolongation, a broken utterance, or unusual stress" is observed (15, pp. 42-43). Such a disfluent word is counted only as one word, even though more than one disfluency may be involved in its production. Young's means for this measure for 100 adult male speakers, and for the 50 least and 50 most severe stutterers in the total group of 100, are to be found in Table 55. In addition, as in the case of Sander's disfluent words, approximate norms computed from Tables 37-39 for the indicated types of disfluency, combined, are presented in Tables 46-48.

Regardless of the method you use in each instance, divide the total number of words spoken or read by the number of disfluencies or of disfluent words, as the case may be, and multiply the result by 100 to determine the number of disfluencies, or disfluent words, per 100 words read or spoken. Use Form 11 to record your tabulations and make your computation.

ASSIGNMENTS

Using Form 11 and the procedures for obtaining tape-recorded samples of oral reading and speaking described in the preceding pages:
1. Obtain from one adult stutterer and one adult nonstutterer a tape-recorded

sample of oral reading (use Oral Reading Test Passage No. 1) and a 200-word sample of speaking (Job Task). Transcribe the samples; identify and tabulate the disfluencies while listening to the tape; and, using Form 11 determine:

a. *Oral reading:*   Total Disfluency Index, Disfluency Type Indexes, Repetition Index, Sander Disfluent Word Index, and Young Disfluent Word Index.

b. *Speaking:*   Total Disfluency Index, Disfluency Type Indexes, Repetition Index, Sander Disfluent Word Index, Young Disfluent Word Index.

Evaluate the values you obtain against the data summarized in Tables 37-49. Write a report of the information and impressions you obtain by interviewing each subject about the differences and similarities among these performances, and of your observations of the differences and similarities between the two speakers.

2. Perform the same operations, with oral reading and speaking samples obtained from one young stutterer and one young nonstutterer. Use Oral Reading Test Passage No. 2. Obtain a 200-word speech sample, using the CAT (*1*) pictures or other suitable pictures as stimulus materials. Evaluate the values you obtain against the data summarized in Tables 51-53. Write a report of the information and impressions you obtain by interviewing each subject about the differences and similarities among these performances, and of your observations of the differences and similarities between the two speakers.

3. With the cooperation of a classmate or friend tape record your own reading of "Your Rate of Oral Reading" (Oral Reading Test Passage No. 1) and 200 words of speaking about your future job; and then perform the same operations as for Assignment 1, above, computing your own disfluency indexes. Evaluate the values you obtain against the data summarized in Tables 37-49. Write a report of your observations and impressions of the differences and similarities among these performances.

MEASURES OF AMOUNT OF SPEAKING

There are two particularly meaningful ways in which you can gauge the amount of speaking a person does. You can have him keep a speaking-time log or you can observe or measure his verbal output in given situations. The speaking-time log is a record made by the individual himself of the amount of time he spends in talking to specified persons or in particular situations (see below). The sorts of measurement you can make of verbal output in designated situations are represented by the data summarized in Tables 54 and 55. The data in these tables are to be used as norms in only a very gross sense. They do provide, in the absence of the more adequate and precise norms that future studies will undoubtedly yield, a general indication of the order of individual differences in verbal output in the indicated types of situations. By comparing your own measurements of verbal output, obtained from comparable speakers by like means under like conditions, with the values shown in Tables 54 and 55 you can sharpen your sense of the usual and unusual in amount of verbal response in such situations.

Speaking-Time Log

A log of the amount of time a person spends in speaking reveals important kinds of information about him:

1. The total amount of time he spends in speaking each day for which he keeps a log, and his average speaking time per day over the period, or periods, sampled.
2. The specific situations in which he speaks and the persons with whom he speaks in these situations.
3. The degree of variability in the individual's speaking situations, the persons with whom he speaks, and his total speaking time, from day to day.

There are many reasons why it is important to determine the amount of speaking done each day by any stutterer, or any person with a voice disorder or any other type of communicative problem.

1. A person's speaking time is a fundamental indicator of the degree to which he is handicapped by his communicative difficulty. A stutterer or a cerebral palsied person who speaks less than two minutes per day, for example—and there are some who do no more speaking than this—is allowing his speech problem to affect him much more than one who speaks as much as a half-hour or more per day. The one who does very little speaking is probably the more handicapped, even though the person who talks much more may not speak as well as he does. After all, the importance of a particular individual's speech problem is felt by him in a peculiarly basic way in the extent to which it restricts or inhibits his communication with other people.

2. A person's speaking time is an indicator of his social adjustment. In planning therapy, you necessarily take account of the speaker's relationships with other people. You would proceed differently with someone who has no close friends and few acquaintances and who spends most of his time by himself with nonsocial hobbies and private daydreams, from the way you would work with a sociable person whose relationships with other people are generally good.

3. An individual's speaking-time log amounts to a particularly meaningful account of how he spends his time. By examining a log covering several days, you can see much more clearly than you could otherwise the person's basic pattern of relationships with others.

Such a record provides, in fact, information for an essentially socio-metric study of the person, an identification of the individuals whom he seeks out more and less and who seek him out often and seldom for the sorts of association that are represented by a sharing of speaking time. So far as truth lies in the old saying that a person is known by the company he keeps, it may be said that a person can become known by the speaking-time log he keeps. This means that a person's speaking-time log can be of value to you in your counseling of him, and it can clarify for him much that is important about himself.

4. The speaking-time log of an individual also helps to bring into focus his needs for various kinds of speech practice, and his unrealized opportunities to obtain that practice in his daily comings and goings. You can spot speaking situations that he meets more or less regularly, judge their probable degree of difficulty for him, and evaluate their suitability for particular retraining purposes. By studying the person's speaking-time logs with him you can help him recognize ways of increasing the amount of speaking he does and of expanding the number and variety of the situations in which he does it. In view of the generally valid rule that the more a person in need of speech improvement talks the better, the uses that you can make of the log in raising a speaker's verbal output to an optimal level for him can be very important.

There are no adequate speaking-time norms. Data obtained informally from normally speaking students at the University of Iowa suggest that the average of them has about 45 minutes per day of what might be called solid speaking time. The average student probably spends considerably more time than that, of course, in conversational or other speech situations; the figure of 45 minutes is meant to represent actual speaking time. It has been our clinical experience that those stutterers who turn in speaking-time records of as much as one hour per day seem to be doing somewhat more speaking than is done by most other persons, stutterers or nonstutterers, of comparable age and circumstance. Such observations can provide, of course, only a rough basis for evaluating the performance of a given speaker. The major value of a speaking-time log is as a record of changes in amount of speaking from month to month, perhaps, or from one time to another, and therefore as a basis for counseling in meaningful relation to the planning of therapy and the evaluation of its effectiveness.

How to Keep a Speaking-Time Log

Since most of the log entries are for less than one minute, speaking time should always be recorded in seconds. It takes one second or less to say "Hello" or "Good-by." It takes most individuals less than 4 seconds to say, "Now is the time for all good men to come to the aid of the party." In a 30-minute conversation between two persons who share the talking about equally, each would speak about 12 minutes or so. If one does most of the talking, the time might be split 24 and 2 minutes perhaps, or 20 and 6, but the total will never be 30 minutes. A person should practice timing himself quite accurately with a stop watch or the second hand of a wrist watch in making various common remarks and typical contributions to conversation or discussion in order to sharpen his ability to estimate his speaking time. By engaging in this sort of practice yourself you can improve your ability to judge the validity of specific entries in the speaking-time logs turned in to you by the speakers with whom you work clinically.

At first the person is almost sure to overestimate his speaking time. What he is to record for each instance or situation is an estimate of his actual speaking time—what may be called "solid yap yap."

An actual speaking-time log (Form 12, completed—with real names disguised) is shown on page 218 as a general model. The speaker should make log entries often enough during the day to insure reasonable accuracy and completeness. If he makes entries as often as three times a day—at midmorning, midafternoon, and just before bedtime— he can readily recall the persons he talked with and the situations in which he talked with them, and estimate fairly closely the times involved.

Entries should be numbered, and each one should be identified by a brief description of the situation, such as "Buying movie ticket," or the name of the listener, "Sally," for example, or both, as in "Telephoned Bob about exam."

The estimates for each day should be totaled, and the total expressed in hours, minutes, and seconds. In addition to showing the total speaking time, the record should indicate (1) the total number of speaking situations; (2) the number of these that involved (a) one other person, (b) two or three other persons, and (c) four or more other persons; (3) the number of situations in which the other persons were (a) members of the speaker's own family, (b) close friends or associates, such as sweetheart, persons with whom he shares a car pool, landlady or house mother, close classmates, etc., (c) others with whom the person has previously spoken, and (d) those spoken with for the first time; (4) the number of situations in which the other persons were (a) members of the speaker's own sex, (b) members of the opposite sex, and (c) members of both sexes; (5) the number of situations in which the other persons were (a) mostly of the same age as the speaker (generally within a couple years or so, but with allowance for the difference between "same age" at 12 and at 45), (b) mostly older, (c) mostly younger, or (d) mixed; (6) the number of

situations in which the other persons were (a) associated with the
speech clinic as students or patients or staff members, or (b) not asso-
cited with the speech clinic.

Provision is made for these classifications on Form 12. You may
break down the data in other ways, of course, in accordance with your
particular purposes.

Example of a Speaking-Time Record for One Day
(Names Disguised)

SPEAKING-TIME LOG

Name _____George Doe_____   Age ___19___ Sex___M___

Clinician _____Harry Roe_____   Date ___February 23, 1962___

Situations	Time (seconds)	Situations	Time (seconds)
1. Herb	180	16. Bud	12
2. Betty	18	17. Jim, returned book	12
3. Waitress	12	18. Bert	18
4. Dr. Bern for test score	180	19. Bud	24
5. Vivian, arranging date	720	20. Mary, telephone	30
6. Ralph	18	21. Bob	36
7. Vivian, telephone	24	22. Pete	12
8. Bud	30	23. Bud	30
9. Stutterers' Group	18	24. Clerk in store	6
10. Ed	18	25. Fern	18
11. Vivian, Bud, Art	18	26. Ann, compared class notes	180
12. Stranger	6	27. Waitress	6
13. Waitress	6	28. Martha	24
14. Bob, argument	120	29. Herb	24
15. Sam	24	30. Herb, bedtime snack	120

Speaking time in seconds   1944

Speaking time in minutes = total seconds divided by 60:   32.4

Total number of situations	30	with others of same age	24
with 1 other person	28	with others mostly older	5
with 2-3 other persons	1	with others mostly younger	0
with 4 or more other persons	1	with others both older and younger	1

Total number of situations

with members of own family	0	with others associated with clinic	9
with close friends or associates	13	with others not associated with clinic	21
with others previously spoken to	14		
with others spoken with first time	2		

with others of own sex	18
with others of opposite sex	10
with others of both sexes	2

Oral Reading Time

Time spent in oral reading is not to be included in the speaking-time log. In connection with therapy you may want to obtain oral reading-time logs, provided they would be relevant to your purposes in specific cases. The diagnostic or evaluative significance of the speaking-time log would be blurred, however, if time spent in reading aloud, either for clinical purposes or for pleasure or study, were included.

ASSIGNMENTS

1. Keep a speaking-time log for yourself for each of three successive days and record the results on Form 12.
2. Obtain three successive daily speaking-time logs for one of your normally speaking friends and for each of two individuals assigned to you as persons with clinically significant speech problems. Provide each person with a copy of Form 12 on which to record his data.

TABLE 34. Ranges and Deciles of Distributions of Values for Speaking and Reading Rates in Words Per Minute, for Each of Three Specified Tasks for Adult Subjects

Task	N	Range	Decile[a]								
			1	2	3	4	5	6	7	8	9
Job[b]											
Male stutterers	50	24.7–184.4	39.3	67.1	81.4	92.5	102.0	105.5	121.0	133.0	139.4
Female stutterers	50	12.9–183.3	44.1	64.8	70.6	81.0	98.9	103.1	120.0	148.3	170.2
Male nonstutterers	50	42.3–201.2	105.4	112.6	120.3	129.7	136.2	141.5	146.6	158.1	160.0
Female nonstutterers	50	94.7–198.4	121.8	131.1	135.7	140.9	147.0	150.0	154.8	164.7	185.1
TAT[c]											
Male stutterers	50	18.3–148.6	29.4	48.9	68.2	78.6	86.1	91.8	102.0	119.9	135.7
Female stutterers	50	9.9–177.2	31.7	44.7	56.6	70.4	78.6	84.0	104.7	113.2	141.4
Male nonstutterers	50	72.5–197.8	99.6	101.6	112.3	114.7	119.2	127.2	130.9	138.0	148.6
Female nonstutterers	50	58.6–202.7	108.8	117.1	119.9	122.9	130.5	138.2	144.3	151.4	162.4
Reading[d]											
Male stutterers	50	31.9–200.0	55.4	76.5	102.4	116.7	123.5	131.6	142.9	162.2	181.8
Female stutterers	50	20.3–200.0	53.6	67.7	84.1	92.3	109.8	128.6	146.5	155.2	181.8
Male nonstutterers	50	104.9–217.4	151.5	160.4	164.8	171.4	176.5	179.6	181.8	187.5	202.7
Female nonstutterers	50	135.1–219.0	155.4	163.9	171.4	173.4	176.5	181.6	184.1	187.5	197.4
Normal speakers[e]	200	129–222	148	155	159	162	166	170	175	181	190

[a] Computed from ungrouped data.
[b] Speaking for about three minutes about future job or vocation.
[c] Speaking for about three minutes about Card No. 10 of the Thematic Apperception Test (11).
[d] Reading aloud the 300-word reading passage, "Your Rate of Oral Reading," which is reproduced on page 000 of this manual.
[e] Darley's (5) 200 college-age normal speakers, 120 men and 80 women.
SOURCE: Johnson, 7; Darley, 5.

TABLE 35. Measures of Over-all Rate and Rate for Nonstuttered Intervals in Words Per Minute of 30 Adult Stutterers, in the Oral Reading of the 300-Word Test Passage, "Your Rate of Oral Reading"

	Over-all Rate	Nonstuttering Rate
Range	42.4–193.3	89.2–191.3
Mean	122.7	144.7
Standard deviation	40.3	24.4
Median	133.4	146.1
25th percentile	88.7	128.6
75th percentile	144.3	155.3

[a] Twenty-seven males and 3 females, 17 to 42 years of age (average age, 24 years).
SOURCE: Bloodstein, 2.

TABLE 36. Summary of Measures of Rate Obtained in Two Performances, Sessions I and II, of 40 Adult Stutterers,[a] in Speaking 250 Words About Future Job and in Reading the 300-Word Test Passage, "Your Rate of Oral Reading"

	Session I	Session II
Speaking		
Mean time	242.4	237.3
Standard deviation	207.3	167.4
Range	86–1235	90–852
Mean words per minute	74	76
Range, words per minute	15–209	21–196
Oral Reading		
Mean time	218.4	198.7
Standard deviation	206.9	141.0
Range	89–1028	85–782
Mean words per minute	82	91
Range, words per minute	17–208	22–212

[a] Thirty-four males and 6 females.
SOURCE: Sander, 12.

TABLE 37. Ranges and Deciles of Distributions of Values for Number of Disfluencies of Each Specified Type Per 100 Words for the Job Task (Speaking for About Three Minutes About Future Job or Vocation) for 200 Adult Subjects

Type	Range	Decile[a]								
		1	2	3	4	5	6	7	8	9
Interjections										
MS[b]	1.0–80.0	2.2	3.5	4.4	4.9	7.3	10.3	12.1	15.5	23.5
FS[c]	0–52.1	2.4	3.1	4.9	5.9	7.5	9.3	11.1	15.8	22.9
MN[d]	0–13.7	1.2	2.3	3.2	3.8	4.4	5.6	6.7	8.2	9.3
FN[e]	0.4–6.6	0.7	1.6	1.8	2.2	2.8	3.1	3.6	4.5	5.6
Part-word repetitions										
MS	0–44.6	1.0	1.4	2.3	3.4	3.7	6.0	7.3	12.8	34.5
FS	0–59.5	0.5	0.8	1.6	2.4	4.8	6.5	8.9	11.8	19.9
MN	0–2.2	0	0	0	0	0	0.2	0.3	0.5	1.0
FN	0–1.0	0	0	0	0	0.2	0.2	0.3	0.4	0.6
Word repetitions										
MS	0–15.5	0.4	0.8	1.5	2.0	2.7	3.4	4.0	5.4	6.6
FS	0–14.9	0.3	0.6	1.3	1.9	2.4	3.1	4.3	5.5	8.4
MN	0–2.9	0	0	0.3	0.5	0.7	0.9	1.1	1.3	1.5
FN	0–2.4	0	0	0.2	0.3	0.4	0.5	0.7	0.9	1.6
Phrase repetitions										
MS	0–8.5	0	0	0.3	0.5	0.6	1.0	1.5	2.0	2.9
FS	0–3.8	0	0	0.3	0.4	0.7	0.9	1.1	1.3	2.2
MN	0–2.2	0	0	0	0	0	0.2	0.3	0.4	0.6
FN	0–0.6	0	0	0	0	0	0.2	0.3	0.3	0.5
Revisions										
MS	0–5.5	0	0.5	0.7	0.8	0.9	1.2	1.5	2.1	2.8
FS	0–1.4	0	0	0	0	0.3	0.5	0.6	0.9	1.1
MN	0–4.3	0.5	0.6	0.8	0.9	1.1	1.3	1.7	2.0	2.2
FN	0–2.7	0	0.2	0.4	0.5	0.6	1.0	1.2	1.5	1.8
Incomplete phrases										
MS	0–5.9	0	0	0	0	0	0	0	0	0.5
FS	0–2.3	0	0	0	0	0.2	0.4	0.6	1.0	1.7
MN	0–0.8	0	0	0	0	0	0	0	0	0.3
FN	0–1.3	0	0	0	0	0	0	0	0.3	0.5
Broken words										
MS	0–28.2	0	0	0	0	0	0.2	0.6	0.9	2.1
FS	0–5.7	0	0	0	0	0.3	0.4	1.1	1.7	3.2
MN	0–0.5	0	0	0	0	0	0	0	0	0
FN	0–0.3	0	0	0	0	0	0	0	0	0.2
Prolonged sounds										
MS	0–21.8	0	0	0	0.5	0.7	1.4	2.7	4.4	9.8
FS	0–25.7	0	0	0	0	0.5	1.2	2.2	4.5	10.6
MN	0–1.7	0	0	0	0	0	0	0	0	0.3
FN	0–0.4	0	0	0	0	0	0	0	0	0.2

[a] Computed from ungrouped data.
[b] MS=50 male stutterers.
[c] FS=50 female stutterers.
[d] MN=50 male nonstutterers.
[e] FN=50 female nonstutterers.
SOURCE: Johnson, 7.

TABLE 38.   Range and Deciles of Distributions of Values for Number of Disfluencies of Each Specified Type Per 100 Words for the TAT Task, Speaking for About Three Minutes About Card No. 10 in the TAT Test (11), for 200 Adult Subjects

Type	Range	Decile[a]								
		1	2	3	4	5	6	7	8	9
Interjections										
MS[b]	0–71.6	1.0	2.7	3.3	5.8	7.2	8.9	11.8	18.2	27.7
FS[c]	0.2–79.6	1.6	5.4	6.5	7.5	8.8	10.8	13.6	16.6	24.8
MN[d]	0–15.3	0.8	1.1	1.7	2.2	2.6	3.7	6.4	7.1	9.4
FN[e]	0–11.6	0.3	0.6	1.0	1.4	2.0	3.1	4.3	5.0	7.5
Part-word repetitions										
MS	0–52.2	1.0	1.6	2.2	3.5	4.2	5.0	8.2	10.7	33.6
FS	0–57.3	0.4	0.8	1.0	3.1	5.2	6.9	12.3	14.1	25.4
MN	0–1.2	0	0	0	0	0.2	0.3	0.4	0.4	0.6
FN	0–1.2	0	0	0	0.1	0.2	0.2	0.3	0.5	0.6
Word repetitions										
MS	0–13.5	0.6	1.1	1.4	1.7	3.1	3.8	4.6	5.9	9.9
FS	0–17.7	0.5	1.2	1.6	2.0	2.9	3.7	5.0	6.7	8.6
MN	0–2.5	0	0.2	0.4	0.6	0.6	0.7	1.0	1.3	1.9
FN	0–4.5	0	0.2	0.3	0.3	0.4	0.5	0.7	1.0	1.5
Phrase repetitions										
MS	0–5.5	0	0.2	0.4	0.6	0.9	1.3	1.5	2.2	3.1
FS	0–2.9	0	0	0.3	0.6	0.8	1.2	1.4	1.7	2.3
MN	0–1.3	0	0	0	0	0.2	0.2	0.4	0.7	1.1
FN	0–1.5	0	0	0	0	0.1	0.2	0.3	0.5	0.6
Revisions										
MS	0–5.4	0.3	0.8	1.0	1.1	1.2	1.4	1.7	2.4	2.6
FS	0–2.2	0	0	0	0	0.3	0.4	0.8	1.2	1.7
MN	0.3–4.3	0.6	0.7	0.8	1.0	1.2	1.4	1.7	2.4	2.8
FN	0–3.1	0.2	0.4	0.6	1.0	1.1	1.2	1.5	1.6	1.8
Incomplete phrases										
MS	0–26.6	0	0	0	0	0	0	0	0.2	0.6
FS	0–5.4	0	0	0	0.2	0.3	0.5	0.8	1.0	1.5
MN	0–1.3	0	0	0	0	0	0	0	0.2	0.3
FN	0–1.2	0	0	0	0	0	0.1	0.2	0.3	0.6
Broken words										
MS	0–3.5	0	0	0	0	0	0	0.3	1.1	1.9
FS	0–7.0	0	0	0	0	0.3	0.7	1.0	1.2	2.1
MN	0–0.6	0	0	0	0	0	0	0	0	0.2
FN	0–0.9	0	0	0	0	0	0	0	0	0.2
Prolonged sounds										
MS	0–17.6	0	0	0.3	0.7	1.1	2.0	2.9	4.4	11.0
FS	0–23.9	0	0	0	0.5	0.6	0.9	2.4	5.7	11.7
MN	0–0.6	0	0	0	0	0	0	0	0.2	0.2
FN	0–0.3	0	0	0	0	0	0	0	0.1	0.2

[a] Computed from ungrouped data.
[b] MS=50 male stutterers.
[c] FS=50 female stutterers.
[d] MN=50 male nonstutterers.
[e] FN=50 female nonstutterers.
SOURCE: Johnson, 7.

223

TABLE 39. Ranges and Deciles of Distributions of Values for Number of Disfluencies of Each Specified Type per 100 Words for the Reading Task (Oral Reading of the 300-Word Passage "Your Rate of Oral Reading") for 200 Adult Subjects

| Type | Range | Decile[a] | | | | | | | | |
		1	2	3	4	5	6	7	8	9
Interjections										
MS[b]	0–85.5	0	0	0	0.3	0.3	0.7	1.0	2.0	9.7
FS[c]	0–84.6	0	0	0	0.3	0.7	1.3	2.0	2.7	12.8
MN[d]	0–1.0	0	0	0	0	0	0	0	0	0
FN[e]	0–1.3	0	0	0	0	0	0	0	0	0.3
Part-word repetitions										
MS	0–47.8	0.7	1.0	1.3	2.3	4.0	5.3	7.0	12.3	16.7
FS	0–88.0	0.7	1.0	1.3	2.0	3.0	5.7	12.3	19.3	25.3
MN	0–2.0	0	0	0	0.3	0.3	0.3	0.7	1.0	1.0
FN	0–1.3	0	0	0	0	0	0.3	0.3	0.3	0.7
Word repetitions										
MS	0–6.7	0	0	0	0.3	0.3	0.7	1.0	2.0	2.7
FS	0–13.9	0	0	0	0.3	0.3	1.0	1.3	2.0	2.7
MN	0–1.0	0	0	0	0	0	0	0.3	0.3	0.7
FN	0–0.7	0	0	0	0	0	0	0	0.3	0.3
Phrase repetitions										
MS	0–7.7	0	0	0	0.3	0.3	0.7	0.7	1.0	1.7
FS	0–6.7	0	0	0	0.3	0.3	0.3	0.7	1.3	1.7
MN	0–0.7	0	0	0	0	0	0	0	0.3	0.3
FN	0–0.3	0	0	0	0	0	0	0	0	0
Revisions										
MS	0–1.3	0	0	0	0.3	0.3	0.7	0.7	0.7	1.0
FS	0–2.3	0	0	0	0	0.3	0.3	0.3	0.7	1.0
MN	0–2.0	0	0	0.3	0.3	0.7	0.7	0.7	1.0	1.3
FN	0–3.0	0	0	0.3	0.3	0.3	0.3	0.7	0.7	1.0
Incomplete phrases										
MS	0–0	0	0	0	0	0	0	0	0	0
FS	0–0.7	0	0	0	0	0	0	0	0	0
MN	0–0	0	0	0	0	0	0	0	0	0
FN	0–0	0	0	0	0	0	0	0	0	0
Broken words										
MS	0–9.7	0	0	0	0	0	0	0.3	0.3	2.7
FS	0–19.3	0	0	0	0	0	0.7	0.7	1.3	3.1
MN	0–0.7	0	0	0	0	0	0	0	0	0
FN	0–0.7	0	0	0	0	0	0	0	0	0
Prolonged sounds										
MS	0–27.7	0	0	0	0.3	0.7	1.0	2.7	4.7	8.7
FS	0–14.3	0	0	0	0.3	0.3	0.7	1.3	4.3	10.7
MN	0–0.3	0	0	0	0	0	0	0	0	0.3
FN	0–0.3	0	0	0	0	0	0	0	0	0

[a] Computed from ungrouped data.
[b] MS=50 male stutterers.
[c] FS=50 female stutterers.
[d] MN=50 male nonstutterers.
[e] FN=50 female nonstutterers.
SOURCE: Johnson, 7.

TABLE 40. Ranges and Deciles of Distributions of Values for Total Numbers of Disfluencies Per 100 Words for Each of the Three Tasks, for 200 Adult Subjects

Task	Range	Decile[a]								
		1	2	3	4	5	6	7	8	9
Job										
MS[b]	2.7–127.3	8.2	12.8	13.9	15.1	19.0	25.7	29.6	44.9	57.7
FS[c]	0.8–101.3	8.3	12.4	13.8	16.6	17.9	22.7	32.3	42.7	62.5
MN[d]	1.6–20.1	4.2	5.0	5.8	6.2	7.0	8.1	9.0	10.8	12.3
FN[e]	0.4–9.1	2.3	2.7	3.1	3.8	4.9	5.9	6.4	7.4	7.9
TAT										
MS	4.6–135.8	8.3	10.5	14.7	18.4	22.6	26.6	33.3	47.3	66.1
FS	1.8–109.3	8.5	13.8	16.2	19.2	22.3	27.7	38.5	49.0	73.7
MN	0.7–19.9	2.2	2.9	3.9	5.3	6.6	8.0	8.8	9.7	12.6
FN	0.5–17.1	1.4	2.0	3.0	3.7	4.6	5.7	7.1	8.4	10.4
Reading										
MS	0–141.5	1.7	2.3	4.0	6.3	8.3	15.7	17.3	26.3	38.0
FS	0–112.8	1.3	2.7	3.7	6.3	9.7	18.7	21.3	35.5	57.0
MN	0–4.0	0.3	0.7	0.7	1.0	1.0	1.3	1.7	2.3	3.0
FN	0–4.0	0	0.3	0.3	0.7	0.7	1.0	1.3	1.7	2.3

[a] Computed from ungrouped data.
[b] MS=50 male stutterers.
[c] FS=50 female stutterers.
[d] MN=50 male nonstutterers.
[e] FN=50 female nonstutterers.
SOURCE: Johnson, 7.

TABLE 41. Ranges and Deciles of Distributions of Values for Number of Part-Word, Word, and Phrase Repetitions, Combined, Per 100 Words for all Three Tasks for 200 Adult Subjects

Task	Range	Decile[a]								
		1	2	3	4	5	6	7	8	9
Job										
MS[b]	0.3–62.0	2.4	3.9	5.1	6.3	7.9	10.1	13.5	21.6	38.4
FS[c]	0.3–60.7	2.6	3.6	4.5	7.4	8.3	10.4	13.5	16.8	28.3
MN[d]	0–3.7	0	0.4	0.7	0.8	1.1	1.4	1.8	2.3	2.9
FN[e]	0–2.9	0.2	0.3	0.5	0.6	0.8	0.9	1.2	1.4	2.2
TAT										
MS	1.7–65.2	2.7	3.3	5.2	7.1	9.4	10.6	14.1	18.3	42.7
FS	0.8–68.4	1.8	2.8	4.5	8.4	12.0	13.1	16.7	23.4	29.9
MN	0–3.6	0	0.6	0.8	1.0	1.2	1.5	1.9	2.3	2.7
FN	0–5.3	0.4	0.4	0.6	0.8	0.9	1.0	1.5	1.9	2.4
Reading										
MS	0–51.0	1.0	1.6	2.7	4.0	5.6	7.0	9.9	14.4	23.7
FS	0–88.6	1.0	1.7	2.3	2.7	4.7	9.3	15.3	22.7	31.0
MN	0–2.7	0	0.3	0.4	0.5	0.6	0.7	0.8	1.2	2.0
FN	0–2.0	0	0	0	0	0.4	0.5	0.6	0.7	0.9

[a] Computed from ungrouped data.
[b] MS=50 male stutterers.
[c] FS=50 female stutterers.
[d] MN=50 male nonstutterers.
[e] FN=50 female nonstutterers.
SOURCE: Johnson, 7.

225

TABLE 42. Ranges and Deciles of Distributions of Values for Number of Sander Disfluent Words (*12*) Per 100 Words, Computed by Combining the Values in Table 37 for the Categories Part-Word Repetitions, Word Repetitions, Broken Words, and Prolonged Sounds, for the Job Task

| | Range | Decile | | | | | | | | |
		1	2	3	4	5	6	7	8	9
MS	0–110.1	1.4	2.2	3.8	5.9	7.1	11.0	14.6	22.5	53.0
FS	0–105.8	0.8	1.4	2.9	4.3	8.0	11.2	16.5	23.5	42.1
MN	0–7.3	0	0	0.3	0.5	0.7	1.1	1.4	1.8	2.8
FN	0–4.1	0	0	0.2	0.3	0.6	0.7	1.0	1.3	2.6

SOURCE: Johnson, 7.

TABLE 43. Ranges and Deciles of Distributions of Values for Number of Sander Disfluent Words (*12*) Per 100 Words, Computed by Combining the Values in Table 38 for the Categories Part-Word Repetitions, Word Repetitions, Broken Words, and Prolonged Sounds, for the TAT Task

| | Range | Decile | | | | | | | | |
		1	2	3	4	5	6	7	8	9
MS	0–87.8	1.6	2.7	3.9	5.9	8.4	10.8	16.0	21.5	56.4
FS	0–105.9	0.9	2.0	2.6	5.6	9.0	12.2	20.7	27.7	47.8
MN	0–4.9	0	0.2	0.4	0.6	0.8	1.0	1.4	1.9	2.9
FN	0–6.9	0	0.2	0.3	0.4	0.6	0.7	1.0	1.6	2.5

SOURCE: Johnson, 7.

TABLE 44. Ranges and Deciles of Distributions of Values for Number of Sander Disfluent Words (*12*) per 100 Words, Computed by Combining the Values in Table 39 for the Categories Part-Word Repetitions, Word Repetitions, Broken Words, and Prolonged Sounds, for the Reading Task

| | Range | Decile | | | | | | | | |
		1	2	3	4	5	6	7	8..	9
MS	0–91.9	0.7	1.0	1.3	2.9	5.0	7.0	11.0	19.3	28.8
FS	0–135.5	0.7	1.0	1.3	2.6	3.6	8.1	15.6	26.9	41.8
MN	0–4.0	0	0	0	0.3	0.3	0.3	1.0	1.3	2.0
FN	0–3.0	0	0	0	0	0	0.3	0.3	0.6	1.0

SOURCE: Johnson, 7.

TABLE 45. Means, Standard Deviations, and Ranges of Total Disfluencies and Sander Disfluent Words for Two Performances, Sessions I and II, of the Oral Reading of the 300-Word Test Passage, "Your Rate of Oral Reading," and of the Job Task (Speaking of 250 Words About Future Job) for 40 Adult Stutterers, 34 Males and 6 Females

	Speaking			Oral Reading		
	Mean	SD	Range	Mean	SD	Range
Total disfluencies						
Session I	78.1[a]	55.4	8–230	48.2[b]	64.3	0–270
Session II	81.2	56.6	15–255	46.0	54.7	1–210
Disfluent words						
Session I	38.2[c]	33.4	1–134	29.0[d]	38.7	0–184
Session II	40.0	32.0	3–122	29.1	35.4	0–160

[a] The approximate mean for both sessions is 32 disfluencies per 100 words.
[b] The approximate mean for both sessions is 16 disfluencies per 100 words.
[c] The approximate mean for both sessions is 16 disfluent words per 100 words.
[d] The approximate mean for both sessions is 10 disfluent words per 100 words.
SOURCE: Sander, 12.

TABLE 46. Ranges and Deciles of Distributions of Values for Number of Young Disfluent Words (15) Per 100 Words, Computed by Combining the Values in Table 37 for the Categories Part-Word Repetitions, Broken Words, and Prolonged Sounds, for the Job Task

		Decile								
	Range	1	2	3	4	5	6	7	8	9
MS	0–94.6	1.0	1.4	2.3	3.9	4.4	7.6	10.6	17.1	46.4
FS	0–90.9	0.5	0.8	1.6	2.4	5.6	8.1	12.2	18.0	33.7
MN	0–4.4	0	0	0	0	0	0.2	0.3	0.5	1.3
FN	0–1.7	0	0	0	0	0.2	0.2	0.3	0.4	1.0

SOURCE: Johnson, 7.

TABLE 47. Ranges and Deciles of Distributions of Values for Number of Young Disfluent Words (15) Per 100 Words, Computed by Combining the Values in Table 38 for the Categories Part-Word Repetitions, Broken Words, and Prolonged Sounds for the TAT Task

		Decile								
	Range	1	2	3	4	5	6	7	8	9
MS	0–73.3	1.0	1.6	2.5	4.2	5.3	7.0	11.4	16.2	46.5
FS	0–82.0	0.4	0.8	1.0	3.6	5.9	8.5	15.7	21.0	39.2
MN	0–2.4	0	0	0	0	0.2	0.3	0.4	0.6	1.0
FN	0–2.4	0	0	0	0.1	0.2	0.2	0.3	0.6	1.0

SOURCE: Johnson, 7.

TABLE 48. Ranges and Deciles of Distributions of Values for Number of Young Disfluent Words (*15*) Per 100 Words, Computed by Combining the Values in Table 39 for the Categories Part-Word Repetitions, Broken Words, and Prolonged Sounds, for the Reading Task

	Range	1	2	3	4	Decile 5	6	7	8	9
MS	0–85.2	0.7	1.0	1.3	2.6	4.7	6.3	10.0	17.3	26.1
FS	0–121.6	0.1	1.0	1.3	2.3	3.3	7.1	14.3	24.9	39.1
MN	0–3.0	0	0	0	0.3	0.3	0.3	0.7	1.0	1.3
FN	0–2.3	0	0	0	0	0	0.3	0.3	0.3	0.7

SOURCE: Johnson, *7*.

TABLE 49. Means, Ranges, and Standard Deviations of Measures of Disfluency Based on 200 Words Spoken by 50 Adult Males with the Problem of Stuttering

Disfluency Category	Mean Number of Disfluencies	Mean Number of Disfluencies Per 100 Words	Percentage of Total Disfluencies	Range of Numbers of Disfluencies	SD
Interjections	19.2	9.6	36.7	2–95	16.8
Part-word repetitions	14.4	7.2	27.5	0–79	16.1
Word-phrase repetitions	5.5	2.8	10.6	0–28	5.1
Prolongations	10.5	5.3	20.0	0–70	15.5
Revisions	2.7	1.4	5.1	0–8	1.8
Total[a]	52.3	26.2	100.0	4–223	40.8

[a] Sum of measures for all disfluency categories.
SOURCE: Young, *15*.

TABLE 50. Mean Frequencies of Designated Types of Repetition Per 100 Words in the Speech of Preschool Children 2 to 5 Years Old in Free-Play and Speech Test Situations

	Free-Play (N=105)[a]	Speech Tests (N=106)[b]
Syllable repetitions	0.69	0.72
Word repetitions	1.65	1.91
Phrase repetitions	2.41	0.96
Total repetitions	4.88	3.64
Number of words involved in all repetitions[c]	23.50	9.85

[a] 55 boys, 50 girls.
[b] 41 boys, 65 girls.
[c] The difference between the two types of situation in this measure is due mainly to the greater number of phrase repetitions per 100 words in the free-play situation.
SOURCE: Branscom, Hughes, and Oxtoby, *3*, Tables 7 and 8, pp. 173-174.

TABLE 51. Range and Decile Distribution of the Indexes of Disfluency (Number of Disfluencies Per 100 Words) for Each of the Eight Disfluency Categories and for all Categories Combined for the Male Clinical (Stuttering) and Control Group Children[a]

Disfluency Category and Group	Lowest Index	Deciles									Highest Index
		1	2	3	4	5	6	7	8	9	
Interjections											
Clinical[b]	.00	.33	1.15	1.85	2.19	2.89	3.41	4.52	6.09	7.10	15.25
Control[b]	.00	.39	.67	1.20	1.63	2.04	2.71	3.98	5.31	8.40	12.71
Sound and syllable repetitions											
Clinical	.00	.43	.93	1.50	2.41	3.13	4.07	5.70	7.94	13.09	36.43
Control	.00	.00	.00	.22	.40	.55	.60	.79	.91	1.51	2.42
Word repetitions											
Clinical	.00	.90	1.66	2.65	3.00	3.23	3.88	5.39	6.11	8.26	14.50
Control	.00	.20	.31	.49	.65	.97	1.17	1.42	1.73	2.03	4.62
Phrase repetitions											
Clinical	.00	.00	.37	.54	.87	.95	1.18	1.59	1.85	1.98	7.07
Control	.00	.00	.00	.23	.40	.47	.64	.80	.99	1.54	2.52
Revisions											
Clinical	.00	.00	.43	.58	.68	1.08	1.36	1.79	2.18	2.78	4.41
Control	.00	.29	.49	.74	.95	1.11	1.41	1.84	2.32	2.66	7.47
Incomplete phrases											
Clinical	.00	.00	.00	.00	.00	.00	.22	.40	.68	.93	2.45
Control	.00	.00	.00	.00	.00	.00	.00	.21	.50	.88	1.65
Broken words											
Clinical	.00	.00	.00	.00	.00	.00	.00	.00	.15	.43	.54
Control	.00	.00	.00	.00	.00	.00	.00	.00	.00	.12	1.09
Prolonged sounds											
Clinical	.00	.00	.00	.18	.43	.64	.97	1.36	1.98	3.95	19.60
Control	.00	.00	.00	.00	.00	.00	.00	.16	.31	.53	1.95
All categories											
Clinical	3.30	6.48	8.27	10.74	12.77	13.62	14.64	22.12	27.15	34.43	46.51
Control	.60	2.05	3.42	4.20	4.97	7.14	8.55	9.74	10.81	13.76	18.28

[a] Ranging in age from about 2.5 to 8.5 years, with an average age of approximately 5 years.
[b] N=68
SOURCE: Johnson et al., 8, p. 206.

TABLE 52. Range and Decile Distribution of the Indexes of Disfluency (Number of Disfluencies Per 100 Words) for Each of the Eight Disfluency Categories and for all Categories Combined for the Female Clinical (Stuttering) and Control Group Children[a]

Disfluency Category and Group	Lowest Index	Deciles									Highest Index
		1	2	3	4	5	6	7	8	9	
Interjections											
Clinical[b]	.81	1.07	1.77	2.38	3.24	3.38	4.23	5.91	6.03	8.64	14.66
Control[b]	.00	.24	.50	1.04	1.52	1.62	3.33	3.97	5.51	8.46	15.22
Sound and syllable repetitions											
Clinical	.00	.50	.64	1.38	2.13	2.29	3.43	4.42	5.20	8.91	16.61
Control	.00	.22	.25	.26	.29	.53	.55	.74	1.10	1.44	6.09
Word repetitions											
Clinical	.00	.32	.81	1.88	2.39	3.45	3.78	4.88	5.74	7.45	9.23
Control	.00	.25	.28	.51	.58	.73	1.21	1.42	1.67	2.61	3.47
Phrase repetitions											
Clinical	.00	.00	.15	.32	.38	.50	.62	.86	1.30	2.16	3.11
Control	.00	.00	.00	.00	.29	.44	.50	.53	1.04	1.30	2.51
Revisions											
Clinical	.00	.32	.42	.75	.81	1.16	1.19	1.72	2.11	2.78	3.34
Control	.00	.36	.67	.88	1.24	1.28	1.46	1.93	2.05	2.25	3.29
Incomplete phrases											
Clinical	.00	.00	.00	.00	.00	.00	.15	.21	.28	.30	2.41
Control	.00	.00	.00	.00	.00	.00	.24	.25	.26	1.05	1.74
Broken words											
Clinical	.00	.00	.00	.00	.00	.00	.00	.13	.30	.56	7.76
Control	.00	.00	.00	.00	.00	.00	.00	.05	.25	.40	.51
Prolonged sounds											
Clinical	.00	.00	.00	.15	.25	.51	1.04	1.46	1.79	2.48	7.25
Control	.00	.00	.00	.00	.00	.00	.00	.16	.25	.53	.87
All categories											
Clinical	4.16	5.68	8.23	9.51	11.38	16.31	17.27	17.47	18.72	32.03	46.55
Control	2.61	2.74	3.31	4.36	4.69	5.01	6.87	8.30	11.06	13.53	28.70

[a] Ranging in age from about 2.5 to 8.5 years, with an average age of approximately 5 years.
[b] N=21
SOURCE: Johnson et al., 8, p. 207.

TABLE 53. Average Percentage of the Disfluencies Classified in Each Category for Clinical (Stuttering) and Control Group Boys and Girls

Nonfluency Category	Experimental Group[a][b]		Control Group[a][b]	
	Male	Female	Male	Female
Interjections	20.2	27.3	43.0	43.7
Sound and syllable repetitions	30.4	24.2	8.4	10.5
Word repetitions	23.9	22.5	14.7	14.4
Phrase repetitions	6.4	5.7	8.4	7.3
Revisions	7.3	8.0	19.6	17.5
Incomplete phrases	1.9	1.5	3.2	3.5
Broken words	0.7	3.9	1.4	1.3
Prolonged sounds	9.3	7.6	1.9	1.8

[a] N = 89
[b] Ranging in age from about 2.5 to 8.5 years, with an average age of approximately 5 years.
SOURCE: Johnson et al., 8, p. 211.

TABLE 54. Summary of Measures of Verbal Output, Defined as Number of Words Spoken, in Responding to the Pictures in the Children's Apperception Test (1) by 178 Children[a]

Group	N	Range	Mean	SD	Median	90th Percentile
Clinical boys[b]	68	31–1,158	499.8	293.0	452.5	955.7
Clinical girls	21	116 1,296	556.0	351.6	389.0	1,156.4
Control boys[c]	68	65–1,229	475.3	234.1	445.5	909.7
Control girls	21	211–2,044	526.5	385.5	402.7	824.4

[a] Age about 2.5 to 8.5 years, with an average age of approximately 5 years.
[b] The clinical groups were regarded by their parents as stutterers.
[c] The control groups were regarded by their parents as normal speakers.
SOURCE: Johnson et al., 8, p. 201.

TABLE 55. Summary of Measures of Verbal Output, Defined as Number of Words Spoken, for the Job Task and TAT Task for 200 Adult Subjects

Task	Range	Mean	Standard Deviation	10th Percentile	Median	90th Percentile
Job[a]						
MS[b]	55–570	280.4	108.5	136	276	430
FS[c]	48–553	248.1	118.3	94	228	400
MN[d]	60–689	359.4	107.7	247	358	498
FN[e]	174–687	392.6	108.7	258	398	550
Tat[f]						
MS	83–766	378.6	175.1	160	381	700
FS	54–960	293.5	179.7	118	264	594
MN	158–1064	518.2	161.0	339	524	703
FN	129–996	565.7	186.7	376	578	828

[a] Speaking for about 3 minutes about future job or vocation.
[b] MS = 50 male stutterers.
[c] FS = 50 female stutterers.
[d] MN = 50 male nonstutterers.
[e] FN = 50 female nonstutterers.
[f] Speaking for about 3 minutes about Card No. 10 in the TAT (11).
SOURCE: Johnson, 7.

YOUR RATE OF ORAL READING*

Your rate of speech will be adequate if it is slow enough to provide for clearness and comprehension, and rapid enough to sustain interest. Your rate is faulty if it is too rapid to accomplish these ends. The easiest way to begin work on the adjustment of your speech to an ideal rate is to measure your present rate in words per minute in a fixed situation which you can keep constant over a number of trials. The best method is to pick a page of simple, factual prose to be read. Read this page in your natural manner, timing yourself in seconds. Count the number of words on the page, divide by the number of seconds, and multiply this result by sixty to calculate the number of words per minute. As you attempt to increase or retard your rate, repeat this procedure from time to time, using the same reading material, to enable you to check your success.

A common accompaniment of rapid rate is staccato speech, in which the duration of words and syllables is too short, whereas in slow speech the words and syllables frequently are overprolonged. When the person with too rapid rate tries to slow down, he tends to make the error of keeping the duration of his tones short, and of attempting to accomplish the slower rate solely by lengthening the pauses between phrases and by introducing new pauses. On the other hand, the person who is working to speed up his rate tends to do this by shortening the pauses alone and retaining his prolonged tones. It is impossible at the present time to set down in rules the ideal relation between the duration of tones and pauses in speech. Further research is needed before this can be done with any great accuracy.

* Reprinted by permission of the publisher, from Grant Fairbanks, *Voice and Articulation Drillbook*, New York, Harper & Row, 1940, p. 144.

ARTHUR, THE YOUNG RAT

Once, a long time ago, there was a young rat named Arthur who could never make up his flighty mind. Whenever his swell friends used to ask him to go out to play with them, he would only answer airily, "I don't know." He wouldn't try to say yes, or no either. He would always shrink from making a specific choice.

His proud Aunt Helen scolded him: "Now look here," she stated, "no one is going to aid or care for you if you carry on like this. You have no more mind than a stray blade of grass."

That very night there was a big thundering crash and in the foggy morning some zealous men—with twenty boys and girls—rode up and looked closely at the fallen barn. One of them slipped back a broken board and saw a squashed young rat, quite dead, half in and half out of his hole. Thus, in the end the poor shirker got his just dues. Oddly enough his Aunt Helen was glad. "I hate such oozy, oily sneaks," said she.

FORM 10. MEASURES OF RATE OF SPEAKING AND ORAL READING

Name _____ Age _____ Sex _____

Examiner _____ Date _____

Reading passage used: No. 1_____ No. 2_____ Other (specify)_____

Speaking procedure used: Job Task__ TAT Task__ CAT Task__ Other (describe):

I. Oral Reading Rate:

	Passage No. 1	Passage No. 2	Other
A. Number of words	_____	_____	_____
B. Number of sentences	_____	_____	_____
C. Number of sentences	_____	_____	_____
D. Over-all rate in words per minute (OR:WPM)	_____	_____	_____
E. Mean sentence rate in words per minute (MSR:WPM)	_____	_____	_____

II. Speaking Rate:

	Job Task	TAT Task	CAT Task	Other
A. Number of words	_____	_____	_____	_____
B. Number of seconds	_____	_____	_____	_____
C. Number of sentences	_____	_____	_____	_____
D. Over-all rate in words per minute (OR:WPM)	_____	_____	_____	_____
E. Mean sentence rate in words per minute (MSR:WPM)	_____	_____	_____	_____

To compute over-all rate in words per minute: Divide the number of words by the number of seconds and multiply the result by 60, the number of seconds in one minute. Under either I or II, above, use the formula $A/B \times 60 = OR:WPM$.

To compute mean sentence rate in words per minute: Under either I or II, above, carry out the following operations: (a) count the number or words in each sentence; (b) time the speaking of each sentence in seconds; (c) for each sentence, divide the number of seconds by the number of words to find the time in seconds consumed in speaking the average word; (d) divide 60 seconds by the result obtained in (c) and the quotient will be the rate in words per minute at which the sentence was uttered;

(e) sum the rates, in words per minute, for all the sentences and divide the total by the number of sentences to determine the mean sentence rate in words per minute; enter this value in E.

Name _____ Age _____ Sex_____

Examiner _____ Date _____

Reading passage used: No. 1_____ No. 2_____ Other (specify)_____

Speaking procedure used: Job Task___ TAT Task___ CAT Task___ Other (describe)___

	Reading Passage			Speaking Task			
	No. 1	No. 2	Other	Job	TAT	CAT	Other
A. Number of words	___	___	___	___	___	___	___
B. Number of Sander disfluent words	___	___	___	___	___	___	___
per 100 = B/A × 100	___	___	___	___	___	___	___
C. Number of Young disfluent words	___	___	___	___	___	___	___
per 100 = C/A × 100	___	___	___	___	___	___	___
D. Number of disfluencies							
a. Interjections	___	___	___	___	___	___	___
per 100 words = a/A × 100	___	___	___	___	___	___	___
b. Part-word repetitions	___	___	___	___	___	___	___
per 100 words = b/A × 100	___	___	___	___	___	___	___
c. Word repetitions	___	___	___	___	___	___	___
per 100 words = c/A × 100	___	___	___	___	___	___	___
d. Phrase repetitions	___	___	___	___	___	___	___
per 100 words = d/A × 100	___	___	___	___	___	___	___
e. Revisions	___	___	___	___	___	___	___
per 100 words = e/A × 100	___	___	___	___	___	___	___
f. Incomplete phrases	___	___	___	___	___	___	___
per 100 words = f/A × 100	___	___	___	___	___	___	___
g. Broken words	___	___	___	___	___	___	___
per 100 words = g/A × 100	___	___	___	___	___	___	___
h. Prolonged sounds	___	___	___	___	___	___	___
per 100 words = h/A × 100	___	___	___	___	___	___	___
i. Total repetitions (b+c+d)	___	___	___	___	___	___	___
per 100 words: i/A × 100 =							
Repetition Index (RI)	___	___	___	___	___	___	___
j. Total disfluencies = a+b+...h)	___	___	___	___	___	___	___
per 100 words = j/A × 100 =							
Total Disfluency Index (TDI)	___	___	___	___	___	___	___

Additional copies of this form may be obtained from the Interstate Printers
and Publishers, 19-27 North Jackson Street, Danville, Illinois.

FORM 12. SPEAKING-TIME LOG

Name _____ Age _____ Sex _____

Clinician _____ Date _____

Situations	Time (seconds)	Situations	Time (seconds)
1. _____	_____	26. _____	_____
2. _____	_____	27. _____	_____
3. _____	_____	28. _____	_____
4. _____		29. _____	_____
5. _____	_____	30. _____	_____
6. _____	_____	31. _____	_____
7. _____	_____	32.	_____
8. _____	_____	33. _____	_____
9. _____	_____	34. _____	_____
10. _____	_____	35. _____	_____
11. _____	_____	36. _____	_____
12. _____	_____	37. _____	_____
13. _____	_____	38. _____	_____
14. _____	_____	39. _____	_____
15. _____	_____	40. _____	_____
16. _____	_____	41. _____	_____
17. _____	_____	42. _____	_____
18. _____	_____	43. _____	_____
19. _____	_____	44. _____	_____
20. _____	_____	45. _____	_____
21. _____	_____	46. _____	_____
22. _____	_____	47. _____	_____
23. _____	_____	48. _____	_____
24. _____	_____	49. _____	_____
25. _____	_____	50. _____	_____

Speaking time in seconds: _____
Speaking time in minutes = total seconds divided by 60: _____

Total number of situations:

with 1 other person _____   with others of same age _____
with 2-3 other persons _____   with others mostly older _____
with 4 or more other persons _____   with others mostly younger _____

with members of own family _____   with others both older and
with close friends or associates _____   younger _____
with others previously spoken to _____   with others associated with
with others spoken to for first   clinic _____
    time _____
     with others not associated with
with others of own sex _____   clinic _____
with others of opposite sex _____
with others of both sexes _____

Additional copies of this form may be obtained from the Interstate Printers and Publishers, 19-27 North Jackson Street, Danville, Illinois.

REFERENCES

1. Bellak, L., *The Thematic Apperception Test and the Children's Appercep-tion Test in Clinical Use*, New York: Grune and Stratton, 1954.
2. Bloodstein, O. N., "The relationship between oral reading rate and se-verity of stuttering," *Journal of Speech Disorders*, 1944, *9*:161-173.
3. Branscom, Margaret E., Jeannette Hughes, and Eloise Tupper Oxtoby, "Studies in the speech of preschool children," in *Stuttering in Children and Adults: Thirty Years of Research at the University of Iowa*, edited by W. Johnson with the assistance of R. Leutenegger, Minneapolis: Uni-versity of Minnesota Press, 1955, pp. 157-180.
4. Cotton, J., "Syllabic Rate: a new concept in the study of speech rate variation," Speech Monographs, 1936, *3*:112-117.
5. Darley, F. L., "A normative study of oral reading rate," unpublished M.A. thesis, University of Iowa, 1940.
6. Franke, P., "A preliminary study validating the measurement of oral reading rate in words per minute," unpublished M.A. thesis, University of Iowa, 1939.
7. Johnson, W., "Measurements of oral reading and speaking rate and dis-fluency of adult male and female stutterers and nonstutterers," *Journal of Speech and Hearing Disorders*, Monogr. Supp. 7, 1961, 1-20.
8. Johnson, W., et al., *The Onset of Stuttering: Research Findings and Implications*, Minneapolis: University of Minnesota Press, 1959.
9. Kelly, J. C. and M. D. Steer, "Revised concept of rate," *Journal of Speech and Hearing Disorders*, 1949, *14*:222-226.
10. Lumley, F. H., "Rates of speech in radio speaking," *Quarterly Journal of Speech*, 1933, *19*:393-403.
11. Murray, H. A., *Thematic Apperception Test*, Cambridge, Mass.: Harvard University Press, 1943.
12. Sander, E. K., "Reliability of the Iowa Speech Disfluency Test," *Journal of Speech and Hearing Disorders*, Monogr. Supp. 7, 1961, 21-30.
13. Skalbeck, O. M., "A statistical analysis of three measures of word length," unpublished M.A. thesis, University of Iowa, 1938.
14. Thorndike, E. L., *Teachers' Word Book of 20,000 Words*, New York: Teachers College, Columbia University, 1932.
15. Young, M. A., "Predicting ratings of severity of stuttering," *Journal of Speech and Hearing Disorders*, Monogr. Supp. 7, 1961, 31-54.

9 THE PROBLEM OF STUTTERING

Stuttering is a problem in which many factors and many persons interact in complex ways. It is a problem that involves not only a speaker but his listeners as well. Indeed, it may be said with peculiar validity that in the beginning stuttering is not so much a problem for the speaker, who is nearly always a small child, as it is for his most important listeners, who are nearly always his parents. After the speaker, the child, takes on the problem he makes it more and more a part of himself as he grows older with it; but it remains a kind of trouble that he shares with those around him who never abandon their investment in it—and each newcomer borrows from him that part of it which serves his own need to be responsive to the stutterer's distress.

In order, then, to evaluate the problem of stuttering you need to give attention to how the one who is said to be the stutterer speaks, and to what he says about the way he speaks, and to the feelings he has because of it and because of what he tells himself about it. You need to find out also what his listeners say about his mode of speaking and how they feel about it. And you need to discover where and when the speaker does what he and the others take to be his stuttering, and what they do because he does these things at the times and in the places where he does them, and what he does because they do what they do.

Some background information will help to give meaning to the various things there are to be done in examining the problem of stuttering.

THREE GENERAL MEANINGS OF "STUTTERING"

We use the word "stuttering" in three main ways: we use it to refer to what the speaker does; we use it as a name for the category in which the listener classifies what the speaker does; and we refer by means of it to the problem that ensues when listeners classify what a speaker does as stuttering and evaluate it as undesirable, and the speaker senses their evaluations and reacts to them with tension and concern, confirming and intensifying their evaluations, and in the bargain further deepening his own concern—in an ever-outreaching spiral of distress.

"Stuttering" as a Name for Something a Speaker Does

We commonly employ the word "stuttering" with the intention of describing certain things that are done by a speaker. When we use it in this way it usually turns out to be rather vague and ambiguous. For example, a series of studies on the onset of stuttering (30) has indicated that when parents begin to feel that their children are "stuttering" they use the word to refer largely to hesitation forms and repetitions that other parents do not regard as stutterings. Although we commonly define stuttering as referring to repetitions, hesitations, and other speech disfluencies, normative studies of the speech of both children (30) and adults (20) have shown that some persons who are regarded as normal speakers are more disfluent than some speakers who are classified by themselves and others as stutterers. Tuthill (45) presented recorded samples of the speech of adult stutterers and non-stutterers to groups of speech clinicians, stutterers, and lay listeners and found within each of these groups of listeners marked disagreement over which specific words were and were not stuttered. For all three groups the number of agreements was only about 37 percent of the number of agreements there would have been had the listeners agreed completely on which words to mark as stuttered.

Boehmler (10) found that listeners agreed most highly in classifying as stutterings those disfluencies which they rated as severe or extreme. He also reported that sound or syllable repetitions were classified as stutterings by his observers more often than were other kinds of disfluency. Williams and Kent (53) found that their laboratory observers, in judging disfluencies, classified syllable repetitions and sound prolongations primarily as "stuttered" and revisions primarily as "nonstuttered." Young (56) had listeners rate the severity of stuttering of speech samples; he also counted the disfluencies in the samples. He found that the severity ratings were highly correlated with frequencies of part-word repetitions, sound prolongations, and broken words, but not with frequencies of revisions, interjections, incomplete phrases, and word and phrase repetitions. (See descriptions of these types of disfluency on pages 209-210.)

The reasons why listeners disagree in classifying disfluencies as stuttering have been identified in a number of studies. Tuthill (45) found that disagreement was related to experience with the problem; in reacting to recorded samples of speech, stutterers classified the greatest number of words as stuttered, speech clinicians the next highest number, and lay listeners (college freshmen) the lowest number. Boehmler (10) asked his listeners to classify as an example of either stuttering or nonstuttering each of 804 tape-recorded disfluencies— 402 selected from the speech of stutterers and 402, of comparable severity, as rated, selected from the speech of normal speakers. Two of his groups of listeners were speech clinicians who had been professionally trained at two different universities, and one of his groups was made up of laymen. One of the groups of clinicians classified significantly more of the disfluencies as stutterings than did the other, and both groups of clinicians regarded significantly more of the disfluencies—from the speech of both the stutterers and normal speakers, incidentally—as stutterings than did the lay listeners.

Bloodstein, Jaeger, and Tureen (8) tape recorded 12 2-minute samples of speech from children, some of whom were regarded by their parents as stutterers, some as normal speakers. They played the tapes to parents (not parents of the children whose speech was recorded on the tapes). They found that parents who had previously come to regard their own children as stutterers classified more of the speech samples as stuttered than did parents who thought of their own children as normal speakers.

Williams and Kent (53) tape recorded a specially contrived sample of speech containing 52 speech interruptions distributed by design among six different kinds of disfluency. They presented the tape recordings three times to each of two groups of lay listeners. Group I was told, first, to mark on mimeographed copies each *stuttered* interruption in the speech. On new copies they were then asked to mark *all* interruptions. Finally, again on new mimeographed copies, they were told to mark the *normal* interruptions. The subjects in Group II were instructed first to mark *normal* interruptions, second to mark *all* interruptions, and third to mark *stuttered* interruptions.

The authors stated, "The group of subjects instructed to mark stuttered interruptions first marked more interruptions as stuttered than they subsequently marked as normal. Conversely, the group instructed to mark normal interruptions first marked more as normal than they subsequently marked as stuttered."

Of particular interest was the inconsistency or confusion of the listeners. As the investigators explained, "Under instruction to mark stuttered interruptions, a subject might mark a particular interruption as stuttered, and later under instruction to mark normal interruptions, might judge the same interruption to be normal. Under instructions to mark stuttered interruptions, subjects in both groups tended to show the fewest inconsistent responses in judging syllable repetitions and prolongations and the most in reacting to revisions. When instructed to mark normal interruptions, they made the fewest inconsistent responses on revisions and the most on syllable repetitions and prolongations. The indicated confusion was observed, however, in degrees varying from pronounced to relatively slight for all six types of disfluency."

The authors, referring to the fact that syllable repetition is the type of disfluency most likely to be thought of by listeners as stuttering, raised the fundamental question of whether a child repeats syllables because he is evaluated as a stutterer or is considered to be a stutterer because he repeats syllables. They offered this answer: "On the basis of this study, it is suggested that the cause and effect relationship may work to a degree in both directions. Apparently, he could became known as a stutterer *because* he repeats syllables. Once, however, he is identified as a stutterer, then his word and phrase repetitions, interjections and even revisions, to a certain extent, also come to be considered as stuttering, seemingly for no other reason than *because* he is now thought of as a stutterer."

In a footnote, Williams and Kent then made this observation: "One of the objectives in counseling the parents of a child who is considered to be stuttering is to help them re-evaluate some of the child's speech interruptions. It has proved profitable to the present authors, at least, first to acquaint the parents with the concept of normal speech and then to ask them to pay particular attention to and to keep track of the normal interruptions in their child's speaking behavior. Often, the parents, when faced with the task of listening for and noting normal interruptions, not only become more interested in what constitutes a normal interruption, but begin classifying more of the interruptions as normal. As a consequence, the number of interruptions reacted to as stuttering is reduced."

A general conclusion to be drawn from the research represented by these studies is that there is considerable variation among listeners in classifying disfluencies as either stutterings or normal breaks in fluency, that many speech disfluencies are not regarded by most professional and lay listeners as stutterings, and that there is more to the stuttering problem than speech disfluencies.

"Stuttering" as a Name for a Classification Made by a Listener

A second use we make of the term "stuttering" is as a name for a category, or, as we may say, for a judgment. That is, when we say of something done by a speaker that "it is stuttering," we are making a judgment, or an evaluation, of what the speaker is doing. We are saying that in our judgment what the speaker is doing should be classified as stuttering. We are implying that "stuttering" is the name of a category, and that we regard what the speaker is doing as belonging in that category. In such a sense, then, we may say that we use "stuttering" as the name of a category, or that we use it to refer to our own judgment that what the speaker is doing is to be classified in that category.

This may be put another way by saying that if Mrs. Jones were to tell you that her little boy Robert is beginning to stutter, and later you were asked by someone else what Robert is beginning to do, you would be unable to say. You would know only how Mrs. Jones had classified whatever it was that she had decided Robert was beginning to do—but she would not have told you what he was doing that she had classified. As the name for a category, then, we use the word "stuttering" to refer, not to what is done by a speaker, but to the classification, made by ourselves or some other listener, of something or other that is done by a speaker. The theoretical and practical significance of this kind of use of the term is discussed in considerable detail by Johnson (*21, 30*).

"Stuttering" as a Name for a Problem

The third way in which we use the term "stuttering" is as the name for a *problem*. As we have said, it is a problem that involves not only a speaker but also his listeners, and not only certain of the speaker's disfluencies but also the ways in which he and his listeners react to them—and interact with one another with respect to them. When we use the word as the name for the problem that we call stuttering, then, we use the term to refer to much more than the hesitations and repetitions and tensings of a speaker, and to more than the evaluations made of them by his listeners. We refer also to the ways in which the listeners react to the speaker's disfluencies. Moreover, we include the listeners' reactions to what the speaker says, as they are affected by the way he says it. We refer to the listeners' reactions to the speaker as a person, and to the speaker's reactions to himself—and his reactions to his listeners' evaluations of him and their reactions to him. We refer to the differences that the speaker's way of speaking—and all the reactions made to it by himself and by others—make to him socially, educationally, economically, emotionally, and otherwise. And we refer to much more besides. Used as the name for a problem, "stuttering" means a great deal, indeed—much more than you would be prepared to expect if you had been used to thinking of it only as a term that meant "a disturbance in the rhythm or fluency of speech."

For a much more fully developed discussion of the stuttering problem along the lines of the foregoing statement, see especially *The Onset of Stuttering (30)*, particularly Chapters 9 and 10, and *Stuttering and What You Can Do About It (21)*. Additional information about stuttering and the various theoretical and clinical approaches to the problem is to be found in books by Ainsworth (2); Barbara (4); Bloodstein (5); Eisenson (15); Hejna (18); Johnson (21, 22, 25, 30); Murphy (33); Van Riper (46); West, Ansberry, and Carr (50); and in past and current issues of the *Journal of Speech and Hearing Disorders* and the *Journal of Speech and Hearing Research* published by the American Speech and Hearing Association.

EXAMINATION OF THE STUTTERING PROBLEM

Procedures for examining the stuttering problem, as defined above, are appropriately selected and designed to reveal significant aspects of (1) the attitudes and reactions of designated listeners to the speaker and his speech, (2) the attitudes and reactions of the speaker to those of his listeners and to himself and his own speech, and (3) the speech behavior of the speaker.

The case study interview, as described in Chapter 2, is your basic means of obtaining information about the significant interactions between the speaker and his listeners—(1) and (2), above. Their more important relevant evaluations and ways of reacting are indicated meaningfully, for the most part, by the case history data supplied by the speaker himself, if he is old enough to be interviewed, and by other informants, especially the parents, wife or husband, teachers, or other associates. The "Supplementary Case History Outline: The Stuttering Problem" in Chapter 2 is of fundamental importance in the investigation of any case of stuttering.

The information you obtain in the case history interviews may be extended and clarified by means of the techniques described in the following pages. These have been selected from a variety of procedures developed and tested over the past several years in laboratory and clinical work with the stuttering problem. They include the Iowa Scale of Attitude Toward Stuttering; the Stutterer's Rating Scale of Speech Situations; Check List of Stutterer's Disfluencies and Related Reactions; Rating Scale of Severity of Stuttering Reactions; Procedure for Measuring Adaptation of Stuttering Reactions; and Procedure for Measuring Consistency of Stuttering Reactions. In examining the speech behavior of stutterers you may also use the procedures, described in Chapter 8, for measuring rate and disfluency of speaking and oral reading and for gauging amount of speaking. Moreover, you may employ the other examination methods described in this manual in the clinical study of the stuttering problem, as your judgment dictates. In some cases you would want to consider referral to audiologists, physicians, or psychologists for reasons to be specified; principles of referral are discussed in Chapter 10.

In the following three sections we shall discuss uses to be made in the examination of stutterers of the measures of disfluency and rate of oral reading and speaking, and of speaking-time, previously described in Chapter 8. We shall also consider certain background information against which the measures are to be evaluated.

MEASURES OF DISFLUENCY OF SPEAKING AND ORAL READING

The procedures employed for measuring disfluency are particularly useful in the examination of stutterers. It is not necessary to repeat here the information about the procedures that is to be found in Chapter 8, but some discussion of their use in evaluating the speech behavior of persons classified as stutterers is in order.

The common tendency to take for granted that disfluency and stuttering are one and the same thing is properly to be noted and reexamined. Several studies have served to make clear that the problem of stuttering encompasses much more than disfluency and that disfluency, per se, does not constitute the problem called stuttering. One of the more fundamental and conspicuous findings from our investigations of the onset of the stuttering problem is the lack of a clear difference between children classified by their parents as stutterers and children classified by their parents as normal speakers so far as disfluency is concerned (30). Parents who regarded their children as stutterers were asked to indicate what, in each case, the child was doing when they began to think of him as a stutterer; control group parents, who regarded their children as normal speakers, but who said that their children were sometimes disfluent in speaking, were also asked to describe the disfluencies displayed by their children when they "began to speak disfluently." The answers of the parents are summarized in Table 56. The data in this table make clear that the various forms of disfluency are of unequal significance in differentiating the two groups of children.

First of all, both groups were reported by their parents to speak disfluently. More of the clinical, or stuttering, group children were said to have been repeating syllables—that is, the first sounds or syllables of words—and prolonging sounds when first regarded as stutterers. Not very many in either group had prolonged sounds, however. More of the children in the control group were reported to have repeated phrases, paused noticeably, and interjected into their speech such sounds and words as "uh uh" and "well uh" and the like. About the same proportion in each group had repeated whole words. It is clear from these data that it is not enough to say that the beginning of the problem of stuttering is marked by repetitions and hesitations and other disfluencies in speech. In any given case it is desirable to find out as much as you can—and to take duly into account that all too often there is not much you can find out—about the particular details of the child's speech behavior that the parents singled out to classify as stuttering in the first hours, days, or weeks when they were beginning to think that the child was starting to stutter.

The data in Table 56 may be used as norms in evaluating case history information and, of course, in counseling parents who are concerned over the question of whether their child has developed or may develop stuttering. The interview used in obtaining the data summarized in Table 56 is contained, together with a tabulation of the responses to each item made by the clinical and control group parents, in the Appendix of *The Onset of Stuttering* (Johnson et al., *30*). The interviewing procedure is described in Chapter 1 of the same book.

You will find it advantageous to tape record and analyze samples of the speech of children brought to you as stutterers. Procedures for doing this are described in Chapter 8 of *The Onset of Stuttering* and also in Chapter 8 of this manual (pp. 201-212). You will find it desirable to familiarize yourself with the normative data presented in *The Onset of Stuttering*. The following is a summary of some of the more important details.

Samples of the speech of the clinical and control group children were tape recorded 18 months on the average after the problem of stuttering was said to have started for the children in the clinical group. The two groups of children were matched for sex, socioeconomic status of family, and age; they ranged in age from about 2.5 to 8.5 years, with an average age of approximately 5 years. The data resulting from analysis of the tapes are summarized in Tables 51-53 (pp. 229-231). The tables show that from 20 to 30 percent of the children regarded by their parents as normal speakers spoke with more disfluencies than did 20 to 30 percent of the children who had been for an average period of 18 months regarded by their parents as stutterers. This was true even for syllable repetitions, word repetitions, and sound prolongations, the types of disfluency for which there were statistically significant group differences for both boys and girls, and for phrase repetitions for which there was a significant group difference for the boys but not for the girls. Interjections, revisions, and incomplete phrases did not serve to differentiate the two groups significantly.

Normative data for representative preschool children, 2 to 5 years old, obtained in several studies by Johnson and his associates (22), were summarized in Table 50 (p. 228). The children represented in Table 50 were presumably normal, from families in the lower middle and upper middle socioeconomic levels for the most part, and many of their parents were in educational or other professional occupations. Their general level of intelligence was somewhat above average for the comparable population as a whole. All were attending the University of Iowa Preschools in the Iowa Child Welfare Research Station. None of the children was considered a stutterer at the time the speech samples were obtained.

Tables 50-53 (pp. 228-231) may be used as normative in evaluating disfluency measurements of specific children at the appropriate age levels. The information they contain is especially relevant in the counseling of parents who are concerned about disfluencies in the speech of their children.

Disfluency norms for adults were presented in Tables 37-41 (pp. 222-225). The data in these tables are taken from an investigation by Johnson (20) in which two samples of speaking and one of oral reading were obtained from each of 200 adult speakers of college age generally, 100 of whom were stutterers and 100 nonstutterers, 50 in each group being male and 50 female. The procedures employed in obtaining and analyzing the samples, which have been described in detail elsewhere (20), were essentially the same as those described in this manual (Chapter 8). The disfluency categories used are those described on pages 209-210. In general, these data show that adult stutterers are considerably more disfluent than adult nonstutterers. The extent of overlap of the distributions and the frequencies of zero values in most of the disfluency distributions of both groups, however, are to be considered in evaluating the differences between the groups.

Tables 37-41 represent 60 different distributions of disfluency measures for the nonstutterers, 30 for the males and 30 for the females, and 60 corresponding distributions for the stutterers. In most of the 60 pairs of distributions there is substantial overlapping. Considering the data in Table 37 for the Job task (speaking for 3 minutes about future job), for example, the overlap of the stutterers' and nonstutterers' distributions of scores is virtually complete for the category of revisions and it is rather extensive for interjections, incomplete phrases, and for both word and phrase repetitions. Because of the proportions of both groups presenting no broken words or prolonged sounds, approximately half of the stutterers were indistinguishable from most of the nonstutterers with respect to these types of disfluency. With regard to word repetitions, roughly 20 percent of the stutterers were more fluent than 30 to 40 percent of the nonstutterers. The most disfluent 30 percent of the nonstutterers performed more phrase repetitions than did 30 percent of the stutterers. Half of the male nonstutterers were no more fluent than 30 percent of the male stutterers, and 40 percent of the female nonstutterers were no more fluent than 20 percent of the female stutterers, as far as interjections were concerned. There is only about a 10 percent overlap of the two distributions, however, for part-word repetitions. Essentially the same statements are to be made concerning the data in Table 38 for the TAT task.

The main differences between the distributions for the speaking tasks and the reading task are to be seen in the large proportions of zeroes, each zero indicating that no disfluencies of the designated type were performed, and the relatively smaller number of disfluencies in oral reading than in speaking. The obviously greater frequencies of disfluency in speaking than in oral reading, as shown in Table 40, were, for both groups and both sexes, statistically significant. Sander (38) reported like differences between speaking and oral reading for adult stutterers (see Table 45, p. 227). You will be well advised to exercise caution accordingly in judging the speaking of a stutterer on the basis of disfluency measurements for oral reading and vice versa. Correlations between oral reading and speaking disfluency measures were generally quite low for the nonstutterers, and although they were somewhat higher for the stutterers nevertheless they were moderate to low for most measures. The coefficients of correlation for total disfluencies were, for the stutterers, .67 between oral reading and the Job task and .75 between oral reading and the TAT task; and, for the nonstutterers, .13 between oral reading and the Job task and .45 between oral reading and the TAT task. There was little difference between the two speaking tasks for either group.

Sander (38) has reported data bearing on the question of the reliability of disfluency counts and the variability of measures for the same speakers from one performance to another. He tape recorded two administrations, 24 hours apart, of the Job task and the oral reading test passage, "Your Rate of Oral Reading," to 40 adult stutterers, 34 males and six females. He performed two analyses of 12 sets of the tape-recorded samples and obtained an index of self-agreement of .96 in identifying disfluencies. That is, "For the 12 reading tasks there was a total of 557 agreements and 23 disagreements; for the speaking tasks, 767 agreements and 35 disagreements. In both instances the coefficient of agreement was .96."

Sander made verbatim transcripts of the tape-recorded samples. He used the first 250 words of the speaking task in each case, not counting repeated words and phrases and revisions. He used the complete 300-word reading passage. He replayed each recording at least three times in identifying and classifying the disfluencies. His samples contained a total of 10,150 disfluencies. He employed the eight categories of disfluency described on pp. 209-210. In addition to tabulating the total number in each of these categories, Sander designed a measure which he called "number of disfluent words." He also measured rate. In computing the number of disfluent words, he defined a disfluent word as follows: "A word was considered to be disfluent if it involved prolonged sounds, was classified as a broken word, was involved in a sound, syllable, or word repetition, or was interrupted by an interjection. Words preceded by interjections or involved in phrase repetitions were not counted as disfluent words."

Sander's disfluency measurements were summarized in Table 45. Converting the mean values in Table 45, we see that Sander's stutterers performed approximately 32 disfluencies and had 16 disfluent words per 100 words in speaking and 16 disfluencies and 10 disfluent words per 100 words in oral reading. The coefficients of correlation between his first and second recording sessions, represented in Table 45, were, for oral reading and speaking, respectively, .94 and .91 for total number of disfluencies and .97 and .94 for number of disfluent words. Thus, very considerable consistency over a 24-hour period was demonstrated by Sander's stutterers.

Sander used the disfluency norms in Tables 37-39 (pp. 222-224) in gauging the variation from the first to the second speaking and oral reading performances of his individual subjects. Approximately one-half of his stutterers scored at the same deciles for both speaking and reading in the two performances that were separated by 24 hours. Either no change or shifts no greater than one decile were shown by four-fifths of the subjects. The extremely mild or severe stutterers showed the least relative changes in performance over the 24-hour period.

Coefficients of correlation between total disfluencies and disfluent words, as defined above, were .87 for speaking and .86 for oral reading. Sander concluded, "These results suggest the feasibility of employing, for certain purposes, a relatively simplified method of disfluency analysis consisting of the counting of disfluent words, as defined in this study, and the measurement of the rate of utterance." He included the measurement of the rate of utterance because he found that total disfluencies and rate correlated .81 for speaking and .86 for reading.

Young (56) investigated disfluency in the speech of adult male stutterers, especially in relation to ratings of the severity of their stuttering. Some of his disfluency data were summarized in Table 49 (p. 228). Young obtained a multiple correlation coefficient of .91 between rated severity of stuttering, using the rating method described on page 259, and the following six measures: rate (time required to speak 200 words), numbers of interjections, part-word repetitions, repetitions of words and phrases, sound prolongations, and revisions. Successively eliminating all but three of these measures, he obtained a multiple correlation of .90 between rated severity of stuttering, on the one hand, and, on the other, rate, part-word repetitions, and sound prolongations. He defined "sound prolongations" somewhat differently from the way the term is defined on page 210; he included in this category "sounds or parts of words that were prolonged, broken words, and words spoken with unusual stress." In other words, he found that listener ratings of stuttering severity depended chiefly on (1) rate of utterance and (2) "the number of words in relation to which a part-word repetition, a sound prolongation, a broken utterance, or unusual stress was observed, a word being counted only once no matter how many or how often these types of behavior were observed during its production" (56, pp. 42-43). He called the disfluency category which he defined in this way "repetitions." It is much like Sander's category of "disfluent words." Young reported correlations between repetitions, as he defined disfluent words, and speaking rate of .59 for both of two investigations each of which involved 50 adult stutterers. He obtained correlations, in the two samplings, of .87 and .85 between rated severity of stuttering and number of repetitions and correlations of .68 and .67 between rated severity of stuttering and speaking rate.

The data reviewed in the foregoing paragraphs serve to make clear that the word "stuttering" is not to be used as a synonym for "disfluency." Listeners react differently to the various forms of disfluency. Boehmler (10) found that sound or syllable repetitions were classified by laboratory observers as stuttering more often than were other kinds of disfluency; revisions and interjections were judged to be stuttering less often than were other disfluencies. Williams and Kent (53) reported that their laboratory observers, in judging disfluencies to be stuttered or nonstuttered, classified syllable repetitions and prolongations primarily as stuttered, and revisions primarily as nonstuttered. In a second study, concerned with the reactions of kindergarten and second-grade children to two different types of disfluency employed systematically by teachers in telling stories, Giolas and Williams (17) found that syllable repetitions appeared to be less acceptable to the children than were interjections of vowel sounds such as "ah."

In analyzing speech samples of stutterers, you have the problem of deciding which specific measure to employ. You can count all disfluencies and classify them in the categories defined on pages 209-210. If you do this you can make direct use of Tables 37-39 and 51-52 in evaluating your measurements for any given stutterer. If you tabulate repetitions of syllables, words and phrases, you can use as reference values the measurements summarized in Tables 41 and 50-53. If you make your disfluency analysis in accordance with Sander's "disfluent words," you may refer to Table 45 for comparison of your values with Sander's means and ranges and you can assume that roughly two-thirds of Sander's scores fell between the points one standard deviation below and one standard deviation above the mean in the case of each of his distributions. Thus, about two-thirds of his subjects performed between 8 and 72 disfluent words in his Session II for speaking, and between 0 and 64.5 disfluent words in his Session II for reading. You may also use Tables 42-44 (page 226) in evaluating scores in terms of Sander disfluent words.

Sander's standard deviations have some interesting implications, by the way. The fact that some of them are larger than their corresponding means indicates that the distributions of scores were considerably skewed or "long-tailed" in one direction; there was in each such case a piling up of scores toward the low end of the distribution, with a few scores falling at the high end of the distribution a relatively great distance away from the bulk of the measures. From these and other data, we may draw the generalization that there are more relatively mild than relatively severe stutterers—that is, most stutterers are "less severe than average." Bloodstein (7), for example, analyzed samples of the oral reading of 30 stutterers and found that whereas the average subject stuttered 10.8 percent of the words, half the subjects stuttered only 6.7 percent of the words, or less. That is, the median was 6.7, considerably below the mean of 10.8. As a matter of fact, nearly three-fourths of Bloodstein's readers stuttered fewer words than the mean reader did. This general type of finding has been reported by several investigators. It highlights a fact that is to be kept in mind in rating the severity of stuttering and in evaluating the results of your disfluency analyses of stutterers' speech samples. More stutterers are mild than severe—in relation to the mean stutterer, that is. Another way of saying this is that the median tends to be lower than the mean, as we have seen in the case of Bloodstein's study, referred to above.

You may prefer to make the type of disfluency analysis suggested by Young who, as we have seen, ended up with a single category made

up of what he called repetitions. If you use Young's single category
you will, in fact, simply count the words "in relation to which a part-
word repetition, a sound prolongation, a broken utterance, or unusual
stress" is observed. What you can use for normative data in that case
is to be found in Tables 49 and 46-48. Additional data from Young's
study are summarized in Table 57.

MEASURES OF RATE OF SPEAKING AND ORAL READING

Early investigators of stuttering behavior noted the generally inhibitory quality and the reduced rate of utterance which tends to be
characteristic of it. As work on the problem has progressed, the relationship between these two facets of stuttering has come to be increasingly well understood. Among the first laboratory studies bearing
on this matter was one carried out in 1932 by Lois Hickman Adams
(1) under the direction of Lee Edward Travis, in which adult stutterers were found to exhibit a narrower range of vocal pitch and less
pitch inflection than "good" and "trained" normal speakers, suggesting
a cautious or restrained mode of utterance. Johnson (19) in 1933 in
his original conceptualization of "the moment of stuttering," and,
with Knott (27) in 1936 in a further development of this basic idea,
pointed up the essentially inhibitory and conflicting character of stuttering behavoir as reflected in part in the speaking rate associated
with it. In 1935 Bluemel (9) published an inhibition theory of stuttering.

The expectation of stuttering has long been regarded as an integral
part of stuttering behavior or, by some writers, as a psychological or
emotional reaction associated with it. Johnson and Knott (27, 28) related the experience of expectancy to overt inhibitory or avoidant
speech reactions—by which they meant reactions carried out with
the intent of avoiding expected, and dreaded, stuttering. Johnson
(25) defined stuttering as "an anticipatory, hypertonic, apprehensive avoidance reaction." In a quantitative study of "expectation of
stuttering in relation to the occurrence of stuttering," Knott, Johnson,
and Webster (31) found that "expectation of stuttering was followed
by stuttering significantly more frequently than was definite expectation of no stuttering." Van Riper and Milisen (48) also reported a
notably consistent relationship of this kind, although they raised a
question about apparent exceptions, and Van Riper (47) concluded
that there is a high degree of correspondence between what he called
expectation and occurrence of block.

Two early studies, one by Johnson and Solomon (29) and the other
by Johnson and Ainsworth (23), were concerned primarily with ex-

pectancy as a form of response to specified words. Johnson and Solomon instructed stutterers to read a passage silently, marking the words on which they felt that they would stutter if they were later to read the passage aloud; later in reading the passage aloud they tended strongly to stutter on the same words they had previously marked as "expectancy words." Johnson and Ainsworth had stutterers follow the same procedure, with the exception that they only read silently, marking "expectancy words," and never read the passages aloud; in the second silent reading of a passage the stutterers tended significantly to expect stuttering on the same words on which they had expected stuttering from two to six weeks previously. Consistency in the words on which stuttering is expected in successive silent readings of a passage has also been demonstrated recently by Peins (35). In general, the relevant data indicate that expectation of stuttering is characterized by apprehensiveness and is integrally related to the stutterer's speech behavior, contributing heavily to its inhibitory quality.

The effect of expectancy of stuttering, together with the associated dread or anxiety or uneasiness, on the stutterer's rate of oral reading and speaking is a question of practical importance. The data published by Johnson (20) and summarized in Table 34 (p. 220) show that rate of utterance is slower for stutterers than for nonstutterers, and similar findings have been reported by other investigators. In 1944 Bloodstein (7) reported a significantly slower rate of oral reading for stutterers, even during nonstuttered intervals, than for nonstutterers; these rate data are summarized in Table 35 (p. 221). Bloodstein, in the same investigation, found a relationship between oral reading rate and severity of stuttering, represented by the data in Table 58. He found, for example, a correlation of −.88 between over-all reading rate and frequency of stuttering and a correlation of −.77 between nonstuttering reading rate and frequency of stuttering. In more recent research Young (56) found a correlation of .68 between the speaking rate of stutterers and the severity of their stuttering as rated by laboratory listeners. He also reported a correlation of .59 between rate of speaking and number of specified disfluencies. Sander (38) found correlations between number of disfluencies and rate of .81 for speaking and .86 for oral reading.

One possible approach to the dynamics involved in the relationship between expectancy as well as severity and rate was suggested by Robbins (36) who, in reporting a study in 1935, stated that "bad stammerers tend either to hold unduly the syllable before a difficult syllable, or to pause before the difficult syllable." In 1936 Van Riper (47) reported an investigation of the speech of stutterers in which he demonstrated changes in breathing, including increased relative duration of inspiration, occurring in anticipation of stuttering. Among the theoretical treatments of the expectancy factor are those of Van Riper (*46*), Wischner (*54, 55*), Sheehan (*39*), Bloodstein (*6*), Johnson and Knott (*27, 28*), and Johnson (*19; 21; 30*, pp. 233-264). They relate expectancy of stuttering to the phenomena of anxiety concerning expected stuttering, adaptation of the stuttering response, and consistency of the stimuli in relation to which the reactions of stuttering and the expectation of stuttering are made.

Williams (*51, 52*) has given particular emphasis to the practical clinical significance of the stutterer's inhibitory reactions, signalized notably by depressed rate of utterance and related phenomena, during the fluent, or at least nonstuttered, segments of his speech. In a study stimulated substantially by Williams' clinical orientations, Wendahl and Cole (*49*) have further quantified and extended the observation that the nonstuttered speech of stutterers is significantly different as perceived and judged by listeners from the speech of nonstutterers; one criterion used by the judges in differentiating samples of the speech of stutterers and of nonstutterers was "normalcy of rate." Roe, Derbyshire, and Sedroski (*37*) have developed a method of analyzing speech that makes possible a more intensive study of this general aspect of stuttering behavior. Their method involves measurements of "pause time" or nonphonated segments of continuous speech. Their findings also suggest that there is an inhibitory or "heel-dragging" quality in the speech of stutterers. Williams and his associates at Iowa are currently developing electronic computer equipment that will make possible extensive and systematic investigation of what might be called the "silence in speech" and its role in stuttering as well as nonstuttering speech behavior (*52*).

The implications of the data under review lend point and significance to the clinical evaluation of the stutterer's rate of oral reading and speaking. A major implication of these data is that severity of stuttering is, in part, a function of the inhibitory or avoidant behavior represented by depressed rate of utterance. This suppression of rate is due not only to the moments of overt stuttering but also to the general lack of expressiveness and spontaneity and the tendency to proceed apprehensively and cautiously, "looking for trouble," during the periods between stutterings. It follows that speech improvement for the stutterer is to be sought to an important degree through increased spontaneity, expressiveness, communicative desire or drive, a growing willingness to get going and keep moving ahead in speaking regardless of accustomed expectations of the stuttering that might occur. In large part this avenue of improvement is opened up and maintained by a change in the stutterer's basic understanding of stuttering as something he does himself rather than something that happens to him. So long as he thinks stuttering might happen to him at any moment he is oriented to be on guard against it; he is motivated to do his best to contend with it and to try to control it. So oriented and motivated, he proceeds hesitantly, reluctantly, uneasily, cautiously, and relatively slowly. To the degree that he comes to believe, to the contrary, that stuttering is nothing more nor less than his own avoidant and inhibitory reactions, the expectation of stuttering takes on an entirely different meaning and the grounds for apprehensiveness shift radically. This transformation, discussed elsewhere in this chapter, provides an apparently substantial approach to the stutterer's improvement. It may be encouraged considerably by the stutterer's change from what we have called a "have and am" language to a "do" language in his manner of thinking and talking, particularly to himself, about the problem. Your measurements of the stutterer's rate of utterance, in accordance with the procedures used in connection with Form 10 (p. 234), can be used to advantage in laying a foundation for clarifying and motivating this general approach to his improvement.

In view of the basic importance of rate measurements in evaluating the problems of the stutterers with whom you work, it is to be recommended that these measurements be made at the beginning of therapy and periodically thereafter. While you will want to make judicious use of the norms provided in Tables 34-36 (pp. 220-221) each rate measurement for a given stutterer is to be compared most fundamentally with his own previous measurements. Changes in his own rate of utterance are more important than any shifts of his position in the distribution of measurements for other stutterers, or for nonstutterers. Due consideration is to be given to the obvious fact that the same rate and the same amount of rate change can have very different meanings for two different stutterers. Each stutterer's past performance provides the most basic standard against which to evaluate his present or future performance in oral reading and speaking, so far as rate is concerned.

Form 10 provides for the computation of over-all rate and mean sentence rate in words per minute; instructions are presented in Chapter 8. The form does not provide for computation of rates of utterance for nonstuttered intervals of oral reading or speech. If you are interested in determining these rates, you may do so by following the same procedure that you use for measuring over-all rate, with the difference, of course, that you will need to eliminate the intervals that you judge as stuttered. A practical procedure consists of timing each of the successive nonstuttered segments of the tape by means of a stop watch. Sum the several times in seconds, and count the number of nonstuttered words. Then compute the rate in the usual way by dividing the number of words by the number of seconds and multiplying the result by 60.

MEASURES OF AMOUNT OF SPEAKING

Speaking-Time Log

The sheer amount of speaking that a stutterer does is one of the most important aspects of his speech behavior. For most stutterers improvement consists, in a peculiarly basic sense, in an increase in the amount of talking they do. It is advisable, therefore, to have any stutterer who enters a clinical program keep a speaking-time log for a few days soon after he comes into the clinic and about once a month thereafter. A sampling of three consecutive days each time a log is kept is sufficient for ordinary purposes. The stutterer may keep his log by using Form 12 (p. 237) and the procedure that goes with it which is described in Chapter 8.

It has been our experience that, during their first few days, even their first week in the clinic, most stutterers do not do an amount of talking that is typical for them. A stutterer is likely to give you a more valid speaking-time log, therefore, if you wait to have him begin keeping the log until he seems to have settled into the situation. The first log should not be so long delayed, however, that it will reflect the first notable effects of therapy. As a general rule, the stutterer should keep his first three-day log either during the last three days of his first week or the first three days of his second week in the Clinic. He should keep his subsequent logs for the same days of the week; that is, if he makes his first log for a Monday, Tuesday, and Wednesday he should keep all subsequent logs on Mondays, Tuesdays, and Wednesdays. The logs will be more highly comparable if he follows this rule; his speaking behavior will vary more or less from one part of the week to another.

If the stutterer is seen only for examination and does not remain in the clinic for therapy, at least on an outpatient basis, no fruitful use can be made of a speaking-time log. In any such case the Stutterer's Self-Ratings of Reactions to Speech Situations (Form 16), which may be used routinely in clinical examinations, affords a means of obtaining an estimate of the frequency with which the stutterer enters a sampling of common speaking situations.

Verbal Output in Test Situations

The data summarized in Tables 54 and 55 (p. 231) make very clear that in response to one and the same pattern of stimuli one person is likely to talk more or less than another. Such data suggest the possible significance of the verbal output (number of words spoken) of any stutterer from whom you obtain a tape-recorded speech sample by means of the procedures described in Chapter 8. This type of observation is of special interest in any case in which you obtain a series of tape-recorded speech samples over a period of several months in the course of a therapy program. While there are as yet no norms specifically designed for this type of evaluation, the observations of this sort that you are able to make will be likely to add to your over-all appreciation of the speaker's problem.

DESCRIPTION OF STUTTERING BEHAVIOR

Since we do not classify every speech disfluency we hear as stuttering, we need, particularly in our work as diagnostic clinicians, to be clear about those disfluencies and related reactions that we do, and do not, classify as stuttering. By using Form 13 to record your observations of what you regard as the speaker's stutterings, you can sharpen your awarenss of just what he does in speaking that you think he should, so far as possible, modify or eliminate. You can help the stutterer become more aware of these things he does—and that you feel he should work on—if you use the check list in Form 13 to point them up for him. He, too, can use the check list to sharpen his own perception of his speech-disrupting behavior. By using a tape recorder and watching himself in a mirror while speaking he will be able to observe his stuttering reactions better, and he can use his own observations, as noted on Form 13, as a basis for analysis and discussion. They will be especially helpful as a guide in modifying in desirable ways, or eliminating, the things that he does which interfere with his speaking.

It is particularly important that the stutterer ponder the question of whether the reactions listed on Form 13 are things that he does in trying to keep from stuttering. Stuttering, as we have noted, has been defined as an "anticipatory, apprehensive, hypertonic avoidance reaction" (25). A less polysyllabic way of saying this is that the things a stutterer does trying to keep from stuttering are the stuttering he does. If this is granted, it follows, of course, that if he were not to do the things that he does trying not to stutter, he would not do anything that he or anyone else would regard as stuttering. It is very important, therefore—so far as this explanation may be considered acceptable— that the stutterer become keenly conscious of just what it is that he is doing that keeps him from talking more smoothly. These are the particular things he does in speaking that he will want to work at changing—and he will want to test and cultivate his ability just to go ahead and talk without doing them at all.

Form 13 has spaces for recording observations of six stuttered words —words, that is, that you, or the stutterer himself, or some other observer regards as stuttered. It is not necessary, of course, to observe six consecutive stuttered words. Indeed, this would not always be possible. Instead, choose words separated in time so that you can be relatively thorough in noting details and in recording your observations.

ASSIGNMENT

Use Form 13 to record your observations of two stutterers. Ask each of these stutterers to record his own observations of himself, also, using Form 13. The stutterer should watch himself in a mirror while talking to you. He should also, if possible, use a tape recorder and observe the audible aspects of his stuttering behavior by listening to the tape. Write a concise summary of your observations of each stutterer, together with the two or three most important suggestions you have to make concerning the reactions to be modified or eliminated first, and how the stutterer might go about making these changes. Ask each stutterer to write a similar statement. Compare your statements with theirs.

RATING OF SEVERITY OF STUTTERING

The rating scale is one of the most widely used means of evaluating the speech of stutterers. Such a scale and the procedure employed in using it may be simple or elaborate. The method which we present here for routine clinical use is quite simple. You will use it with a more cultivated sense of its limitations and its practical value if you first examine such discussions of scaling theory and procedure, together with research methods and findings, as those of Lewis and Sherman (*32*), Sherman (*40*), and Young (*56*). Meanwhile, it will serve to clarify the problem somewhat if we consider briefly the procedure employed by Young in securing severity ratings of tape-recorded samples of the speech of 50 adult male stutterers. He employed three groups of listeners (stutterers, speech clinicians, and laymen).

The listeners in each session attended to the 50 tape-recorded speech samples, taking four short rest periods while the experimenter changed the test tapes, and rated the severity of stuttering of each sample on the basis of a nine-point equal-appearing intervals scale. Two short samples of speech were chosen to represent the extremes on this scale and were incorporated as part of the instructions to the raters. These segments were chosen from the tape-recorded speech samples of the two speakers who exhibited the highest and lowest total numbers of disfluencies (*56*, p. 37).

Young gave the raters these instructions:

"You are about to hear some samples of speech from speakers who consider themselves to be stutterers. Your task will be to make an over-all rating of the severity of stuttering in each sample. You will do this on a nine-point scale on which a rating of 1 means no stuttering. (You may or may not judge any given sample to contain stuttering.) A rating of 2 means very mild stuttering and a rating of 9 means very severe stuttering. A rating of 5, in the middle of this scale, indicates an average severity of stuttering. The other values on the scale, 3, 4, and 6, 7, 8, represent equal intervals between these scale points. Before you start, however, you will hear a few segments of speech arbitrarily chosen to represent extremes on this nine-point scale. Now we will begin the judging procedure. Remember, a rating of 1 means no stuttering and a rating of 9 indicates very severe stuttering, while a rating of 5 is to be considered a middle point between these two extremes. Please be sure to rate every sample, giving only one rating. Each sample is numbered, and the number of each sample will be announced just before the sample is presented. Write your rating in the space provided in each case. You will be allowed a short pause after each sample to record your rating. Are there any questions?"

"Twenty-four hundred ratings of severity of stuttering were obtained from the 48 experimental listeners. The mean rating of severity of stuttering for all 48 listeners was 3.84, with the means for G1 (stutterers), G2 (clinicians), and G3 (laymen) being 4.01, 3.88, and 3.68, respectively."

It may be that in an occasional clinical situation or, more likely, in the laboratory, you will prefer to use the relatively precise and elaborate scaling methods represented by this quotation; but probably you would not often employ them for general clinical purposes. This description of Young's procedure, however, should serve to bring into focus the question of how best to rate the severity of stuttering in routine clinical situations where procedures of the type described by Young are not feasible. In recommending the gross rating method presently to be described, we are at pains to call attention to its limitations, and to urge that you regard the ratings obtained by means of it as rough measures only. It is to be taken for granted that you and others who work with you will make judgments of the severity of the problem of every stutterer you serve clinically. The major virtue of the rating procedure here presented is that it insures a certain degree of uniformity and comparability of the judgments that you and others make of particular stutterers. For all these precautions, however, it is by no means to be overlooked or underemphasized that the sorts of listener judgments represented by ratings, however rough and even wildly unscientific they may be, are among the most substantial facts of life that stutterers face hour after hour day in and day out. They are, therefore, extremely important—regardless of their precision or reliability as gauged by laboratory standards. It is, for all practical purposes, impossible to disregard them in working with stutterers clinically.

A scale of severity can provide for distinguishing mild from severe stuttering, or mild from moderate or severe stuttering, or for still finer distinctions. The accompanying scale, Form 14, represents a continuum from 0 (no stuttering) through 1 (very mild stuttering) to 7 (very severe stuttering). You should think of the intermediate degrees of severity between 1 and 7 as falling at equally spaced intervals, with the midpoint of the scale, or 4, representing average or moderate stuttering. The various scale values are defined for the purpose of making the ratings of different observers as comparable as possible. It is not assumed that any one of these definitions will necessarily fit exactly the speaking performance of any specific stutterer on any particular occasion; the definitions are intended simply as guide lines.

It is desirable that each stutterer be rated by more than one clinician if possible and by a number of his lay associates and friends. He should also rate himself. Discrepancies among these ratings can be analyzed and discussed to advantage.

You may base your rating of a stutterer on more than one sample of his speech, and the more samples of his speech you observe the more valid your rating is likely to be. If you base your rating on a single sample be sure to describe the sample and situation clearly enough to indicate whether or not your rating might be comparable with another one made by you or someone else. If you use the rating sheet for evaluating more than one sample of speech, or for making a general rating on the basis of all observations made of the stutterer's speech during a stated period of time, supply the information called for at the end of the rating sheet accordingly. Comparison of ratings based on oral reading and speaking can sometimes provide a basis for worthwhile analysis of factors related to variations in severity of a given speaker's stuttering. A similar use can be made of ratings made by different observers or in different situations.

Ratings might well be made once each month or so during therapy. Two or more observers should make these ratings, since some disagreement among raters is to be expected, and a consensus is more valid than a single judgment.

Using Form 14, rate the severity of the stuttering of two stutterers. Place each one at a point on the scale by making a check mark beside that point. Ask each of these two stutterers to rate himself on Form 14. Give a copy of Form 14 to each of three friends of each stutterer and ask each of them to rate the severity of his stuttering. Be sure that each rater indicates whether each rating was made while observing the stutterer read aloud, or speak, and whether it was meant to cover one or more speech samples, or all of the stutterer's speaking and oral reading observed by the rater over an extended period of time. Write a brief summary of these several ratings, and if there are discrepancies among the ratings try to explain them and discuss their possible implications. Is it more likely that differences among the ratings represent variations in severity of the stuttering or differences in the rating behavior of the observers? In either case, how would you explain the differences?

IOWA SCALE OF ATTITUDE TOWARD STUTTERING

A further part of the analysis of the stuttering problem is an assessment of the speaker's feelings about his own speech and about stuttering and stutterers in general. In many cases you will also want to investigate the attitudes toward stuttering of the stutterer's parents and perhaps of some of his other important listeners.

The Iowa Scale of Attitude Toward Stuttering, developed by Ammons and Johnson (*3*), is designed to be used in this connection. The scale consists of 45 statements about stutterers and what they should or should not do or feel in various speaking situations. The person to whom the scale is administered is asked to indicate his opinion about each statement, to state whether he strongly agrees with it, moderately agrees, moderately disagrees, strongly disagrees, or is undecided. The numerical score yielded by the scale is intended to throw some light on the respondent's attitude toward stuttering, specifically his tolerance or intolerance of stuttering. The authors, using a split-half technique, estimated the reliability of the scale to be .89.

In Table 59 data having a certain degree of normative value are summarized. The table shows mean, median, and quartile values for an Iowa Speech Clinic sampling of 162 parents of stutterers and for 36 of their children who were old enough to respond to the scale. Ammons and Johnson administered an original 160-item form of the test to four different groups, 63 stutterers, 61 speech clinicians and advanced students of speech pathology, 40 university freshmen, and

40 townspeople of Iowa City. The clinicians' mean of 1.37 represented the best attitude; the stutterers scored a mean of 1.53, the freshmen a mean of 1.58, and the townspeople indicated the least tolerance of stuttering with a mean of 1.73. The authors emphasize, however, that all groups bunched their scores toward the low or "good" end of the scale. The skewness of the distribution of all scores combined was almost certainly too great to be attributed to chance. The authors suggest that it might indicate a cultural value of acceptance of stuttering that is not applied consistently in actual practice. In other words, it is well to interpret responses to the scale with due consideration of the common tendency of people to give verbal expression to somewhat better attitudes than they live by.

You may give this questionnaire to any person who is able to read it and follow instructions in responding to it. Anyone with at least junior high school reading ability should be able to understand the marking system employed and to grasp the point of each statement without help.

Note that the stutterer is asked on the face sheet of the questionnaire to indicate his judgment as to the severity of his own stuttering. This self-rating provides one more indication of the severity of the problem and may be compared with the ratings which you and others make of his stuttering in using the Scale for Rating Severity of Stuttering (Form 14).

In administering the Iowa Scale of Attitude Toward Stuttering, present it to the person who is to fill it out and explain it briefly to him. Ask him to read the statements on the first page and to fill in the blanks that apply to him. Then ask him to respond to each of the 45 items of the scale, circling the response to each which best reflects his own attitude.

Although there can be no absolute right or wrong responses to statements such as those that comprise the Scale of Attitude Toward Stuttering, certain responses appear to reflect a more healthful attitude toward the problem than do others. In scoring the scale, the most preferred answers are given a weight of 1. Responses which indicate increasingly lesser degrees of tolerance are weighted 2, 3, and 4. Responses of "Undecided" are given a weight of 0. The five possible responses to each item are, then, scored as follows:

Response	Weights
Strongly agree	4
Moderately agree	3
Moderately disagree	2
Strongly disagree	1
Undecided	0

In scoring the scale, indicate the value of each response made by writing the appropriate number in the margin after each item. Total the values so indicated. In order to derive a mean value, which you will use as the respondent's score on the scale, divide the total by the number of items answered minus the number of items marked "Undecided." For example, a person might have made a total score of 118. Of the 45 items, he omitted two and marked three "Undecided." To obtain his mean score you would divide 118 by 40—that is, $45 - (2 + 3)$. His mean score would be 2.95. Enter the mean score in the blank marked "Score" at the top of the first page of the scale.

The lower the score, the better the attitude toward stuttering. The following roughly defined categories, used judiciously, may be useful in evaluating the scores obtained:

1. Scores between 1.0 and 1.4 represent very good attitudes, considerable tolerance of stuttering.
2. Scores between 1.4 and 2.2 represent average or moderate attitudes.
3. Scores above 2.2 represent poor attitudes, considerable intolerance of stuttering.

The score itself is of limited value, largely because it is obviously easy for the subject, if he is so inclined, to make responses that "look good"—or that "look bad"—rather than responses that reflect his attitude in an honest or valid fashion. The responses are probably most valid when the scale is filled out by stutterers or other persons who are essentially uninformed about the problem. After a stutterer has spent a few weeks in the speech clinic with you he may very well know how he should respond to the scale items, and you will need to decide as best you can in such a case whether the attitude the person expresses is his own or a reflection of your attitude which he has not really made his own and does not live by for the most part. You will probably use the scale mainly as a means of exploring for leads that you will want to follow up in your counseling sessions with the stutterer or his parents or teachers. Even if the answers seem to be the right ones, you will do well to determine as best you can whether they are valid, and so far as they seem not to be you may want to give attention to them in counseling.

ASSIGNMENT

Administer the Iowa Scale of Attitude Toward Stuttering (Form 15) to two individuals assigned to you as stutterers and to two persons who are

important to one of the two stutterers. These might be his parents, or a room-
mate, close friend, sweetheart, husband or wife, brother or sister, or teacher
perhaps. Give each of these two persons a copy of the scale, explain it briefly,
and ask him to read the statements on the first page and fill in the blanks
that apply to him. Then ask him to complete the scale. Finally, complete the
scale yourself.

THE STUTTERER'S SELF-RATINGS OF REACTIONS TO SPEECH SITUATIONS

By filling out Form 16, Stutterer's Self-Ratings of Reactions to
Speech Situations, a stutterer indicates four aspects of his adjustment
to a sample of 40 common types of speech situations. The responses
he makes to the rating scales are especially useful in providing indications of trouble spots and of his possible need for counseling with
respect to certain aspects of the problem.

Shumak (42) analyzed the responses made to this test by 95 adult
male stutterers between approximately 17 and 30 years of age in the
University of Iowa Speech Clinic. By correlating the scores made on
the four parts of the test, she found that to some degree ($r = .52$) the
more frequently the subject stuttered in specified types of speech situations the more he tried to avoid entering these situations. She also
reported that the more the stutterer disliked the speech situations the
more he avoided going into situations ($r - .84$). Moreover, the more
the speaker stuttered in the situations the more he disliked speaking
in them ($r = .57$). As these findings suggest, you can use a stutterer's
responses to this test as a means of helping him to understand some
of the more important interactions among the different facets of his
total problem.

In administering the test, present it to the stutterer and ask him to
read the instructions. In scoring his responses, add the numbers written by him in each column and write the sum in the space provided
as the Total. Divide this sum by the number of items answered, carry
to one decimal place, and enter the quotient in the space provided for
Average. The lower the average the better—that is, low scores represent better reactions than high scores.

Evaluate the average for each column with reference to the values
shown in Table 60, based on the work of Shumak (42). The values
shown in Table 60 are for adults, mostly college-age, and for the most
part stutterers who are college or university students. In the absence
of norms for younger age levels, use those given in Table 60 with all
due caution in evaluating scores. The rating sheet can be administered
to junior or senior high school stutterers, but it can hardly be used for
most subjects below 14 or 15 years of age.

With these considerations in mind, then, you may use Table 60 in this general way: a score of 2.8 for Avoidance, for example, would place the stutterer who makes it at the 75th percentile for Shumak's college-age stutterers; this would mean that 75 percent of Shumak's subjects made lower scores than his—and low scores are good scores. A score of 2.8 for Avoidance, therefore, is not very good.

You may also interpret the average in a general way by reference to the descriptions of the five numbered responses for each column. Thus, you might fairly interpret an average of 2.8 for Avoidance as showing that the stutterer probably does not try to avoid speaking situations "on the average," though sometimes he would like to and occasionally actually does try to avoid them.

Of more importance than the average, however, which is clearly a rather abstract bit of information in this instance, is the number of items rated 1, 2, 3, 4, and 5, respectively, in each column. If, for example, 25 of the 40 items are rated 4 or 5 under Frequency, you would doubtless conclude that one of the important objectives of therapy would be to increase the frequency with which the person enters into common speech situations. In general, the more often the stutterer talks the better, and the greater the variety of situations in which he does his talking the better. After all, in a very important sense, the working time for a stutterer working on his speech is his *speaking* time. For this reason a measure of the frequency with which a stutterer meets representative speech situations such as this rating sheet affords, is of value from a clinical point of view. It is a measure that you may well make periodically during therapy. Moreover, an examination of the response made to each item will often suggest to you specific activities or goals to be attempted during remedial training.

The stutterer's responses in the Stuttering column yield practical information concerning the specific types of situations to which he needs particularly to make a better speech adjustment—and from them you may also draw possible tentative generalizations as to the common denominators in his hard and easy situations, respectively. These common denominators—which may be such things as the age or status of listeners, audience or group situations, etc.—are helpful in suggesting specific needs for counseling and additional speaking experience and specific types of practice.

The responses made in the Reaction and Avoidance columns should be compared with those in the other two columns. They indicate motivational tendencies to be developed (such as those suggested by 1's and 2's in both the Reaction and Avoidance columns), eliminated, or reversed (such as those implied by the 4's and 5's especially).

avoidance
Reaction
Stuttering
Frequency

Administer Form 16 to at least two individuals assigned to you as stutterers. Check in each case to see that the subject understands the instructions and the nature of the aspects of adjustment that are surveyed by the rating sheet.

THE ADAPTATION OF STUTTERING

Since the adaptation effect was first reported and named in 1937 by Johnson and Knott (*26*), it has been observed repeatedly that when a stutterer makes several successive oral readings of a passage there is a tendency for the number of words that are judged as stuttered to decrease from reading to reading. In additional studies done at Iowa by Donohue (*14*), Shulman (*41*), Wischner (*54*), Cohen (*13*), and others it has been found that there is also statistically significant, though less, adaptation of stuttering during continuous oral reading of changing, or nonrepeating, material. Cohen (*13*) and Newman (*34*) found still less, but some, adaptation during extemporaneous speaking.

On Form 17 provision is made for computation of the adaptation of frequency of stuttering and also the adaptation of oral reading rate. As was noted in Chapter 8, there is a considerable relationship between frequency of stuttering (or of disfluency) and rate of oral reading or of speaking. As a general rule, a *decrease* in the number of stuttered words during oral reading goes along with an *increase* in the rate of reading as measured in words per minute.

Procedures employed to measure adaptation in frequency of stuttering can also be used, if desired, to measure adaptation in frequency of disfluency, as defined in Chapter 8. In measuring adaptation of stuttering, of course, you must decide with respect to each disfluency whether or not to classify it as stuttering, whereas in measuring the adaptation of disfluency you need not make this sort of decision. If you do not classify all the disfluencies in a reading sample as stuttering, your measures of adaptation for disfluency and for stuttering, respectively, may be different, of course.

You may wonder whether there is some hard and fast rule to be followed in deciding whether or not a particular disfluent word is to be classified as a stuttered word. No, there does not exist in the Bureau of Standards in Washington, or anywhere else, a sample of disfluency that "is stuttering" and another sample of disfluency that "is not stuttering." You must unavoidably use your own judgment, with or without comparing notes with other clinicians, as to whether or not a specific disfluency is to be regarded as stuttering. For further discussion of this matter, together with relevant data, see Johnson (*20, 25, 30*), Young (*56*), Williams (*51*), Tuthill (*45*), Boehmler (*10*), and Bloodstein, Jaeger, and Tureen (8).

The stuttering adaptation effect is important mainly because a stutterer's improvement usually consists, in part, in a decrease in the frequency of his stuttering reactions. Adaptation, therefore, may be viewed *within limits and with due qualifications* as a sort of miniature "model of improvement." It is to be emphasized, however, that adaptation is less variable as a group phenomenon than as an individual characteristic, and that due caution is to be exercised in generalizing from the adaptation exhibited by a given stutterer in a specific situation on a particular day. Whether or not a stutterer's adaptation during successive readings of a test passage may be usefully compared to long-term improvement in his speech, you are interested in two chief kinds of observation that you can make of such adaptation, or by means of it. First, you can observe the amount of adaptation in the test situation and, second, you can explore to some extent the conditions under which adaptation is increased or decreased.

The following statements represent some of the possible interpretations of the sorts of data that are to be obtained from adaptation readings.

1. If a speaker stutters more rather than less frequently from reading to reading, the reason might be that to him stuttering is more fearful or unpleasant than his anticipation of it. Each time he stutters, therefore, he becomes a little more rather than a little less anxious about whether or not he might stutter again. The more anxious he becomes the more he does the things that he feels he must do in order to keep from stuttering—and when he does these things he experiences them—and others regard them—as his stuttering. If he dreads stuttering a little more each time he reads the passage he will try a little harder to keep from stuttering, and so he will do more of the things that he, and you, regard as stuttering.

2. If the stutterer does not adapt appreciably, but stutters about the same number of words in one reading as another, one assumption you can make is that he is more or less like the sort of stutterer just discussed. Another possibility, of course, is that he was, to begin with, so well adapted to the reading passage and the situation and to you that there was, in effect, no room for improvement.

3. If the speaker adapts, stuttering fewer and fewer words from reading to reading, one interpretation is that the stuttering is less anxiety producing than the speaker's anticipation of it. It may be less anxiety producing because your reactions to it are not fearful to the

reader, or because with each rereading he feels that he is communicating less and less to you, and so whether or not he stutters may seem less important to him.

You may sometimes want to instruct the stutterer to do his best to read without stuttering.[1] If he stutters more frequently and adapts less or not at all under this condition, it is a possibly reasonable assumption that in trying to keep from stuttering he is doing the things that constitute his stuttering behavior. The demonstration is one that you may want to use in some cases to help the stutterer appreciate more clearly the nature of his problem. If he stutters less or adapts more under this condition, you will want to discuss with the stutterer which of these two explanations seems the more likely: (1) the stutterer employs some technique or pattern of speech behavior, such as speaking very slowly or in a rhythm, by means of which he keeps going, or (2) he has learned to speak more fluently as a result of therapy designed to enable him to develop his inclination to go ahead and speak without indulging in the reactions that formerly disrupted his speech (and that still do whenever he performs them). Artificial patterns of speech such as those involving slow rate or exaggerated rhythms are to be evaluated with a view to their longterm advantages, if any, or disadvantages, as the case may seem to be.

Investigations have been made of variation in adaptation from one reading passage to another, from one listener to another, with number of listeners, with length of reading passage, with amount of time between readings, and other conditions (*13, 14, 26, 31, 34, 41, 54*). If you are interested in making other relevant clinical uses of adaptation tests you should consult the reports of these and related studies.

Theoretical issues raised by the various possible definitions of adaptation, the methods of measuring it, and the data obtained under a variety of experimental conditions have been discussed by Wischner (*54, 55*), and by Tate, Cullinan, and Ahlstrand (*44*).

Procedure for Measuring Adaptation of Stuttering

Using the procedure described on page 204, obtain a sample of the oral reading of a stutterer. When he has finished ask him to read the passage a second time, and when he has finished ask him to read it a third time, and a fourth time, and a fifth. Time each reading carefully by means of a stop watch or a watch with a second hand.

During the first reading of the passage, follow along on your own copy and write the numeral 1 above each word you judge to be stuttered. During the second reading write a 2, during the third read-

---

[1] This general type of instruction was employed in a pilot study done as an M.A. thesis by Marjorie Ann Ahlstrand at the University of Iowa under the direction of Dean Williams in 1962.

ing a 3, during the fourth a 4, and during the fifth reading a 5, above each word classified by you as stuttered. You may do this while the stutterer is reading, or if you use a tape recorder you may mark the stuttered words—and also time each reading—later while listening to the tape recording.

Count the words you judged as stuttered and enter your totals for the different readings in the appropriate spaces on Form 17. Enter the time in seconds for each reading in the spaces provided. Then complete Form 17.

You may use the data obtained by means of this procedure to obtain a measure of adaptation based on a somewhat different method of computation. For this purpose use the chart in Figure 3, and proceed as follows. Find the point on the horizontal axis that represents the percentage of words stuttered by the subject during the first reading and project a vertical line upward from this point. Locate the point on the vertical axis that corresponds to the percentage of words stuttered during the fifth reading, and project a horizontal line to the right of this point. The score on the curved line nearest the intersection of the vertical and horizontal lines is the adaptation score. If the point is closer to the point midway between two curved lines than to either line, add 1.0 to the score indicated by the upper line.

Tate, Cullinan, and Ahlstrand (44), who devised the chart, found that it appeared to give reasonably good adaptation scores for subjects other than those from whose data it was derived—good in the sense that the scores correlated highly with other more general and exact measures. It is to be considered, even so, that the chart was constructed by analyzing data obtained from one particular sample of stutterers, and you must always weigh the degree to which a given speaker tested by you is a member of the population sampled. You should familiarize yourself with the details of the report by Tate, Cullinan, and Ahlstrand (44) in order to safeguard your interpretations based on the chart in specific instances.

ASSIGNMENTS

Using Form 17 and the procedure described above, do the following assignments:

1. Tape record five successive readings by a stutterer of the passage "Your Rate on Oral Reading" on page 232, or "Arthur, the Young Rat" on page 233. Mark and tally the words you judge as stuttered in each reading of the passage and enter your tallies on Form 17. Also time each reading and

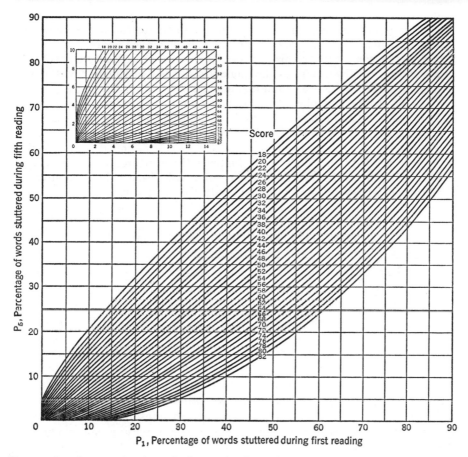

FIGURE 3. A reproduction of chart of adaptation scores independent of initial frequency of stuttering. Directions for use of the chart, printed lower right, are as follows: "Enter chart at P_1, the percentage of words stuttered during first reading. Go vertically up to the point directly opposite P_5, the percentage of words stuttered during the fifth reading. The curved line nearest the point gives the adaptation score. If the point is closer to midway between two lines than to either line, add one to the score given by the upper line. If $P_1 < 15$, $P_5 < 10$, refer to inset figure at upper left of chart. Examples: if $P_1 = 7$, $P_5 = 4$, the score is 46; if $P_1 = 50$, $P_5 = 32\frac{1}{2}$, the score is 57. The adaptation scores given by the curved lines are standard scores, mean 50, standard deviation 10. They were obtained from the residuals about the line of regression of P_5 on P_1, after an arc line sine transformation of the Ps, in a group of 89 college students enrolled in the University of Iowa Speech Clinic during the years 1955-1959. The students read the 180-word passage 'Arthur the Young Rat.'" (Copies of this chart may be obtained from the Interstate Printers and Publishers, Inc., 19-27 North Jackson Street, Danville, Illinois.) From the *Journal of Speech and Hearing Research*, 1961, *4* (4): 321-339.

enter the time of each reading in seconds in the space provided. Complete the computations called for on Form 17. Compute the adaptation score also by using Chart A, following the instructions given above.

2. Using the same tape recording and the same procedures, measure the adaptation of disfluency, as disfluency is defined in Chapter 8. Compute adaptation scores for (a) total disfluencies; (b) interjections; (c) repetitions of words and phrases combined; and (d) part-word repetitions, broken words, and prolonged sounds combined. Compare these adaptation scores with that for words you judged as stuttered.

3. After a minimal interval of 24 hours, repeat Assignment 1 and Assignment 2(a), with this difference: instruct the stutterer to do his best to read without stuttering. Compare results and discuss their possible implications with your supervisor and with the stutterer.

THE CONSISTENCY OF STUTTERING

Several investigators (25, 22) have observed that when a stutterer reads the same passage two or more times in succession, he tends to stutter on the same words from reading to reading. This finding was first reported by Johnson and Knott (26), who named it the consistency effect.

The consistency effect indicates that stuttering is something the speaker *does*, rather than something like a disease or a disorder or a trait that he *has*, or a disfunction that *occurs* in a random or hit-or-miss fashion. It suggests that what we call a speaker's stuttering consists of responses that he makes to certain cues or stimuli, such as specific words. Some of the possible reasons why some words are stuttered more consistently than other words have been indicated by Johnson and Brown (24), who found that words which begin with consonants are stuttered by most stutterers more often than words which begin with vowels. Brown (12) reported also that the stuttering response is more often made to long words than to short ones; to words at the beginnings of sentences; and to nouns, verbs, adverbs, and adjectives than to conjunctions, prepositions, pronouns, and articles. He found, too, that meaningful words elicit the stuttering response more frequently than do nonsense words or syllables (11); a similar finding has been reported also by Eisenson and Horowitz (16). In other research it has been observed that the stuttering response is more frequently made in some situations, or to certain listeners, or in reacting to certain other conditions—even the color of the paper from which the stutterer reads—than in other situations, with other listeners, etc. (22, 25, 54, 55).

The importance of a consistency measure for an individual stutterer is that, in general, it may indicate how strongly his stuttering responses are associated with the stimuli or cues to which they have, presumably, been conditioned. You can use this information in helping the stutterer to understand that his stuttering is something that he does, rather than something that mysteriously happens to him. It can be an impressive and very enlightening discovery for the stutterer that he makes his stuttering responses in a more or less orderly relationship to certain words and other cues. Relevant analysis and discussion are likely to suggest to the stutterer that he is, indeed, singling out certain words as those on which he expects to have trouble. Peins (35) observed that when she asked stutterers to read a passage silently five times in succession on each of four consecutive days and to underline words on which they expected they would stutter if they were reading orally to the group, "more than half the words expected to be stuttered on a given reading were expected to be stuttered on a previous reading." And essentially similar findings were obtained in earlier studies by Johnson and Solomon (29) and Johnson and Ainsworth (23).

The stutterer's expectations, of course, may be so fleeting and subtle as to seem to him all but unconscious. The consistency effect implies that he expects trouble on the words with which he has had trouble before. He appears to react to his expectation of trouble by getting ready to avoid it, to keep it from happening, as he might say; or to control it if he cannot avoid it. It is important for him to consider the view that what he does trying to avoid the stuttering he expects, and to control or stop the stuttering he is doing, is precisely nothing more nor less than what he calls his stuttering. In other words—and for him they are tremendously significant words—his stuttering consists of what he does trying not to stutter again, or any longer.

After you have determined a stutterer's Consistency Index you may contribute to his working understanding of the nature of his problem by discussing with him his degree of consistency. He may gain a clearer sense of purpose in therapy by giving due consideration to the implication that his stuttering is his own doing, that it is something he has learned to do—without meaning to, of course—in the very act of trying not to do it. He may be well advised to ponder the possibility that he is as consistent as he is in doing it in response to certain words because they are the words on which he has done it before. What he has done in the past he remembers as stuttering and as trouble, and the words associated with trouble in the past are, therefore, the words on which he expects to have trouble again. The implication is that he does what he feels he must do in order to avoid the stuttering that he expects to occur—and what he does to avoid the stuttering *is the stuttering he does.*

It follows from these observations and considerations that if he would do nothing to avoid stuttering there would be no stuttering—simply because he would not do the things that constitute stuttering. And if he would not do those things, presumably they would not occur by themselves, without his doing them. The stutterer's contemplation of the consistency effect, therefore, goes far to bring into clear focus for him just what he must learn to do in order to improve his speaking. He must learn to talk without doing the various things he has been doing in his misguided effort to keep from stuttering. He must learn, that is, just to go ahead and talk. This is not to say that it will necessarily be easy for him to learn this, or that he can learn it in a short time.

Tate and Cullinan (*43*) have evaluated the several different methods proposed for computing the degree or strength of the consistency effect. See their article and the additional publications to which they refer for further information about the various technical problems involved in research on the consistency effect.

A relatively simple procedure for measuring consistency is presented here. It is designed to serve essential purposes in most clinical situations. As computed by means of this procedure, degree of consistency is expressed as a Consistency Index. In using this method, you compute in each case the percentage of the words which you have judged as stuttered in a given reading of a passage that are words which you also judged as stuttered in one or more specified previous readings of the passage. For example, suppose that you have a subject read a 100-word passage twice, and that you judge him to stutter on 20 words, or 20 percent of all the words, in the first reading and on 15 words in the second reading. (In Form 18, the 20 percent would be entered as *A*.) Suppose, further, that of the 15 words stuttered in the second reading 12, or 80 percent, were among the 20 words stuttered in the first reading. His Consistency Index, therefore, is 80 percent. (In Form 18, the 80 percent would be entered as *B*.)

Relevant studies (*22, 26*) have shown that in a series of successive readings of a passage the average adult stutterer is about 65 to 70 percent consistent—that is, of the words he stutters in any given reading about two-thirds are words that he had stuttered in the preceding reading.

Concerning Form 18: In making out Form 18 you divide *A* by *B*—that is, you divide the percentage of words stuttered in the first reading, for example, by the percentage of words stuttered in the second reading that were also stuttered in the first reading. The value you obtain in dividing *A* by *B* provides a general comparison between the consistency of stuttering that could have occurred by chance and the consistency of stuttering that actually did occur. When this value is 1.0 or less it represents an absence of consistency; it shows that the stutterer was no more consistent, or even less consistent, in stuttering on words previously stuttered than on other words. The term "chance" as used here has the meaning suggested in the following explanation. Suppose, for example, one stutters 10 percent of all the words in the first reading of a passage. Now, in the second reading of the passage he is no more likely *by chance* to stutter on one word than on any other word. Therefore, *by chance* 10 percent of the words he stutters in the second reading will be among the 10 percent that he stuttered in the first reading and 90 percent will be among the 90 percent he did not stutter in the first reading. If more than 10 percent of the words he stutters in the second reading are among the words that he stuttered in the first reading, he is more consistent than he would have been by chance. In that case the value you obtain in dividing A by B will be greater than 1.0.

In general, the higher the value obtained by dividing A by B, the greater the degree of consistency it represents—the more, that is, the observed consistency exceeds chance consistency. This statement needs to be duly qualified by consideration of the magnitude of B in each case. If, for example, 80 percent of all words in the passage were stuttered in the first reading, then even if 100 percent of the words that are stuttered in the second reading were also stuttered in the first, A divided by B—in this case, 100 divided by 80—would give a value of only 1.25. If, on the other hand, 10 percent of all words were stuttered in the first reading, and 100 percent of all words stuttered in the second reading were also stuttered in the first reading, then A divided by B would be 100 divided by 10, which would give a value of 10. The value obtained is to be evaluated, therefore, by reference to the magnitude of the B term in each case.

Procedure for Measuring Consistency of Stuttering

Using the procedure described on page 204, obtain a sample of oral reading from a stutterer. When he has finished, ask him to read the passage a second time; and, again, when he has finished, ask him to read it a third time. Tape record the readings if possible. (You may, if you prefer, use the first three readings you tape recorded in doing Assignment No. 1 on page 270.)

During the first reading of the passage, follow along on your own copy and write the numeral 1 above each word you judge to be stuttered. During the second reading write a 2 and during the third reading a 3 above each word classified by you as stuttered. You may do this while the stutterer is reading, or if you use a tape recorder you may mark the stuttered words later while listening to the tape recording.

Count the words you judged as stuttered and enter your totals for the three readings in the appropriate spaces on Form 18. Then complete Form 18.

ASSIGNMENTS

Use Form 18 and the procedure described above.
1. Obtain from one stutterer a series of three consecutive readings of "Your Rate of Oral Reading" or of "Arthur, the Young Rat."
2. Mark and tally the words judged by you as stuttered in each reading of the passage, and enter your tallies on Form 18.
3. Complete the computations called for on Form 18. (See p. 292).
4. It is possible also, of course, to measure the consistency of disfluency, as disfluency is defined on page 209, by employing the procedure used here for measuring the consistency of stuttering. In measuring the consistency of disfluency, do not sort the disfluencies into those to be classified as stuttering and those not to be so classified.

TABLE 56. Percentages of Control and Clinical Group Fathers and Mothers Who Reported That the Child Was Performing Each of the Indicated Speech Reactions When They First Thought the Child Was Stuttering (Control Group Parents Answered with Reference to the First Time They Thought the Child's Speech Was Disfluent)

| Group and Item | Repetition | | | | | Other Disfluency | | | |
	Combined[a]	Only[b]	Syllable	Word	Phrase	Sound Prolongations	Silent Intervals, Pauses	Interjections	"Complete Blocks"[c]
Control									
Fathers (N=69)	79	42	4	59	23	3	36	30	0
Mothers (N=80)	61	35	10	41	24	4	41	21	0
Clinical									
Fathers (N=143)	85	72	57	48	8	15	7	8	3
Mothers (N=146)	90	77	59	50	8	12	3	9	3

[a] Children for whom repetitions of any kind were reported, alone or in combination with one or more other types of reaction.

[b] Children for whom the only reactions reported were repetitions (and interjections such as "uh uh," which are also usually repeated, provided they were combined with one or more of the categories of repetition—sound or syllable, word or phrase).

[c] Defined liberally with possible error on the side of including rather than excluding specific instances in this category; this general type of report was given for nine children, but in no case did both parents agree in this kind of description.

SOURCE: Johnson et al., 30.

TABLE 57. Summary of Measures of Disfluency and Time in Seconds Required to Speak 200 Words About Future Job, Together with Ratings of Severity of Stuttering for 100 Adult Male Stutterers

| | Severity | | Repetitions[a] | | Time | | Words Per Minute |
	Mean	SD	Mean	SD	Mean	SD	
100 speakers							
Tapes 1 and 2	4.23	2.30	26.49	26.94	161.52	108.51	74
50 speakers with lowest severity ratings	2.27	0.80	8.60	6.77	109.58	24.52	110
50 speakers with highest severity ratings	6.19	1.52	44.38	27.67	213.48	132.47	56

[a] Number of words in relation to which a part-word repetition, a sound prolongation, a broken utterance, or unusual stress was observed.

SOURCE: Young, 56, p. 49.

TABLE 58.   Coefficients of Correlation Between Various Measures of Oral Reading
Rate and Severity of Stuttering of 30 Adult Stutterers

Measures	r
Frequency of stuttering and mean duration of stutterings	.17
Frequency of stuttering and total duration of stuttering	.95
Total duration of stuttering and mean duration of stutterings	.38
Over-all rate and nonstuttering rate	.88
Over-all rate and frequency of stutterings	−.88
Over-all rate and mean duration of stutterings	−.46
Over-all rate and total duration of stuttering	−.85
Nonstuttering rate and frequency of stuttering	−.77
Nonstuttering rate and mean duration of stutterings	−.33
Nonstuttering rate and total duration of stuttering	−.72

SOURCE: Bloodstein, 7.

TABLE 59.   Mean, Median, and Quartile Scores on the Iowa Scale of Attitude
Toward Stuttering for Mothers and Fathers Who Were Spouse Pairs and
Parents of Stutterers, and for Their Stuttering Children

	N	Mean	Median	25th Percentile	75th Percentile
Mothers[a]	81	1.91	1.96	1.58	2.30
Fathers[b]	81	1.94	1.94	1.50	2.23
Children[c]	36	2.17	2.28	1.78	2.58

[a] Median age=38 years
[b] Median age=40 years
[c] Aged 10 to 20 years, with a median age of 13.5 years: 27 males and 9 females.
SOURCE: University of Iowa Speech Clinic.

TABLE 60.   Means, Standard Deviations, Ranges, and Indicated Percentile
Values for Each of the Four Modes of Response to the Stutterer's Self-
Ratings of Reactions to Speech Situations for 95 Adult Male Stutterers

Mode of Response	Mean	SD	25th Percentile	50th Percentile	75th Percentile	Range of Scores
Avoidance	2.31	.66	1.82	2.20	2.80	1.02–4.20
Reaction	2.57	.62	2.10	2.56	2.97	1.41–3.97
Stuttering	2.54	.60	2.08	2.53	2.98	1.20–3.92
Frequency	3.80	.45	3.48	3.88	4.11	2.39–4.72

SOURCE: Shumak, 42.

FORM 13. CHECK LIST OF STUTTERING REACTIONS

Name _____ Age _____ Sex _____

Observer _____ Date _____

INSTRUCTION TO OBSERVER

Observe the stutterer as he speaks or reads aloud. Focus your attention on such of his disfluencies and related reactions as you would classify as stuttering. Observe these reactions as they are associated with the speaking of specific words. Write each such word at the top of a column and make a check mark in the appropriate space to indicate each type of disfluency or other reaction noted. Under "Supplementary Observations" add descriptive details concerning any of the numbered items checked, and comment on apparent emotionality of the speaker, general degree of tension, relevant remarks made by the speaker, etc.

Types of Reaction	Word 1	Word 2	Word 3	Word 4	Word 5	Word 6
1. Repeating part of word	_____	_____	_____	_____	_____	_____
2. Repeating whole word	_____	_____	_____	_____	_____	_____
3. Repeating this and other word(s)	_____	_____	_____	_____	_____	_____
4. Saying "uh uh" or the like	_____	_____	_____	_____	_____	_____
5. Prolonging sound(s)	_____	_____	_____	_____	_____	_____
6. Pausing in middle of word	_____	_____	_____	_____	_____	_____
7. Failing to complete the word	_____	_____	_____	_____	_____	_____
8. Holding brieath	_____	_____	_____	_____	_____	_____
9. Gasping	_____	_____	_____	_____	_____	_____
10. Inhaling irregularly	_____	_____	_____	_____	_____	_____
11. Exhaling irregularly	_____	_____	_____	_____	_____	_____
12. Speaking on exhausted breath	_____	_____	_____	_____	_____	_____
13. Delay in starting word	_____	_____	_____	_____	_____	_____
14. Pressing lips together	_____	_____	_____	_____	_____	_____
15. Pressing tongue against teeth or palate	_____	_____	_____	_____	_____	_____
16. Closing eyes	_____	_____	_____	_____	_____	_____
17. Protruding tongue	_____	_____	_____	_____	_____	_____

Types of Reaction	Word 1	Word 2	Word 3	Word 4	Word 5	Word 6
18. Enlarging eyes	_____	_____	_____	_____	_____	_____
19. Opening mouth irrelevantly	_____	_____	_____	_____	_____	_____
20. Dilating nostrils	_____	_____	_____	_____	_____	_____
21. Turning head sideways	_____	_____	_____	_____	_____	_____
22. Bending head downward	_____	_____	_____	_____	_____	_____
23. Moving head up or back	_____	_____	_____	_____	_____	_____
24. Moving hands or fingers	_____	_____	_____	_____	_____	_____
25. Moving legs or feet	_____	_____	_____	_____	_____	_____
26. Moving body	_____	_____	_____	_____	_____	_____
27. Other (specify)	_____	_____	_____	_____	_____	_____
28. _____	_____	_____	_____	_____	_____	_____
29. _____	_____	_____	_____	_____	_____	_____
30. _____	_____	_____	_____	_____	_____	_____

Supplementary Observations:

Additional copies of this form may be obtained from the Interstate Printers and Publishers, 19-27 North Jackson Street, Danville, Illinois.

FORM 14. SCALE FOR RATING SEVERITY OF STUTTERING

Speaker _____ Age _____ Sex _____ Date _____

Rater _____ Identification _____

INSTRUCTIONS:

Indicate your identification by some such term as "speaker's clinician," "clinical observer," "clinical student," or "friend," "mother," "father," "classmate," etc.

Rate the severity of the speaker's stuttering on a scale from 0 to 7, as follows:

0   No stuttering

1   Very mild—stuttering on less than 1 percent of words; very little relevant tension; disfluencies generally less than one second in duration; patterns of disfluency simple; no apparent associated movements of body, arms, legs, or head.

2   Mild—stuttering on 1 to 2 percent of words; tension scarcely perceptible; very few, if any, disfluencies last as long as a full second; patterns of disfluency simple; no conspicuous associated movements of body, arms, legs, or head.

3   Mild to moderate—stuttering on about 2 to 5 percent of words; tension noticeable but not very distracting; most disfluencies do not last longer than a full second; patterns of disfluency mostly simple; no distracting associated movements.

4   Moderate—stuttering on about 5 to 8 percent of words; tension occasionally distracting; disfluencies average about one second in duration; disfluency patterns characterized by an occasional complicating sound or facial grimace; an occasional distracting associated movement.

5   Moderate to severe—stuttering on about 8 to 12 percent of words; consistently noticeable tension; disfluencies average about 2 seconds in duration; a few distracting sounds and facial grimaces; a few distracting associated movements.

6   Severe—stuttering on about 12 to 25 percent of words; conspicuous tension; disfluencies average 3 to 4 seconds in duration; conspicuous distracting sounds and facial grimaces; conspicuous distracting associated movements.

7   Very severe—stuttering on more than 25 percent of words; very conspicuous tension; disfluencies average more than 4 seconds in duration; very conspicuous distracting sounds and facial grimaces; very conspicuous distracting associated movements.

If this rating was based on a single sample of speech, describe the speech sample and the situation in which you made the rating. If the rating was based on two or more specific samples of speech, describe the various speech samples and the situations in which you made the ratings:

If this rating was not based on one or more specific speech samples in one or more specific situations, but covers instead many observations made in a variety of situations over a period of time, indicate the period covered and the main general types of speech samples and situations observed.

Dates: from _____ to _____. Main types of samples and situations:

Additional copies of this form may be obtained from the Interstate Printers and Publishers, 19-27 North Jackson Street, Danville, Illinois.

FORM 15. IOWA SCALE OF ATTITUDE TOWARD STUTTERING

Name _____Age _____ Sex _____

Examiner _____ Score _____Date _____

Purpose of Scale: This is not a test or quiz. It is a scale of attitude toward stuttering. In order to help stutterers, we must know their attitudes and the attitudes of other people in connection with stuttering. Please mark this questionnaire as carefully as you can. We went to know your attitude. Don't hesitate to put down what you believe.

First please fill out the following blanks. Disregard any items which do not apply to you.

Extent of education (circle one):   elementary school   high school
college   graduate college

Fields of university major and minor (specify):

Have you ever taken courses in speech correction?   Yes_____   No_____.

What relatives of yours have stuttered?

How severe was the stuttering of each?

With how many stutterers other than relatives have you been acquainted? How severe was the stuttering of each?

Have you ever noticeably stuttered?   Yes   No   If yes, rate yourself on the following scale as to the severity of your stuttering. Indicate your rating of your stuttering severity by circling one of the division bars:

mild		moderate		severe

How many brothers have you?   List ages:

How many sisters have you?   List ages:

Procedure: Now you are ready to begin marking the scale, which begins at the top of the next page. In responding to each item, you are to circle the response which best reflects your own attitude. Work accurately and as rapidly as possible. Don't spend a great deal of time analyzing wording. Mark all statements. If you are not sure what your attitude is, mark the best guess you can and go on. Remember: In responding to each item, circle the answer which best reflects your own attitude.

1. If a person at the family dinner table is about to stutter on a word, he should substitute another word for it and go on.
   Strongly agree   Moderately agree   Undecided   Moderately disagree   Strongly disagree

2. When giving a talk before a group of friends, a person should talk more slowly and prolong sounds in order to put off saying words he thinks he is going to stutter on.
   Strongly agree   Moderately agree   Undecided   Moderately disagree   Strongly disagree

3. A stutterer should not try out for the debating team.
   Strongly agree   Moderately agree   Undecided   Moderately disagree   Strongly disagree

4. A fellow should prefer to sit in silence rather than stutter to a girl he is with at a party.
   Strongly agree   Moderately agree   Undecided   Moderately disagree   Strongly disagree

5. A husband who stutters should try to have his wife answer the doorbell or telephone.
   Strongly agree   Moderately agree   Undecided   Moderately disagree   Strongly disagree

6. If while introducing two friends a person believes he will stutter, he should prolong the final sound of the preceding word or say "a-a-a" until he believes he can get the word out.
   Strongly agree   Moderately agree   Undecided   Moderately disagree   Strongly disagree

7. If he feels he will stutter while doing so, a father should avoid talking to his son about sex and marriage.
   Strongly agree   Moderately agree   Undecided   Moderately disagree   Strongly disagree

8. If a girl goes for an auto ride with a young man she likes and believes she will stutter, she should speak as little as possible.
   Strongly agree   Moderately agree   Undecided   Moderately disagree   Strongly disagree

9. If she stutters, a girl should not apply for a position as salesgirl in a department store.
   Strongly agree   Moderately agree   Undecided   Moderately disagree   Strongly disagree

10. When at a party you should talk as little as possible if you are a stutterer.
    Strongly agree   Moderately agree   Undecided   Moderately disagree   Strongly disagree

11. A person should not be a Boy or Girl Scout leader if he stutters.
    Strongly agree   Moderately agree   Undecided   Moderately disagree   Strongly disagree

12. If you stutter, you should not prepare yourself to be a salesman.
    Strongly agree   Moderately agree   Undecided   Moderately disagree   Strongly disagree

13. A person should be embarrassed if he stutters while telling a casual, chance acquaintance about a book he has read.
    Strongly agree   Moderately agree   Undecided   Moderately disagree   Strongly disagree

284

14. A stutterer should not volunteer to be class secretary.
Strongly agree   Moderately agree   Undecided   Moderately disagree   Strongly disagree

15. You should be embarrassed if you stutter while talking before a school assembly.
Strongly agree   Moderately agree   Undecided   Moderately disagree   Strongly disagree

16. A boy who stutters should not run for class or school president.
Strongly agree   Moderately agree   Undecided   Moderately disagree   Strongly disagree

17. If you feel you are going to stutter when answering the phone, you should try to boost up your courage by telling yourself you won't stutter.
Strongly agree   Moderately agree   Undecided   Moderately disagree   Strongly disagree

18. If one is telling a story at a party and thinks he is going to stutter on a word he should try to find an easier word to take its place.
Strongly agree   Moderately agree   Undecided   Moderately disagree   Strongly disagree

19. If a person believes he will stutter when applying at a certain time for a job as a janitor, he should wait until later to apply, when he believes his speech will cause him less embarrassment.
Strongly agree   Moderately agree   Undecided   Moderately disagree   Strongly disagree

20. When visiting a friend's house for the evening and asked what he would like to do or play, a stutterer should choose a game where he would have little talking to do.
Strongly agree   Moderately agree   Undecided   Moderately disagree   Strongly disagree

21. If a person stutters while talking in class, he should talk more loudly and act more confidently.
Strongly agree   Moderately agree   Undecided   Moderately disagree   Strongly disagree

22. A street car or bus conductor should be embarrassed if he stutters on the name of a street he is calling out.
Strongly agree   Moderately agree   Undecided   Moderately disagree   Strongly disagree

23. A stuttering woman should avoid going into a store to buy a hat if she believes the saleslady will feel sorry for her or secretly laugh at her because of her stuttering.
Strongly agree   Moderately agree   Undecided   Moderately disagree   Strongly disagree

24. If a person stutters while answering a question in class, he should just stop and start over again.
Strongly agree   Moderately agree   Undecided   Moderately disagree   Strongly disagree

25. A person should not try to tell jokes to a person of the opposite sex if he is likely to stutter while doing so.
Strongly agree   Moderately agree   Undecided   Moderately disagree   Strongly disagree

26. A girl should feel embarrassed if she stutters saying her escort's name when introducing him to some of her friends.
Strongly agree   Moderately agree   Undecided   Moderately disagree   Strongly disagree

27. A stutterer should try to be hired for jobs requiring little speaking—for example, janitor or wrapping clerk.
Strongly agree   Moderately agree   Undecided   Moderately disagree   Strongly disagree

28. A salesgirl should be embarrassed if she stutters while trying to sell an article.
Strongly agree   Moderately agree   Undecided   Moderately disagree   Strongly disagree

29. A person should try to avoid leading a prayer at church or Sunday school if he believes he will stutter.
Strongly agree   Moderately agree   Undecided   Moderately disagree   Strongly disagree

30. A stutterer should stay at home and listen to the radio or watch TV rather than go to a discussion group where he would stutter if called on to speak.
Strongly agree   Moderately agree   Undecided   Moderately disagree   Strongly disagree

31. If he feels he will stutter while asking a girl to go with him to a party, a fellow should put off asking, hoping that later on his speech will be more fluent.
Strongly agree   Moderately agree   Undecided   Moderately disagree   Strongly disagree

32. If he believes he will stutter, a husband should avoid embarrassing his wife by talking while at a dinner given by one of her close friends.
Strongly agree   Moderately agree   Undecided   Moderately disagree   Strongly disagree

33. At church, if a person believes he will stutter while introducing friends, he should wait until some time later when he feels less likely to stutter.
Strongly agree   Moderately agree   Undecided   Moderately disagree   Strongly disagree

34. A salesgirl should be embarrassed if she stutters while trying to sell a book to a man.
Strongly agree   Moderately agree   Undecided   Moderately disagree   Strongly disagree

35. A teacher who stutters should conceal this by substituting easy words for the hard ones he feels he will stutter on.
Strongly agree   Moderately agree   Undecided   Moderately disagree   Strongly disagree

36. A stutterer should not plan to be a lawyer.
Strongly agree   Moderately agree   Undecided   Moderately disagree   Strongly disagree

37. A wife who stutters should try to keep it from her husband's notice by speaking slowly or prolonging sounds until she thinks she can say her words better.
Strongly agree   Moderately agree   Undecided   Moderately disagree   Strongly disagree

38. If he stutters, a young man should not prepare himself to be a salesman.
Strongly agree   Moderately agree   Undecided   Moderately disagree   Strongly disagree

39. A teacher generally should not call upon a stutterer in his class for oral recitation.
Strongly agree   Moderately agree   Undecided   Moderately disagree   Strongly disagree

40. A stutterer should not be a bus driver.
Strongly agree   Moderately agree   Undecided   Moderately disagree   Strongly disagree

41. If a person stutters in one of your classes, you should feel sorry for him.
Strongly agree   Moderately agree   Undecided   Moderately disagree   Strongly disagree

42. If acquaintances come to visit the family, a stutterer should leave the talking to them up to non-stuttering members of the family.

   Strongly agree   Moderately agree   Undecided   Moderately disagree   Strongly disagree

43. When asked at a party to choose between a game where he will have to talk a good deal and one where he could keep still, the stutterer should choose the one where he could keep still.

   Strongly agree   Moderately agree   Undecided   Moderately disagree   Strongly disagree

44. A woman who stutters should avoid meeting and talking with her husband's influential friends.

   Strongly agree   Moderately agree   Undecided   Moderately disagree   Strongly disagree

45. A barber who stutters should not stutter while giving haircuts.

   Strongly agree   Moderately agree   Undecided   Moderately disagree   Strongly disagree

Scoring:
   Number "Strongly Agree"   _____ × 4 = _____
   Number "Moderately Agree"   _____ × 3 = _____
   Number "Moderately Disagree"   _____ × 2 = _____
   Number "Strongly Disagree"   _____ × 1 = _____

A. Total   _____
B. Total number of items answered
   "Strongly" or "Moderately" agree
   or disagree   _____

Score = A divided by B   _____

Additional copies of this form may be obtained from the Interstate Printers and Publishers, 19-27 North Jackson Street, Danville, Illinois.

FORM 16. STUTTERER'S SELF-RATINGS OF REACTIONS TO SPEECH SITUATIONS

Name _____ Age _____ Sex _____

Examiner _____ Date _____

After each item put a number from 1 to 5 in each of the four columns.

Start with right-hand column headed Frequency. Study the five possible answers to be made in responding to each item, and write the number of the answer that best fits the situation for you in each case. Thus, if you habitually take your meals at home and seldom eat in a restaurant, certainly not as often as once a week, write the number 5 in the Frequency column opposite item No. 1, "Ordering in a a restaurant." In like manner respond to each of the other 39 items by writing the most appropriate number in the Frequency column. When you have finished with this column fold it under so you cannot see the numbers you have written. This is done to keep you from being influenced unduly by the numbers you have written in the Frequency column when you write your responses to the 40 situations in the Stuttering column.

Now, write the number of the response that best indicates how much you stutter in each situation. For example, if in ordering meals in a restaurant you stutter mildly (for you), write the number 2 in the Stuttering column after item No. 1. In like manner respond to the other 39 items. Then fold under the Stuttering column so you will not be able to see the numbers you have written in it when you make your responses in the Reaction column.

Following the same procedure, write your responses in the Reaction column, fold it under, and, finally, write your responses in the Avoidance column.

Numbers, for each of the columns, are to be interpreted as follows:

A. Avoidance:
  1. I never try to avoid this situation and have no desire to avoid it.
  2. I don't try to avoid this situation, but sometimes I would like to.
  3. More often than not I do not try to avoid this situation, but sometimes I do try to avoid it.
  4. More often than not I do try to avoid this situation.
  5. I avoid this situation every time I possibly can.

B. Reaction:
  1. I definitely enjoy speaking in this situation.
  2. I would rather speak in this situation than not.
  3. It's hard to say whether I'd rather speak in this situation or not.
  4. I would rather not speak in this situation.
  5. I very much dislike speaking in this situation.

C. Stuttering:
1. I don't stutter at all (or only very rarely) in this situation.
2. I stutter mildly (for me) in this situation.
3. I stutter with average severity (for me) in this situation.
4. I stutter more than average (for me) in this situation.
5. I stutter severely (for me) in this situation.

D. Frequency:
1. This is a situation I meet very often, two or three times a day, or even more, on the average.
2. I meet this situation at least once a day with rare exceptions (except Sunday, perhaps).
3. I meet this situation from three to five times a week on the average.
4. I meet this situation once a week, with few exceptions, and occasionally I meet it twice a week.
5. I rarely meet this situation—certainly not as often as once a week.

	Avoidance	Reaction	Stuttering	Frequency
1. Ordering in a restaurant				
2. Introducing myself (face to face)				
3. Telephoning to ask price, train fare, etc.				
4. Buying plane, train, or bus ticket				
5. Short class recitation (10 words or less)				
6. Telephoning for taxi				
7. Introducing one person to another				
8. Buying something from store clerk				
9. Conversation with good friend				
10. Talking with an instructor after class or in his office				
11. Long distance telephone call to someone I know				
12. Conversation with father				
13. Asking girl for date (or talking to man who asks me for a date)				
14. Making short speech (1 or 2 minutes) in familiar class				
15. Giving my name over telephone				
16. Conversation with my mother				
17. Asking a secretary if I can see her employer				
18. Going to house and asking for someone				
19. Making a speech to unfamiliar audience				
20. Participating in committee meeting				
21. Asking instructor question in class				

	Avoidance	Reaction	Stuttering	Frequency
22. Saying hello to a friend going by	___	___	___	___
23. Asking for a job	___	___	___	___
24. Telling a person a message from some-one else	___	___	___	___
25. Telling funny story with one stranger in a crowd	___	___	___	___
26. Parlor games requiring speech	___	___	___	___
27. Reading aloud to friends	___	___	___	___
28. Participating in a bull session	___	___	___	___
29. Dinner conversation with strangers	___	___	___	___
30. Talking with my barber (or beauty operator)	___	___	___	___
31. Telephoning to make appointment, or arrange meeting place with someone	___	___	___	___
32. Answering roll call in class	___	___	___	___
33. Asking at a desk for book, or card to be filled out, etc.	___	___	___	___
34. Talking with someone I don't know well while waiting for bus or class, etc.	___	___	___	___
35. Talking with other players during a playground game	___	___	___	___
36. Taking leave of a hostess	___	___	___	___
37. Conversation with friend while walking along the street	___	___	___	___
38. Buying stamps at post office	___	___	___	___
39. Giving directions or information to strangers	___	___	___	___
40. Taking leave of a girl (boy) after a date	___	___	___	___
Total	___	___	___	___

Average
No. of 1's   _____
 "   " 2's   _____
 "   " 3's   _____
 "   " 4's   _____
 "   " 5's   _____

Additional copies of this form may be obtained from the Interstate Printers and Publishers, 19-27 North Jackson Street, Danville, Illinois.

Name _____ Age _____ Sex _____

Examiner _____ Date _____

Reading Passage Used: _____

ADAPTATION OF STUTTERING

Reading	Number of Words Stuttered	Percentages of Adaptation	
1	a _____		
2	b _____	$(a-b)/a \times 100 =$ _____	
3	c _____	$(a-c)/a \times 100 =$ _____	$(b-c)/b \times 100 =$ _____
4	d _____	$(a-d)/a \times 100 =$ _____	$(c-d)/c \times 100 =$ _____
5	e _____	$(a-e)/a \times 100 =$ _____	$(d-e)/d \times 100 =$ _____

ADAPTATION OF ORAL READING RATE

Reading	Time in Seconds	Percentages of Adaptation	
1	a _____		
2	b _____	$(a-b)/a \times 100 =$ _____	
3	c _____	$(a-c)/a \times 100 =$ _____	$(b-c)/b \times 100 =$ _____
4	d _____	$(a-d)/a \times 100 =$ _____	$(c-d)/c \times 100 =$ _____
5	e _____	$(a-e)/a \times 100 =$ _____	$(d-e)/d \times 100 =$ _____

CHART-COMPUTED ADAPTATION OF STUTTERING

A. Percentage of words stuttered, Reading No. 1 _____
B. Percentage of words stuttered, Reading No. 5 _____
C. Adaptation score, according to Chart in Fig. 3, p. 271 _____

Additional copies of this form may be obtained from the Interstate Printers and Publishers, 19-27 North Jackson Street, Danville, Illinois.

FORM 18. MEASURES OF STUTTERING CONSISTENCY

Name _____ Age _____ Sex _____

Examiner _____ Date _____

Reading Passage Used: _____

CONSISTENCY INDEX: 2-1

Number of words stuttered in Reading No. 2 _____

A. Percent of these words that were stuttered in Reading No. 1
(this percentage is the Consistency Index for Reading 2 relative to Reading 1, or CI:2-1) _____

B. Percent of all words stuttered in Reading No. 1 _____

A divided by B (see pp. 274-275) _____

CONSISTENCY INDEX: 3-2

Number of words stuttered in Reading No. 3

A. Percent of these words that were stuttered in Reading No. 2
(this percentage is the Consistency Index for Reading 3 relative to Reading 2, or CI:3-2) _____

B. Percent of all words stuttered in Reading No. 2 _____

A divided by B (see pp. 274-275) _____

CONSISTENCY INDEX: 3-1

A. Percent of the words stuttered in Reading No. 3 that were
also stuttered in Reading No. 1 (this percentage is the Consistency Index for Reading 3 relative to Reading 1, or CI:3-1)_____

B. Percent of all words stuttered in Reading No. 1 _____

A divided by B (see pp. 274-275) _____

Additional copies of this form may be obtained from the Interstate Printers
and Publishers, 19-27 North Jackson Street, Danville, Illinois.

REFERENCES

1. Adams, Lois Hickman, "A comparison of certain sound wave character-istics of stutterers and nonstutterers," in W. Johnson (Ed.) with the assistance of R. Leutenegger, *Stuttering in Children and Adults: Thirty Years of Research at the University of Iowa*, Minneapolis: University of Minnesota Press, 1955, pp. 398-401.
2. Ainsworth, S., "Integrating theories of stuttering," *Journal of Speech Disorders*, 1945, *10*:205-210.
3. Ammons, R., and W. Johnson, "The construction and application of a test of attitude toward stuttering," *Journal of Speech Disorders*, 1944, *9*: 39-49.
4. Barbara, D. A., *Stuttering: A Psychodynamic Approach to its Under-standing and Treatment*, New York: Julian Press, 1954.
5. Bloodstein, O. N., *A Handbook on Stuttering for Professional Workers*, Chicago: National Society for Crippled Children and Adults, 1959.
6. Bloodstein, O. N., "Hypothetical conditions under which stuttering is reduced or absent," *Journal of Speech and Hearing Disorders*, 1950, *15*:142-153.
7. Bloodstein, O. N., "The relationship between oral reading rate and severity of stuttering," *Journal of Speech Disorders*, 1944, *9*:161-173.
8. Bloodstein, O. N., W. Jaeger, and J. Turcen, "A study of the diagnosis of stuttering by parents of stutterers and non-stutterers," *Journal of Speech and Hearing Disorders*, 1952, *17*:308-315.
9. Bluemel, C. S., *Stammering and Allied Disorders*, New York: Macmillan, 1935.
10. Boehmler, R. M., "Listener responses to non-fluencies," *Journal of Speech and Hearing Research*, 1958, *1*:132-141.
11. Brown, S. F., "An analysis of certain data concerning loci of 'stutterings' from the viewpoint of general semantics," *Papers from the Second Amer-ican Congress of General Semantics*, 1943, *2*:194-199.
12. Brown, S. F., "The loci of stutterings in the speech sequence," *Journal of Speech Disorders*, 1945, *10*:181-192.
13. Cohen, E., "A comparison of oral reading and spontaneous speech of stutterers with special reference to the adaptation and consistency effects," unpublished Ph.D. dissertation, University of Iowa, 1952.
14. Donohue, Irene R., "Stuttering adaptation during three hours of con-tinuous reading," in W. Johnson (Ed.) with the assistance of R. Leu-tenegger, *Stuttering in Children and Adults: Thirty Years of Research at the University of Iowa*, Minneapolis: University of Minnesota Press, 1955, pp. 264-267.
15. Eisenson, J. (Ed.), *Stuttering: A Symposium*, New York: Harper, 1958.
16. Eisenson, J., and E. Horowitz, "The influence of propositionality on stuttering" *Journal of Speech Disorders*, 1945. *10*:193-197.

17. Giolas, T. G., and D. E. Williams, "Children's reactions to nonfluencies in adult speech," *Journal of Speech and Hearing Research*, 1958, *1*:86-93.
18. Hejna, R. F., *Speech Disorders and Nondirective Therapy*, New York: Ronald Press, 1960.
19. Johnson, W., "An interpretation of stuttering," *Quarterly Journal of Speech*, 1933, *19*:70-77.
20. Johnson, W., "Measurements of oral reading and speaking rate and disfluency of adult male and female stutterers and nonstutterers," *Journal of Speech and Hearing Disorders*, 1961, Monogr. Supp. 7, 1-20.
21. Johnson, W., *Stuttering and What You Can Do About It*, Minneapolis: University of Minnesota Press, 1961; New York: Doubleday (Dolphin paperback ed.), 1962.
22. Johnson, W. (Ed.) assisted by R. Leutenegger, *Stuttering in Children and Adults: Thirty Years of Research at the University of Iowa*, Minneapolis: University of Minnesota Press, 1955.
23. Johnson, W., and S. Ainsworth, "Constancy of loci of expectancy of stuttering," *Journal of Speech Disorders*, 1938, *3*:101-104.
24. Johnson, W., and S. F. Brown, "Stuttering in relation to various speech sounds: a correction," *Quarterly Journal of Speech*, 1939, *25*:20-22.
25. Johnson, W., S. F. Brown, J. F. Curtis, C. W. Edney, and Jacqueline Keaster, *Speech Handicapped School Children*, New York: Harper, 1948; rev. ed., 1956.
26. Johnson, W., and J. R. Knott, "The distribution of moments of stuttering in successive readings of the same material," *Journal of Speech Disorders*, 1937, *2*:17-19.
27. Johnson, W., and J. R. Knott, "The moment of stuttering," *Journal of Genetic Psychology*, 1936, *48*:475-480.
28. Johnson, W., and J. R. Knott, "A systematic approach to the psychology of stuttering," in W. Johnson (ed.) with the assistance of R. Leutenegger, *Stuttering in Children and Adults: Thirty Years of Research at the University of Iowa*, Minneapolis: University of Minnesota Press, 1955, pp. 25-33.
29. Johnson, W., and Anita Solomon, "A quantitative study of expectation of stuttering as a process involving a low degree of consciousness," *Journal of Speech Disorders*, 1937, *2*:95-97.
30. Johnson, W., et al., *The Onset of Stuttering: Research Findings and Implications*, Minneapolis: University of Minnesota Press, 1959.
31. Knott, J. R., W. Johnson, and Mary Webster, "A quantitative evaluation of expectation of stuttering in relation to the occurrence of stuttering," *Journal of Speech Disorders*, 1937, *2*:20-22.
32. Lewis, D., and Dorothy Sherman, "Measuring the severity of stuttering," *Journal of Speech and Hearing Disorders*, 1951, *16*:320-326.
33. Murphy, A. T., and Ruth M. FitzSimons, *Stuttering and Personality Dynamics: Play Therapy, Projective Therapy, and Counseling*, New York: Ronald Press, 1960.
34. Newman, P. W., "A study of adaptation and recovery of the stuttering response in self-formulated speech," *Journal of Speech and Hearing Disorders*. 1954, *19*:450-458.

35. Peins, Maryann, "Adaptation effect and spontaneous recovery in stuttering expectancy," *Journal of Speech and Hearing Research*, 1961, *4*:91-99.
36. Robbins, S., "The role of rhythm in the correction of stammering," *Quarterly Journal of Speech*, 1935, *21*:331-343.
37. Roe, A. M., A. J. Derbyshire, and Jo Ann Sedroski, "Qualifying periods of silence and sound in speech," unpublished paper presented at annual meeting of American Speech and Hearing Association, New York, November, 1958.
38. Sander, E. K., "Reliability of the Iowa speech disfluency test," *Journal of Speech and Hearing Disorders*, 1961, Monogr. Supp. 7, 21-30.
39. Sheehan, J. G., "Theory and treatment of stuttering as an approach-avoidance conflict," *The Journal of Psychology*, 1953, *36*:27-49.
40. Sherman, Dorothy, "Clinical and experimental use of the Iowa scale of severity of stuttering," *Journal of Speech and Hearing Disorders*, 1952, *17*:316-320.
41. Shulman, E., "Factors influencing the variability of stuttering," W. Johnson (Ed.) with the assistance of R. Leutenegger, in *Stuttering in Children and Adults: Thirty Years of Research at the University of Iowa*, Minneapolis: University of Minnesota Press, 1955, pp. 207-217.
42. Shumak, Irene Cherhavy, "A speech situation rating sheet for stutterers," in W. Johnson (Ed.) with the assistance of R. Leutenegger, in *Stuttering in Children and Adults: Thirty Years of Research at the University of Iowa*, Minneapolis: University of Minnesota Press, 1955, pp. 341-347.
43. Tate, M. W., and W. Cullinan, "Measurement of consistency of stuttering," *Journal of Speech and Hearing Research*, in press.
44. Tate, M. W., W. L. Cullinan, and Ann Ahlstrand, "Measurement of adaptation in stuttering," *Journal of Speech and Hearing Research*, 1961, *4*:321-339.
45. Tuthill, C. E., "A quantitative study of extensional meaning with special reference to stuttering," Speech Monographs, 1946, *13*(1):81-98. Abstracted in *Papers of American Congress of General Semantics*, 1943, *2*:200-204, and *Journal of Speech Disorders*, 1940, *5*:189-191.
46. Van Riper, C., *Speech Correction: Principles and Methods*, 3rd ed., New York: Prentice-Hall, 1954.
47. Van Riper, C., "Study of the thoracic breathing of stutterers during expectancy and occurrence of stuttering spasm," *Journal of Speech Disorders*, 1936, *1*:61-72.
48. Van Riper, C., and R. Milisen, "A study of predicted duration of the stutterer's blocks as related to their actual duration," *Journal of Speech Disorders*, 1939, *4*:339-345.
49. Wendahl, R. W., and Jane Cole, "Identification of stuttering during relatively fluent speech," *Journal of Speech and Hearing Research*, 1961, *4*:281-286.
50. West, R., M. Ansberry, and Anna Carr, *The Rehabilitation of Speech*, 3rd ed., New York: Harper, 1957.
51. Williams, D. E., "A point of view about 'stuttering,' " *Journal of Speech and Hearing Disorders*, 1957, *22*:390-397.

52. Williams, D. E., in W. Johnson and D. E. Williams, unpublished progress report of Grant RD-319 to U.S. Office of Vocational Rehabilitation, 1962.
53. Williams, D. E., and Louise R. Kent, "Listener evaluations of speech interruptions," *Journal of Speech and Hearing Research*, 1958, *1*:124-131.
54. Wischner, G. J., "An experimental approach to expectancy and anxiety in stuttering behavior," *Journal of Speech and Hearing Disorders*, 1952, *17*:139-154.
55. Wischner, G. J., "Stuttering behavior and learning: a preliminary theoretical formulation," *Journal of Speech and Hearing Disorders*, 1950, *15*:324-335.
56. Young, M. A., "Predicting ratings of severity of stuttering," *Journal of Speech and Hearing Disorders*, 1961, Monogr. Supp. 7, 31-54.

10

SUPPLEMENTARY DIAGNOSTIC PROCEDURES AND REFERRAL PRINCIPLES

Audiol,
Psych.
Medical

Speech pathologists use routinely the investigative and evaluative procedures described in the preceding chapters. For certain purposes they employ other techniques in addition to these, and they also refer some of the persons whom they serve to other professional resources in accordance with their distinctive needs. In this chapter we consider a number of procedures that speech pathologists sometimes use in addition to those previously presented, and we discuss the purposes and principles of referral, together with the patterns of interprofessional relationships within which speech pathologists carry on their clinical activities.

SUPPLEMENTARY DIAGNOSTIC PROCEDURES

The clinical speech pathologist has available to him, or within the reach of his own ingenuity, a number and variety of tests, observational techniques, methods of interviewing, kinds of experimental therapy and counseling, and laboratory procedures that extend far beyond the array of relatively basic procedures included in this manual. Many of these are utilized exclusively, or most appropriately, through

297

referral to such other professional persons as audiologists, otolaryn-gologists and neurologists or other physicians, and clinical psycholo-gists. Others have been developed within the province of speech pathology, or must be fashioned by the individual speech clinician to meet in more or less original ways the unusual evaluational require-quirements that arise impressively often in his day to day work, be-cause the neatness of the diagnostic categories in our textbooks is not matched by the heterogeneity of the individualities, inconsistencies, and unpredictabilities of the men, women, and children who come to speech clinics in real life. In the following pages we describe in detail two tests of handedness, discuss less extensively measures of socio-economic status and social maturity, and consider, in relation to principles of referral and interprofessional relationships, the sorts of evaluational information to be secured as needed by referral of the person being served to other professional specialists.

Handedness

Several years ago it was more or less widely supposed that handed-ness was closely related to the development of speech disorders, particularly stuttering. Regardless of one's point of view regarding the importance or lack of importance of handedness and shifts in handedness in this connection, there are times when it is useful for the speech pathologist to make a determination of a person's handed-ness.

The following are a few of the situations in which an evaluation of handedness may be desirable:

1. The speech problem is related to some organic impairment which may have affected the neuromuscular functioning of the extremeties as well as the speech organs. In cases of cerebral palsy or of cerebro-vascular accident (stroke) associated with dysphasia, for example, hand usage may indicate to some degree the nature and location of the neuropathology. Moreover, previous and present handedness are sometimes to be considered in the over-all planning of rehabilitation in such cases. In a hospital or rehabilitation center it is often the speech pathologist who is depended upon to make the necessary obser-vations and tests in this connection and to inform the rest of the rehabilitation team of the findings. Obviously these should be ade-quately objective and detailed.

2. Parents bring a young child to a speech clinic with the complaint of stuttering, having heard or read something that has made them concerned about the possibility that the cause of the stuttering might lie in the child's apparent or possible lack of a strong preference for one hand or the other. If you are to discuss with these parents the

importance or lack of importance of the alleged possible cause, it may be desirable to determine first what the child's hand usage is in as objective a way as possible, rather than simply to take someone's word for it that he is generally right- or left-handed or ambidextrous. By analogy, a discussion of the importance of high fever in illness has more relevance to a particular patient after it has been determined whether he himself has a fever.

3. Parents and teachers often frankly report that they have taken definite, even drastic, steps at some earlier time to discourage a child from using his left hand, and because the child also has a speech problem, or for some other reason, they have come to worry about what they have done. They ask for advice. Should they now reverse the procedure and reintroduce the strain and tension that might be involved in restricting the use of the hand which the child was earlier pressured into using? You, as the speech pathologist—recognizing that the emotional pressure and the disturbed relationships between the child and his parents or teachers arising from the forced shift in handedness are probably much more important than the shift itself— may want to discourage further pressure of the same sort, especially if the present hand preference appears well established and satisfactory to the child. If, however, the present pattern of hand usage seems to be disorganized and frustrating to the child you will want to investigate the advisability of reversing the earlier attempted shift of handedness. In this type of case also objective information about present hand preference is desirable.

As several recent studies have served to emphasize, it is easy to oversimplify the matter of hand preference and to reach unwarranted conclusions by making insufficient observations. Research conducted over a period of many years indicates, for example, that stutterers and nonstutterers are essentially alike in handedness (*8, 18, 19, 28*) and that much of the population is more ambidextrous than had been supposed (*13, 15, 16, 17, 18*).

Much depends on how handedness is defined operationally and on the specific tests that are employed. In general the investigations referred to above have shown that whereas most individuals are fairly definitely right-handed or left-handed with respect to unimanual activities, such as eating with a spoon or writing, which are definitely taught according to well-established social customs, a considerable degree of ambidexterity is commonly observed with regard to activities that are not uniformly taught. Johnson and Duke (*17*) found, for example, that all of the 50 6-year-olds they tested were consistent in the hand they used for writing, whether the writing was done with a pen, pencil, chalk, or crayon, but that in performing five "put" and eight "take" operations the children were quite inconsistent in hand preference.

The "put" operations are putting pencil in desk, putting scissors in desk, putting crayons in box, placing blocks, and laying down cards. A check of the individual records showed that only seventeen of the 50 children were consistent in the hand used for these five activities. Even with regard to putting pencil in desk and putting scissors in desk, fifteen of the children used one hand for one of these operations and the other hand for the other, or at least used the hands differently for them. Since two performances of each operation were made, it was possible for a subject to perform an operation both times with the right hand, or both times with the left hand, or once with the right and once with the left, or even to complicate the record by using both hands more or less equally for one or both performances. With regard to placing blocks and laying down cards, sixteen children performed inconsistently.

The eight "take" operations were taking articles from desk, taking crayons from box, picking up scissors, picking up blocks to pile, picking up blocks to carry, picking up cards, picking up chalk, and picking up pen. Considering all eight operations together, only five children were consistent in hand usage, although the operations are quite similar in that they all involve prehension. If the six "picking up" items are considered, only twelve of the children performed consistently. One might tend to assume that there would be very little inconsistency in picking up blocks to pile and picking up blocks to carry, but as a matter of fact seventeen of the children were inconsistent. Perhaps the most revealing fact in this connection was the following: It will be remembered that all the children were consistent in hand usage in both writing with a pen and writing with chalk; nevertheless, as between picking up the pen and picking up the chalk, twenty of the fifty children were inconsistent with regard to the hand used for the "picking up."

Here would seem to be evidence indicating that hand usage practices tend to be consistent (involve the same hand) in proportion to the degree that they are formally taught and supervised (17).

After all, the average individual has two good, intact, more or less strong hands, not just one that is good and one that is limp and numb. Moreover, there is no single one-hand activity that can be taken as a safe index of hand preference. Rather, systematic observation and reporting of many manual activities are necessary if conclusions are to be dependable and relevant to most specific clinical purposes.

We present below two tests of handedness selected, from among the many that have been developed, for ease of administration, reliability, and clinical usefulness.

The Iowa Unimanual Hand Usage Questionnaire: The subject himself fills out the questionnaire if he is old enough or able to do so, or a parent or other qualified informant may fill it out for him if he is not. If the speaker is a child and is old enough to follow your instructions, ask him to answer each question orally and also to go through the motions of performing the indicated activity, and fill in the questionnaire yourself in accordance with the child's oral and performed responses to your questions. The questionnaire requires a rating of hand usage in performing 25 different unimanual activities and yields a handedness index, which indicates degree of right- or left-handedness or ambidexterity.

This test can be used for obtaining a detailed statement about the previous hand usage habits of a person who has suffered a stroke with resulting hemiplegia, or an injury or amputation of a hand or arm, or other impairment affecting handedness, by instructing the person to answer the questions with reference to his customary hand usage before the injury or impairment. If he is unable to write, ask him the questions and fill in the blanks yourself on the basis of his answers. If his spoken answers seem unclear ask him to act out his responses. If you are still in doubt, check his answers with an appropriate informant.

In scoring the Iowa Unimanual Hand Usage Questionnaire, proceed as directed on Form 19. Assign a weight of -2 to all items for which the symbol $L+$ is encircled, -1 to items for which the symbol $L-$ is encircled, O for an E response, and $+1$ and $+2$ for $R-$ and $R+$ responses, respectively. Divide the sum of these weights by the number of items actually answered to determine the handedness index. Thus, an index of -2 indicates the maximum degree of left-handedness and an index of $+2$ (usually written without the plus sign) the maximum possible degree of right-handedness that could be represented by the questionnaire responses.

The test was used by Johnson and his associates (19) in an investigation of the onset of the stuttering problem; data were obtained from 294 children and 589 adults who were parents of the children. Davison (4) gave the test to 386 university students and, for a special purpose, selected the 25 who were most right-handed and the 25 who were most left-handed. The average index of the 25 most right-handed individuals was 1.83 and the average for the 25 most left-handed individuals was -1.53. These compare with Johnson's adult means which ranged from 1.3 to 1.5 and his children's means of 1.3 for the control group and 1.4 for the clinical group. Table 61 contains a summary of the data, which can be used as norms, with due regard, of course, to the populations represented by them. The scores summarized in Table 61 demonstrate, incidentally, an absence of any notable difference in handedness, as measured, between stutterers and nonstutterers, and between their respective parents as well. Additional data concerning the handedness of the clinical and control groups represented in Table 61, including reported changes in handedness and family histories of handedness, are to be found in *The Onset of Stuttering* (*19*), Items 94-111 and 775-778, Summary Table, pages 23-32 and 232-235 of Appendix A.

Iowa Performance Test of Selected Manual Activities: This test involves the controlled observation of 64 operations in a person's performance of 32 simple manual activities requiring a minimum of equipment. The test was originally designed for testing the handedness of school children (*15, 16, 17*), and is best adapted to the age levels represented by the early elementary grades. It has been used with high school students (*13*), however, and can be employed in testing adults. Table 62 contains normative data for 6- and 7-year-olds and high school students 13-19 years old.

The test yields a dextrality quotient, a score indicating percentage of right-handedness. The dextrality quotient (*DQ*) is computed by means of the formula

$$DQ = \frac{R + (B/2)}{N},$$

in which R and B represent the number of test operations performed by the right hand and by both hands (neither hand predominating), respectively, and N represents the total number of operations performed.

The materials needed for the test are: a room with a window having a shade which can be easily manipulated by a child; a desk of the type from which articles are taken with equal ease by either hand, such as a desk with an open shelf or drawer under the desk top; a pencil; a small pencil sharpener of the type held in one hand; a tablet of paper of customary school size; a pencil with eraser attached; a box of crayons; scissors in which the finger holes are the same on both sides; five regular flash cards; a blackboard; a piece of chalk; eight alphabet blocks, lettered A to H; a fountain pen with screw top and side lever for filling; a bottle of ink; and a large picture book with pages which can be readily turned. Record the child's responses on Form 20; in the instructions that follow, the words in italics refer to the responses that you are to observe and record on Form 20 as R (performed with the right hand), L (performed with the left hand), or B (performed with both hands).

Before beginning the test, place the tablet, pencil, pencil sharpener, and crayons in the desk. As soon as the child enters the room give him the following directions:

"Will you please *pull down the curtain* a little? That's fine, but will you please *pull it down* a trifle more?" See that the child has taken his hand from the curtain before you instruct him to make the second adjustment. Also, be sure that he approaches the shade so that it can be as readily pulled with one hand as with the other. Record in the appropriate spaces on Form 20 the hand—R (right), L (left), or B (both hands)—the child used each time he pulled down the curtain.

Next, say to the child, "Now will you please *take the articles out of the desk* one at a time and place them on the top of the desk?" Record on Form 20 the first two responses for this item. Pick up the articles and place only the tablet in front of the child, and then say, "Please *tear out* one sheet of paper and *turn over* the paper."

Next put the pencil and pencil sharpener in front of the child, and say, "Please *sharpen the pencil.*" Record the hand that does the turning of the sharpener.

Next place the pencil directly in front of the child and continue, "*Write* your name at the top of the paper. No, please *erase it,* and *write it* at the bottom of the sheet. Now will you please *draw* a picture; and when you are finished, *put the pencil in the desk.*"

Place a box of crayons directly in front of the child and say, "Now *color* the picture." Note which hand is used in *taking out each crayon* (score the first two), in *coloring,* in *placing each crayon* in the box (score the first two), and in *closing the box.* In case the child does not voluntarily use more than one color, you may say, "Let's use another color for this part of the picture." As soon as the child is through and no longer has his hands on the box, say: "Let's look in the box to see if we have all the crayons in it." This gives a second score for *closing the box.*

Next place the scissors directly in front of the child. "Cut off the bottom line, please." Note the hand used in *picking up the scissors.* "Now *put the scissors in the desk.*"

Next arrange the blocks in a straight line from one side of the table to the other, the middle block being directly before the child, and say, "*Point to A; point to G,*" etc. Be sure to see that the child is relaxed and ready to start with neither hand favored before the second letter is named. Call off the first two letters, the only ones scored, in a definite order, calling the sixth from the left first and the third from the left next. "Now pile the blocks one on top of the other to make a pile eight blocks high, being sure to *pick up* only one block at a time." Note the hand used in *picking up,* as well as in *placing,* the second and fourth blocks. Put the blocks on the desk again, and instruct the child by saying, "Please carry these over to that desk one at a time." If there is not a second desk handy, some other surface may be substituted. Record the hand used in *picking up* the first and third blocks. Do not record the hand used in carrying the blocks.

Next place five flash cards on the top of the desk and say, "Please *point* to the cards as I name them." Call first for the second from the left and then for the fourth from the left. "Now please *pick them up* one at a time and now *lay them down* one at a time." (For these last two items, record the first two responses in each case.)

Now place a tablet directly in front of the child, and say, "Please *tear out* another sheet of paper; *turn over the sheet of paper;* and *fold it* in the middle." Record the hand which actually creases the folded edge.

Next, present the pencil sharpener and pencil in the midline again, and instruct the child to *sharpen the pencil.*

Following this activity, present the picture book in the middle of the desk, and say, "Please *turn* to the picture of Casper Carrot." Any picture will do so long as two or more pages are turned. Record the hand used in turning each of the first two pages. Then after presenting the pencil again directly in front of the child, say, "Now *draw* the picture, and when you are through *put the pencil in the desk.*"

Next, remove the book and place the scissors directly in front of the child, and say, "Please cut out your picture, and then *put the scissors in the desk.*" Record the hand used for *picking up* the scissors, for *cutting* with the scissors, and for *putting the scissors in the desk.*

Next place the bottle of ink and the pen directly in front of the child, taking care to see that the pen is placed on neither side of the ink bottle. Then say, "Please *pick up the pen, take off the top,* (record the hand doing the actual turning), put them both down, *take the top off the ink bottle, fill the pen,* and *write your name.* Then *put the top back on the pen.*" While the child is doing these things, put the top back on the ink bottle. Next say, "Please *erase* your name. Now *fold* the paper so that the ink spot will not show. *Pick up* the pen, *take off the top,* put down the pen, *take the top off the ink bottle, fill the pen, write* your name, and *put the top on the pen.*"

The last two activities are concerned with the blackboard. Direct the child to stand squarely in front of it where he can as easily reach the chalk with one hand as with the other. Say "Please write your name." Note the hand used in *picking up the chalk,* as well as in *writing.* Lastly, ask the child, "Will you please *print* your name?" This also gives the second score for *picking up* the chalk. This concludes the test.

Any remarks by the child or your own further directions, in case the child has difficulty in grasping your instructions, need not be curtailed, provided they do not influence hand preference.

The time required to give the test is 20 to 25 minutes per child.

Table 62 contains the lowest and highest scores on the test here described, together with the decile values, for 50 children 6 years old, 100 children 7 years old, and 100 high school students 13 to 19 years of age. Suppose a six-year-old child scores a DQ of .86. By referring to Table 62 you would find that he falls at the 70th percentile for his age group. This means that he is more right-handed than 70 percent and less right-handed than 30 percent of the 6-year-olds tested by Johnson and Duke. In such terms, any child's score may be evaluated. You must keep in mind, of course, that these norms are only for the age levels indicated. The score of a child at some other age level is to be evaluated by reference to Table 62 only by taking into account the difference in age. However, differences between the high-school-age subjects and the two groups of younger subjects represented in Table 62 are not great. Since the activities involved in this test were originally selected by observing actual school-room activities of 6-year-old children, it would seem reasonable to conclude that the hand which an individual has come to use consistently for a given activity at the age of 7 years or so is the hand he will use for the same activity 8 to 10 years later. In other words, the norms shown in Table 62 are probably quite stable.

ASSIGNMENTS

1. Fill out the Unimanual Hand Usage Questionnaire, Form 19, yourself. Also ask at least two other persons, one of high school or college age and one of elementary school age, to fill it out.
2. Administer the Performance Test of Selected Manual Activities to at least two children of elementary school age. Follow the instructions, above, and record responses in each case on Form 20.

Socioeconomic Status

The speech clinician often finds it useful to have as clear a statement as possible about the socioeconomic status of the family of the speaker whose problem he is trying to understand. As we have previously considered, the individual and his communicative attitudes and behavior are importantly influenced by the family to which he belongs and the neighborhood and larger social setting in which he lives. You can appreciate more fully the communicative difficulties of a person and their personal and social implications for him if you take account of the general social and economic level on which he experiences these difficulties and their consequences.

Several ways of measuring and representing socioeconomic status have been developed. Strictly speaking, it is the socioeconomic level of a person's family, of course, rather than that of the person himself, that is determined. We have found the Index of Status Characteristics, developed by Warner, Meeker, and Eells (*31*), easy to calculate, easy to understand, and reliable for general clinical and related research purposes. It proved to be well suited to the requirements of our investigations of the onset of the stuttering problem (*12, 19*), for example.

The Index of Status Characteristics is calculated by taking account of the family breadwinner's occupation, his source of income (not the amount of income), the size and type of the family dwelling place, and the area lived in (for which the level of education of the father of the family may be substituted). You rate the information concerning each of these four factors on a seven-point scale, multiply the number representing each rating by a prescribed weight, and total the resulting values. The possible sums range from 12 to 84, and these are grouped into five socioeconomic class equivalents: upper, upper middle, lower middle, upper lower, and lower lower.

The details of the procedure are as follows:

1. *Factor 1:* Occupation of Breadwinner. Using Chart B, classify the breadwinner first according to *kind* of occupation. Seven kinds of occupation are indicated in the chart, namely, Professionals, Proprietors, Businessmen, White Collar Workers, Manual Workers, Service Personnel, and Landowners-Farmers. Having classified the breadwinner according to occupation, determine the *level* within that occupation. Some occupations have three levels, some five, some six, some seven. Weight: Multiply by 4 the numerical value of the level selected to represent the breadwinner of the family.

2. *Factor 2:* Source of Income. Use Chart C, Part I. Select the number, from 1 to 7, which designates the primary source of the family's income. Weight: multiply this value by 3.

3. *Factor 3:* House Size and Type. Use Chart C, Part II. Use the following definitions, excluding bathrooms, in calculating the number of rooms: small house, up to 6 rooms; medium house, 7 or 8 rooms; large house, 9 or more rooms. Determine the number of rooms and the general condition of the house or apartment and choose the number, from 1 to 7, which corresponds to the appropriate description. Weight: multiply this value by 3.

4. *Factor 4:* Alternative (a): Area Lived in; Alternative (b): Education of Breadwinner. Use Chart C, Part III. If the family lives in an urban community and if you are sufficiently familiar with the characteristics of the various neighborhoods in the community, use Alternative (a), Area Lived in. Choose the number, from 1 to 7, which corresponds to the appropriate description of the neighborhood.

If the family lives in a rural area or if for some reason you find yourself unable to determine reliably the type of neighborhood an urban family lives in, use Alternative (b), Education of Breadwinner. Select the number corresponding to the level of education attained by the breadwinner. Weight: whether you use Alternative (a) or Alternative (b), multiply the number selected by 2.

5. *Total* the four weighted values obtained in steps 1 to 4.

6. From The Index of Status Characteristics (i.e., the total obtained in step 5) determine the socioeconomic class as follows:

Index	Socioeconomic Class
12–22	Upper
23–37	Upper middle
38–51	Lower middle
52–66	Upper lower
67–84	Lower lower

Let us take a hypothetical family and calculate the Index of Status Characteristics. Assume that the father of a child brought to your speech clinic is a high school teacher and coach, a college graduate with a B.A. degree. He is salaried and has no other income. The family lives in a modern, three-year-old, five-room house in a new housing development considered in the community to be "average." *Factor 1:* the father is a Professional, level 2; weighted score, 8. *Factor 2:* the income is from salary, level 4; weighted score, 12. *Factor 3:* the family home is a small house in good condition, level 5; weighted score, 15. *Factor 4:* if you use alternative (a), the area lived in is average, level 4, weighted score, 8; if you use alternative (b), the father is a graduate of a 4-year college, level 2, weighted score, 4. *Totals:* if you use alternative (a), the total score is 45, and if you use alternative (b), the total score is 41. In either case, the family is judged to fall in the lower middle socioeconomic class.

NOTE: In the event that you can make a determination of only three of the four factors, you can still calculate the Index of Status Characteristics by changing the weights of the three factors you have. Use the revised weights indicated below. For example, if the missing factor is occupation, each of the other three factors is given a weight of 5; if the missing factor is source of income, occupation is given a weight of 5 and each of the other factors a weight of 4; etc.

Missing Factor	Usual Weight	Revised Weight If Factor X Is Missing			
		1	2	3	4
1	4	X	5	5	5
2	3	5	X	4	4
3	3	4	4	X	3
4	2	3	3	3	X

SOURCE: Both tables adapted from Warner, Meeker, and Eells (*31*).

Another index, based solely upon the type of occupation of the family breadwinner, is the Minnesota Scale of Parental Occupations (*10*). This scale has been used by several research workers, including Templin (*30*) who employed it in her normative study of speech and language development in children.

Social Maturity

There are times when the speech pathologist desires an estimate of a child's level of social maturity. In evaluating such problems as delayed speech development, or speech and language disorders associated with mental retardation, impaired hearing, cerebral palsy, or emotional insecurity, you will find it advantageous to compare the child's degree of social maturity with that of other youngsters of his chronological age. In addition to the pertinent information you may obtain in the case history interview, you can secure certain items of relevant data by means of the Vineland Social Maturity Scale (5).

The Vineland Social Maturity Scale is not a test in the ordinary sense, since it does not involve the observing and scoring of a prescribed sampling of the child's responses to specified stimuli. The score or rating which this scale makes possible is based, rather, on certain types of information about the child's self-care and social skills as reflected in his day-to-day behavior. This information is provided by an appropriately qualified informant, usually the mother or father. The scale covers self-help in eating and dressing, locomotion, occupation or daily activities, communication, self-direction, and socialization. In scoring the scale, you transform the information you obtain by means of it into a social age, and by relating this to the child's chronological age you arrive at a social quotient. This social quotient is not directly comparable to, nor the equivalent of, an intelligence quotient, or IQ, derived by relating a child's chronological age to his performance on an intelligence test, but it does indicate how a child compares with his peers in the development of skills and activities indicative of social maturity. See the current edition of the Manual (5) for full instructions to follow in administering and scoring the scale.

A more or less similar scale, which is limited in design and purpose to the appraisal of a child's degree of communicative skill, has been developed by Mecham (20).

INTERPROFESSIONAL RELATIONSHIPS AND PRINCIPLES OF CASE REFERRAL

The speech pathologist belongs to the great fraternity of the helping professions and shares the obligations and responsibilities and the ethics and prerogatives common to all who are joined together in dedication to its ancient and honorable purposes. It is his responsibility to maintain effective communication with members of those professions that are closely related to his own—and to do all he can to insure their effective relationships with him in the interests of those persons whom he and they can best serve through joint efforts. When other specialists refer their patients or clients to him, as they are ethically and professionally obligated to do whenever they can assist in providing more effective services by so doing, the speech clinician is obligated to render a report of his findings that is as clear and valid as he can possibly make it. It is equally true that when the speech pathologist refers a person in his clinical charge to another specialist, as he is ethically and professionally obligated to do whenever he can, by so doing, insure more effective services, it is his prerogative to receive from the other specialist a report that is as clear and valid as might reasonably be expected.

It is to be taken for granted, then, that as a clinical speech pathologist, you will invariably respond to the best of your ability to the requests for assistance and collaboration that are addressed to you by members of the other helping professions. This understood, you are fundamentally concerned with fulfilling your obligation to do all you can personally for those persons who seek your services and whom you are qualified to serve, and to secure for them, by referring them to other appropriate specialists, the attentions they need which you are not prepared to provide.

A fundamental principle of case referral is that it should be based upon adequate and clearly stated grounds. It involves an expenditure of time and money for the person referred, it means that a busy physician or other specialist must take time from other important activities in order to render the services requested, and there is always the possibility that the examination or evaluation asked for is irrelevant to the needs of the person for whom you are responsible, or is theoretically relevant but practically nonessential, or is perhaps even harmful under the circumstances, or is something that is needed which you should be able to do yourself with adequate professional training. Any statement of clinical policy that begins with the words "Always refer . . ." is to be viewed critically and evaluated conscientiously. As a clinician you must locate and keep well marked the borderline between the wisdom of meaningful thoroughness and the inconsiderateness and waste of examination without purpose.

A basic rule that goes far to insure desirable and to eliminate pointless referrals is this: State clearly the specific questions you want answered by the specialist to whom you are making the referral. State them not only to the specialist but also to the person whom you are referring to him, unless to do so would intensify rather than alleviate anxiety and bewilderment. By considering the rationale for this rule in serving persons with various kinds of speech problems, we are able to shape up the main generalizations that are useful to us for practical purposes.

We can best begin by discussing the two kinds of special examinations, in addition to those previously described in this manual, for which speech clinicians make the greatest number of referrals, day in and day out. These are audiological and psychological examinations. We discuss referral for these two types of examinations in the following two sections. We consider in a later section the related matters of referral for medical examination by the otologist and otolaryngologist and for psychiatric evaluation.

Referral for Audiological Evaluation

Speech pathologists, clinically certified by the American Speech and Hearing Association, have a basic knowledge of the hearing function, the modes of its impairment, and the kinds of methods used in the measurement of hearing acuity and in the communicative rehabilitation of the hard of hearing. Many of them are qualified to do at least routine hearing testing, and some of them hold ASHA Clinical Certification in audiology as well as in speech pathology. Moreover, speech pathologists and audiologists share the same professional training programs in the universities, belong to the same professional organization—the American Speech and Hearing Association—and very often work side by side in the same clinical programs. Under the circumstances, while evaluations of hearing are generally made by audiologists, frequently the person with a speech problem is not, strictly speaking, referred by the speech pathologist to the audiologist, but rather he is seen by both of them, or by one clinician qualified in both fields, in the course of a single comprehensive clinical examination. In other situations, of course, there is referral to an audiologist in something like the usual sense of that term.

The basic question is whether or not every child or adult who has, or is suspected of having, a speech, voice, or language problem should have an audiological examination. It may be argued, for example, that relevant research has generally failed to demonstrate a functional relationship between hearing impairment and the problem of stuttering. Moreover, hearing loss seems not to be a very important factor in relation to the developmental or functional misarticulations of children. Nevertheless, it is desirable, in our judgment, to include at least a screening test of hearing in the examination of any person with a speech, voice, or language problem. This screening test, whether group or individual, should be done by means of a calibrated audiometer of current design. The major purpose of it is to determine whether a more extensive audiological evaluation is advisable. We believe that this is a service that is reasonably to be expected by everyone who goes to a speech clinic, or participates in a school or college speech and hearing program, primarily because the conservation of hearing and the early detection of hearing impairment are fundamental responsibilities of all speech pathologists as well as audiologists. Indeed, speech and hearing disorders are commonly classified together as communication problems, and speech pathologists and audiologists are sometimes called communicologists because of their common concern with the communication process, of which speech and hearing are discernible but functionally inseparable aspects.

Hearing and speech go together and can be evaluated most adequately in any case only as their interactions are appreciated. Even in respect to stuttering, to which hearing loss as such appears unrelated, as we have noted, a striking observation is that of the virtual elimination of stuttering as distinguished from disturbed speech fluency as such, under conditions of high-level noise received by the stutterer through headphones (24). The marked disturbance of speech occasioned by delayed auditory feedback is another impressive illustration of the intimate relationship between speech and hearing (21). Neelley's (21) findings with respect to the differences between stuttering and the speech disturbances associated with delay of auditory feedback have implications of interest to both audiologists and speech pathologists. There are intriguing implications for both also in the differences as well as the relationships between the perception of pure tones and the perception and interpretation of speech and other patterns of sound having symbolic significance. Again, although hearing loss per se, as we have observed, and even speech sound discrimination ability seem not very significantly related to functional articulatory problems, nevertheless such problems are approached remedially largely through auditory stimulation designed to heighten the speaker's awareness of the acoustic difference between his misarticulations and the correct articulations of specific sounds and patterns of sounds. For this reason, if there is any impairment of hearing it is to be duly considered in planning and administering remedial procedures.

After all, there is no more basic hypothesis concerning speech development than the one which holds that the child learns to speak by responding in kind as best he can to the speech he hears about him. The importance of hearing in relation to the learning of speech is dramatized in the grave difficulty experienced by deaf children in their efforts to learn to speak. A severe loss of hearing after speech has been learned tends to be followed by some degree of deterioration of the individual's ability to monitor his voice and his articulation of speech sounds. In any case of delay of speech development impaired hearing is a possible etiological factor that must be ruled in or out by means of appropriate, and sometimes necessarily elaborate, audiological examination. The status of the auditory functions is to be appraised most carefully in all cases involving neuropathology. The importance of auditory reception in dysphasia has been heavily underscored by Schuell's findings (26). In cases of cleft palate the evaluation of hearing is indicated by the possibility of conductive hearing loss associated with otitis media occasioned by the exposed condition of the pharyngeal openings of the Eustachian tubes with resulting increased susceptibility to middle ear infection.

In these and all other types of clinical speech cases the basic questions to be answered by referral for audiological and related otological evaluation are:

Is there impairment of hearing and, if so, how great is it for what frequencies—that is, what is the pattern of the audiogram?

If there is a loss of hearing, is it conductive (due to obstruction in the external auditory canal, or otosclerosis, or otitis media, or other condition in the middle ear), or sensory-neural (due to pathology or damage in the inner ear, in the auditory branch of the eighth cranial nerve, or in the brain)?

How long has the loss been present?

Is it progressive and, if so, how severe is it likely to become?

Is a hearing aid indicated and, if so, how much gain in hearing acuity will it probably effect, particularly in the perception of speech and the self-monitoring of voice and articulation?

Is surgery indicated and, if so, when and with what predicted result in improvement of hearing, particularly in the speech range?

On the basis of the audiological findings, what are the indications for the use of sound amplification in speech therapy?

Is there need for auditory training or speech-reading instruction?

What should be stressed in counseling?

In what respects is the person's speech or language problem related to the impaired hearing, and in what respects is it not affected by the hearing loss?

Some of these questions are best answered by the audiologist or the otologist, and some of them you must answer with the aid of the information supplied by the audiologist and otologist.

For the reasons indicated, we recommend that audiological assessment be an integral part of the clinical examination in all cases involving speech, voice, or language problems, with acknowledgment, of course, of the circumstances under which it may not be feasible. We do not believe, however, that even the more simple audiometric procedures should be described in this manual. If you have been trained to employ these or other more complex audiological techniques, you do not need to have them described. If you have not been trained to use even the gross screening methods, you are hardly prepared to apply properly any audiometric instructions that we might provide, and you should therefore make referrals for audiological examinations. If that is, in fact, your situation we assume that you will include in your further professional training at least introductory courses in the fundamentals of hearing, audiology, and audiometric techniques. Meanwhile, you may find much of interest and value in such books as those of Davis and Silverman (*3*), Hirsh (*9*), and Newby (*22*) and in articles on hearing and audiology in the *Journal of Speech and Hearing Disorders* and the *Journal of Speech and Hearing Research* as well as the other relevant publications to which you will be directed by reading *dsh Abstracts,* published quarterly by Deafness Speech and Hearing Publications, sponsored jointly by the American Speech and Hearing Association and Gallaudet College, the national college for the deaf in Washington, D.C.

It is to be expected that audiologists, as well as otologists and otolaryngologists, will refer to speech pathologists for testing and evaluation all persons served by them who have apparent speech, voice, or language problems, or who present progressive or substantial impairments of hearing that might be expected to affect eventually speech sound articulation and vocal pitch, volume, quality, and inflectional patterns. The over-all communicative problem of a person with a hearing loss is greater if he also has a speech or language disorder, and vice versa, and clinical evaluations are to be governed accordingly. In responding to referrals made to you in such cases, you will be concerned especially with the questions of need for speech conservation in preparation for the future effects of a progressive or severe hearing loss, therapy for existing speech or voice impairment, and the probable advantages to the person of auditory training and speechreading, as well as counseling designed to improve his understanding of and adjustment to the communicative problem.

Referral for Psychological Evaluation

By virtue of their professional training, speech pathologists, clinically certified by ASHA, are acquainted with the fundamentals of psychodiagnostics. Some of them are prepared to administer such intelligence tests as the Stanford-Binet and Wechsler, the Minnesota Multiphasic Personality Inventory and other "paper and pencil" personality tests, and perhaps various projective tests as well as other diagnostic instruments employed in the area of clinical psychology. A few of them are Diplomates in Clinical Psychology by authority of the

American Board of Examiners in Professional Psychology. In general, however, testing and evaluating of intelligence and personality reaction tendencies are done by clinical psychologists.

Again, the basic question to be considered is whether or not every child or adult who has a communication problem involving speech, voice, or language, should have a psychological examination. Just as the interaction between speech problems and hearing acuity is variable and complex, so the relationship between the various types of speech, voice, and language impairment and psychological aberration or personality maladjustment is inconsistent and not well defined. For example, the assumption, taken for granted in some quarters, that stuttering is a psychoneurosis is to be evaluated against the relatively large accumulation of relevant data which does not support such an assumption. These data have been reviewed by Goodstein (6), Sheehan (27), and Johnson (14, 19). They show that such differences on personality tests as are sometimes found between stutterers and non-stutterers reflect on the whole the reactions to be expected of fundamentally normal persons in response to the frustration, strain, and distress involved in the experience of stuttering—and of being categorized as a stutterer in a society in which the classification of "stutterer" is negatively valued. Meanwhile, there is a problem of differential diagnosis which arises from these three facts: (1) the reactions made by some stutterers to their stuttering are sometimes maladjustive; (2) since approximately 10 percent of the population has need of psychiatric attention at one time or another, it is to be expected that 10 percent of stutterers are persons who, even if they did not stutter, would now and then exhibit psychiatrically notable behavior; and (3) some persons with psychoneuroses speak with blockages and disfluencies that may or may not appear to be much like stuttering reactions.

Spriestersbach (29), in a review of studies concerned with possible relationships between functional articulatory disorders and personality adjustment, concluded that in general children and older subjects with such disorders have not been found to be significantly different from other persons with respect to the aspects of personality investigated.

The interaction between mental and emotional variables and speech, voice, and language problems that are functionally related to cleft palate, laryngectomy, cerebral palsy, cerebrovascular accident (stroke), and other neuropathologies is complicated by the effects on personal and social adjustment of the physical disabilities involved. Cerebral palsy, for example, tends to restrict the child's capacity for moving about and maneuvering himself into speech situations, and, especially during the period of early speech development, this can have a marked effect not only in fashioning the speech problem but also in patterning emotional and social adjustment and in fixing the rate and extent of mental growth. In one segment of Spriestersbach's research on the comprehensive problem centering around cleft palate, Goodstein (7) found that children with cleft palates tend to score higher on the performance than on the verbal parts of the Wechsler intelligence scale. His findings serve to focus attention on the question of the general relationship between intellectual development and the frustration and restriction of oral expression, with the attendant distress or penalty. We have provided in the supplementary case history outlines in Chapter 2 for consideration of emotional reactions to cleft palate, cerebral palsy, laryngectomy, aphasia, and stuttering. In cases involving these problems, tests of intelligence and personality reactions are clearly advisable. It is obviously essential to obtain an objective evaluation of intelligence in any case in which a communication problem is related to apparent mental retardation. In any case of speech, voice, or language impairment in which emotional disturbance or significant personality maladjustment, including neurotic and psychotic tendencies, is noted or suspected, there is no question of the desirability of referral for psychodiagnostic evaluation.

We believe that every speech clinic and every clinical speech program in a school, college, hospital, or rehabilitation center should have at least one clinical psychologist on its staff, or have available the facilities essential for psychodiagnostic evaluation. These facilities are an integral part of many clinical speech programs at the present time. In such programs psychodiagnostic testing is not obtained through referral, in the usual sense, but is part and parcel of a unitary clinical evaluation, along with examinations of speech, voice, language, and hearing. In most public schools intelligence testing is provided, and the cumulative records of the children with whom you work will usually contain a variety of test scores, teacher evaluations, and other information that will be relevant to your purposes.

The main questions to be answered in most cases by the clinical psychologist, or on the basis of information and judgments provided by him, are these:

What is the level of intelligence of the person?
Is the level of intelligence probably related causally in some degree
   to the speech problem?
In what respects is the level of intelligence to be taken into account
   in therapy and counseling?
Is there any evidence in the pattern of mental test responses, or in
   the results of any other tests administered, of brain damage?
If so, what might be its functional relationship to the speech, voice,

or language problem; and in what ways should it be considered in therapy and counseling?

Is there any evidence of neurotic or psychotic, or at least seriously maladjustive patterns of adjustment and, if so, do they indicate a need for psychiatric referral?

Do they suggest a possible need for psychological counseling or psychotherapy over and above the counseling to be included in the program of clinical speech services?

Are they functionally related to, or essentially independent of, the speech, voice, or language problem? Is it likely that their alleviation would result in improved speech, or that improved speech behavior would lead to their alleviation?

In what specific ways should they be taken into account in planning speech therapy?

In any case in which psychodiagnostic evaluations are made of the parents of a child with a demonstrated or alleged speech problem, similar questions concerning their adjustment patterns are to be answered so far as possible.

We believe that it is desirable to include at least intelligence testing and some form of relatively objective evaluation of personality in the routine examination of persons with communication problems involving impaired speech, voice, or language, with acknowledgment—as in the case of audiological assessment—of the circumstances under which these procedures may not be feasible. In our judgment, however, psychodiagnostic methods are not to be appropriately included in this manual. If you have been trained to use them you do not need to have them described here, and if you have not you should make referrals for any psychodiagnostic information you require. In any event, your professional training should familiarize you with the fundamental principles of psychodiagnostic methods and provide you with the background of knowledge you need in order to make effective use of psychodiagnostic facilities. Relevant references are Allen (1) and Rosenzweig (23).

Clinical psychologists, as well as psychiatrists, who appreciate the fact that speech disorders are basic as well as symptomatic (11), recognize their obligation to refer to speech pathologists for appropriate evaluation the persons served by them who have speech, voice, or language disorders, or who present patterns of maladjustment in which a major reaction is that of seriously restricted or disturbed speech, impaired voice, or deviant language behavior. In evaluating the communication problems of such persons who are referred to you, your chief purpose will be to provide a definitive description of the speech, voice, and language deviations, and to help determine so far as possible whether they preceded the personality problem, are independent of it or basic to it, and require speech therapy in addition to, or instead of, psychotherapy.

Referral for Medical Evaluation

A properly organized program of clinical speech services includes available medical evaluation and care. It is not that all speech, voice, and language problems have anatomical or neurological or physiological causes, or that every person with such a problem requires a neurological or metabolic or cardiovascular or general physical examination. Certain communicative disorders, of course, as we have considered, are directly related to such physical conditions as cerebral palsy, cerebrovascular accident, other neuropathology, cleft palate, laryngeal pathology, laryngectomy, anomalies of oral structure, and ear pathology. Persons with communicative problems associated with such conditions have a clear need for appropriate medical examination as well as treatment and surgery perhaps. Moreover, as we indicated in the preceding section, in some cases disorders of communication may interact with personality disturbances which require psychiatric evaluation and possibly psychotherapy.

The questions you want to have answered so far as possible by medical referral are both general and specific. Like any other member of any one of the helping professions, you are, as a speech clinician, concerned about the general health and welfare of everyone you serve. If a child's tongue or gum tissues seem to you off-color, if he appears to have a skin irritation, if a college sophomore referred to you for a voice problem seems overly tired or subject to headaches, if any person seen by you clinically complains of any one of a large number and variety of other common or uncommon indications of possible physical malfunction, you will as a matter of course advise a visit to a physician or actually set up an appointment with an appropriate medical specialist. You will do this, not necessarily to get an answer to a specific question about the person's communication problem, but primarily because you consider his health to be important. It may be that the physician's report in such a case will not be relevant to your clinical interests, but there is always the possibility that it will be.

There are times when you will want to know whether a child or adult for whom you are clinically responsible has a disease or physical weakness or disability—a heart condition, perhaps, or diabetes, or epilepsy, a visual problem, a metabolic disturbance, or some other condition of medical significance—that you should take into account in planning and conducting speech therapy. It is this sort of information that you want to obtain from the physician of a child who is to be enrolled in your summer speech clinic, for example. The medical data in such a case may not bear upon the question of the nature or cause of the speech, or voice, or language problem, of course. Moreover, if the physical impairment is not functionally related to the communication problem, it is important to make sure that the speaker and his family understand that it is not. They may *think* it is, and so long as they do their reactions to speech therapy will be affected accordingly.

This particular consideration suggests another one related to it. There are cases in which a physical examination may not be advisable because of its possible effect on the thinking of those concerned. Brown (2), in reporting his experience as a pediatrician in dealing with speech problems of children, pointed out that the physical examination of a child may arouse or confirm parental fears or suspicions of physical fault of some sort. For example, he stated that he had discontinued the practice of making a routine physical examination of the child whose parents feel that he has begun to stutter, or that he might have a tendency to stutter. He explained that, having made such an examination, he experienced difficulty in convincing the parents that the findings were negative and that the child was physically all right. They found it hard to understand why he had made a physical examination in the first place if he had not assumed he was going to find the cause of the trouble by doing so. As he put it, there is always time to make a physical examination later if, in the course of taking the case history, any reason for doing so is indicated. If it is indicated, the parents can then be told in advance why it is being done. If it is not indicated, the communication problem can be discussed with the parents without inadvertently implying physical causes that are not, in fact, a part of the picture.

Brown's approach to the clinical examniation of children whose parents feel they may be stuttering is consistent with the general view that attention to the physical and medical needs of children, and of adults as well, should be given in such a way that attitudes of health and well-being are encourged. It is not good for a person to feel sicker than he is, to imagine weaknesses he does not have, to assume that he needs more sleep or rest than he requires, or to cultivate the self-attitudes of an invalid. All members of all the helping professions need at all times to be duly sensitive to the unfortunate fact that trouble can sometimes be not only found but also created by looking for it. In providing people with the help they need it is deeply important that we not give them help they cannot receive without losing their sense of wellness and their self-reliance. It is a sound safeguard to explain to anyone who is about to undergo a physical evaluation why he is to be examined.

We have considered medical referrals that you make because (1)

you are concerned in a general way about the health of any person you serve clinically, or (2) you want to determine whether the person has any illness or disability, not necessarily related to the communication problem, that you should take into account in planning and conducting therapy. You also make medical referrals in order to obtain information concerning the presence or absence of physical factors of possible importance in relation to the speech, voice, or language problem. Among the great number of questions that you have to ask of the various medical specialists to whom you make referrals for specific diagnostic reasons are such as these:

Is the hoarseness in this case associated with laryngeal pathology, and, if so, of what type?
Is there evidence of cancer? Polyps? Vocal nodules? Laryngitis? Sinus infection?
Is the pathology temporary or chronic? Should the speaker be put on vocal rest?

Does this person have an ear pathology, and if so what is the nature of it? Is it acute or chronic?
Is it progressive, and if so what is the probable ultimate level of severity?
Is surgery indicated, and if so, what are the results likely to be so far as gain in hearing acuity is concerned?
Is medical treatment indicated, and if so, what is the nature of it and what is its effect likely to be?

Does the palatal and velopharyngeal examination in this case of cleft palate indicate that further surgery is feasible?
Would speech be improved more by surgery or by an appropriate prosthetic appliance?

What is the probable prognosis for this 70-year-old lady who has suffered a stroke, with resulting right-sided hemiplegia?
Is the paralysis of the tongue and facial muscles likely to clear up, or should speech therapy be based on the assumption that it will probably be permanent?

From a psychiatric point of view, what seems to be the interaction between the excessive vocal tension and the speaker's significant personality characteristics?
What would be the most advisable—and feasible—arrangement to work out concerning the relationship between speech therapy and psychotherapy, if this is indicated?

The particular reasons for medical referral vary over a wide range, of course. Sometimes the questions to be asked can be more specific.

and often less so, than those listed above. The main point to be emphasized is that medical referral is to be accompanied by questions that will enable the physician to respond as effectively as possible to your need for information and counsel.

In general, it is desirable for the speech pathologist and audiologist to work together in relationship with the otologist in cases involving ear pathology. It is advisable also, as a rule, for the speech pathologist and psychologist to work together in relationship with the psychiatrist in cases requiring psychiatric attention. It is sound practice, in our judgment, for the speech clinician to work closely with the oto-laryngologist in cases involving voice problems, and with the neurolo-gist in cases involving demonstrated or suspected neuropathology. Frequently, of course, persons with speech, voice, or language problems associated with cerebral palsy, cleft palate, or other medi-cally significant conditions will have been given medical attention before they come to you. They will often be referred to you by their physicians. In any such case you will want to obtain a medical report. You will also make a report of your findings to the referring physician, in accordance with his indicated interests or specific requests for in-formation or clinical judgment. You will work in any case with an informed awareness of your relationship with the family physician, or general practitioner, or internist, or pediatrician who is concerned on a continuing basis with the person whose problems of communication are your responsibility. You will proceed also with a sensitivity to your working relationship with the additional medical specialists whose services are relevant to the person's distinctive needs. Your skill in achieving and maintaining cooperative professional relationships is one of your most essential attributes as a speech clinician.

TABLE 61. Summary of Scores on the Iowa Unimanual Hand Usage Questionnaire Made by Children Regarded by Their Parents as Stutterers (Clinical) or as Normal Speakers (Control) and by the Parents; and the Mean Scores of the Most Right-Handed and Most Left-Handed of 386 University Students

	N	Lowest[a] (Most Left-Handed) Score	Mean	Median	90th Percentile	Highest[a] (Most Right-Handed) Score
Adults						
Control group fathers[b]	150	−1.7	1.3	1.5	2.0	2.0
Control group mothers[c]	150	−2.0	1.5	1.6	2.0	2.0
Clinical group fathers[d]	143	−1.5	1.3	1.5	2.0	2.0
Clinical group mothers[e]	146	−1.1	1.5	1.7	2.0	2.0
Children[f]						
Control group	144	−2.0	1.3	1.6	2.0	2.0
Clinical group	150	−2.0	1.4	1.6	2.0	2.0
University students						
"Most right-handed"	25		1.83			
"Most left-handed"	25		−1.53			

[a] The most left handed score possible is −2.0; the most ambidextrous score possible is 0; and the most right-handed score possible is 2.0. Minus signs are retained, plus signs are deleted.
[b] Aged 25 to 50, with a mean age of 34 years.
[c] Aged 23 to 48, with a mean age of 32 years.
[d] Aged 24 to 55, with a mean age of 36 years.
[e] Aged 21 to 47, with a mean age of 33 years.
[f] Ranging in age from about 2.5 to 8.5, with an approximate mean age of 5 years; approximately two boys to one girl.
SOURCE: Children—Johnson et al., 19, Summary Table Item 788, Appendix A, p. 235. Adults—Johnson et al., 19, Summary Table Item 783, Appendix 9, pp. 233-24. University Students—Davison, 4.

TABLE 62. Lowest and Highest Scores and Percentiles on the Iowa Performance Test of Selected Manual Activities for 6-Year-Old, 7-Year-Old, and High School-Age Subjects

Percentile	6-Year-Olds N=50 (1)	7-Year-Olds N=100 (2)	High School Age[a] N=100 (3)
Lowest Score	.07	.12	.01
10	.52	.63	.43
20	.65	.71	.64
30	.74	.78	.69
40	.80	.81	.74
50	.82	.83	.79
60	.84	.85	.84
70	.86	.88	.87
80	.90	.92	.91
90	.94	.95	.95
Highest score	1.00	1.00	.97

[a] Age 13-19 years.
SOURCE: (1) Johnson and Duke, 17; (2) Johnson and Davis, 15; (3) Johnson and Bissell, 13.

FORM 19. IOWA UNIMANUAL HAND USAGE QUESTIONNAIRE

Name _____ Age _____ Sex _____

Examiner _____ Date _____

Purpose of Administering Questionnaire: _____

Indicate whether responses represent present hand usage (Yes _____ No_____)
or hand usage at some time in the past (specify): _____

Instructions: Please indicate whether you perform each of the following activities
consistently with your right hand, consistently with your left hand, or with either
hand. In responding to each item:

    If you always or very nearly always perform the activity with your right hand,
      circle the symbol R+.

    If you use your right hand most of the time, circle the symbol R−.

    If you always or nearly always perform the activity with your left hand, circle
      the symbol L+.

    If you use your left hand most of the time, circle the symbol L−.

    If you use your right hand and your left hand about equally, circle E.

1. Throwing a baseball	L+	L−	E	R−	R+
2. Writing with a pencil	L+	L−	E	R−	R+
3. Using an eraser at the blackboard	L+	L−	E	R−	R+
4. Using an eraser on the end of a pencil	L+	L−	E	R−	R+
5. Using a fork to raise food to the mouth	L+	L−	E	R−	R+
6. Using a tennis racquet	L+	L−	E	R−	R+
7. Using a hammer	L+	L−	E	R−	R+
8. Pulling down a window shade	L+	L−	E	R−	R+
9. Holding a glass of water to drink	L+	L−	E	R−	R+
10. Placing a postage stamp on an envelope	L+	L−	E	R−	R+
11. Raising hand to ask a question	L+	L−	E	R−	R+
12. Turning a screw driver	L+	L−	E	R−	R+
13. Emptying out an ash tray	L+	L−	E	R−	R+
14. Using a knife to butter bread	L+	L−	E	R−	R+
15. Pouring milk from a bottle into a glass on the table	L+	L−	E	R−	R+
16. Using a salt shaker	L+	L−	E	R−	R+
17. Knocking on a door	L+	L−	E	R−	R+

18. Holding an ice cream cone	L+	L−	E	R−	R+
19. Turning a key in a lock	L+	L−	E	R−	R+
20. Waving good-by	L+	L−	E	R−	R+
21. Using spoon to eat soup	L+	L−	E	R−	R+
22. Combing hair	L+	L−	E	R−	R+
23. Tearing a page off a calendar	L+	L−	E	R−	R+
24. Lifting the lid from a sugar bowl	L+	L−	E	R−	R+
25. Using a spoon to put sugar in a hot drink, or on fruit or cereal	L+	L−	E	R−	R+

Totals: L+ _____ L− _____ E _____ R− _____ R+ _____

COMPUTATION OF HANDEDNESS INDEX

1. Number of items answered L+ _____ $x - 2 = -$ _____
2. Number of items answered L− _____ $x - 1 = -$ _____
3. Number of items answered E _____ $x \ \ 0 = 0$ _____
4. Number of items answered R− _____ $x + 1 = +$ _____
5. Number of items answered R+ _____ $x + 2 = +$ _____

Total   A _____   B _____

Handedness Index $= B/A$ _____

Additional copies of this form may be obtained from the Interstate Printers and Publishers, 19-27 North Jackson Street, Danville, Illinois.

FORM 20. IOWA PERFORMANCE TEST OF SELECTED MANUAL ACTIVITIES

Name _____ Age _____ Sex _____

Examiner _____ Date _____

Purpose of Administering Test: _____

Place a check mark in appropriate space below to indicate whether each activity listed is performed by the right hand (R); the left hand (L); or both hands (B), neither hand predominating.

	R	L	B			R	L	B
1. Pull down curtain	__	__	__	34. Pick up card		__	__	__
2. Pull down curtain	__	__	__	35. Lay down card		__	__	__
3. Take article from desk	__	__	__	36. Lay down card		__	__	__
4. Take article from desk	__	__	__	37. Tearing paper from				
5. Tear paper from tablet	__	__	__	tablet		__	__	__
6. Turn over paper	__	__	__	38. Turn over paper		__	__	__
7. Sharpen pencil	__	__	__	39. Fold paper		__	__	__
8. Write with pencil	__	__	__	40. Sharpen pencil		__	__	__
9. Erase with pencil-tip				41. Turn page of book		__	__	__
eraser	__	__	__	42. Turn page of book		__	__	__
10. Write with pencil	__	__	__	43. Draw a picture		__	__	__
11. Draw a picture	__	__	__	44. Put pencil in desk		__	__	__
12. Put pencil in desk	__	__	__	45. Pick up scissors		__	__	__
13. Take crayon from box	__	__	__	46. Put scissors in desk		__	__	__
14. Take crayon from box	__	__	__	47. Pick up pen		__	__	__
15. Color with crayon	__	__	__	48. Take top off pen		__	__	__
16. Color with crayon	__	__	__	49. Take top off ink bottle	__	__	__
17. Put crayon in box	__	__	__	50. Fill pen		__	__	__
18. Put crayon in box	__	__	__	51. Write with pen		__	__	__
19. Close crayon box	__	__	__	52. Put top on pen		__	__	__
20. Close crayon box	__	__	__	53. Erase with pencil-tip				
21. Pick up scissors	__	__	__	eraser		__	__	__
22. Put scissors in desk	__	__	__	54. Fold paper		__	__	__
23. Point to block	__	__	__	55. Pick up pen		__	__	__
24. Point to block	__	__	__	56. Take top off pen		__	__	__
25. Pick up block to pile	__	__	__	57. Take top off ink bottle	__	__	__
26. Place block on pile	__	__	__	58. Fill pen		__	__	__

	R	L	B			R	L	B
27. Pick up block to pile	—	—	—	59. Write with pen		—	—	—
28. Place block on pile	—	—	—	60. Put top on pen		—	—	—
29. Pick up block to carry	—	—	—	61. Pick up chalk		—	—	—
30. Pick up block to carry	—	—	—	62. Write with chalk		—	—	—
31. Point to card	—	—	—	63. Pick up chalk		—	—	—
32. Point to card	—	—	—	64. Write with chalk		—	—	—
33. Pick up card	—	—	—					

Totals: R _____ L _____ B _____

Dextrality Quotient (DQ) $= \dfrac{R + (B/2)}{N} =$ ___ + ___ $=$ ___ $=$ ___ ___

    R = total for column R
    B = total for column B
    N = total number of items performed

Additional copies of this form may be obtained from the Interstate Printers and Publishers, 19-27 North Jackson Street, Danville, Illinois.

CHART B. Occupational Ratings Used in Determining Index of Status Characteristics

PROFESSIONALS[a]	PROPRIETORS	BUSINESSMEN	WHITE COLLAR WORKERS	MANUAL WORKERS	SERVICE PERSONNEL	LANDOWNERS-FARMERS
Rating						
1. Doctor, dentist, engineer, judge, lawyer, minister, professor, school superintendent, etc.	Investment of $75-100,000 in business or industry; varies by community size	Top management —president; manager; executive of corporation, public utility, bank, etc.	Executive secretary of status organization; C.P.A.; editor of reputable newspaper, magazine; executive level of government			"Gentlemen farmers," landowners not directly supervising operation; the "patrons" of community activities
2. High school teacher, trained nurse, chiropodist, chiropractor, mortician, minister (no college education), veterinarian	Reputed value of $20-70,000; a very good business but not the largest kind	Assistant—department and office manager or supervisor; manager of large branches; manufacturers' agent	Accountant; insurance, stock and bond, real estate men in reputable firms; columnist, editorial writer, etc.			Landowners, operators, and managers of large properties with active urban life
3. Grade school teacher, assistant to undertaker, optician, city veterinarian, pharmacist, any unionized profession	Value or equity reputed $5-20,000 in a "good" but rather small business	Manager of branch stores and businesses (no office staff), buyers and salesmen with "connections," (office and secretary)	Bank and broker's clerks; secretary; senior postal clerk; railroad agent; supervisor in public utilities; county and civic officials; newspaper reporters	Small contractor who works with his men	Commercial air pilot	Owners and operators of good mechanized farms, with hired hands

#	Proprietors	Clerks & Kindred Workers	Manual Workers	Protective & Service Workers	Farmers
4.	Value or equity in business of $2-5,000; few if any employees	Stenographer, bookkeeper, typist, mail clerk; ticket agent; auto, book, cloth-clerk; office employee	Construction, factory, or mine foreman; carpenter, electrician, master mechanic; railroad engineer or trainman; printer	Police captain; butcher, tailor, dry cleaner; railroad and Pullman conductors; "white collar men"	Small landowners and the "forgotten farmer" who owns a "decent place"; operators of good leased property employing hired help
5.	Value or equity $500-2,000; no employees	Drugstore, hardware, grocery, five-and-ten clerks; telephone and beauty operators; dressmaker; practical nurse; etc.	Apprentice to skilled trades; timekeeper; railroad fireman or brakeman; telephone lineman; medium-skill factory workers	Policemen; barber; gas station operator; butcher's apprentice; bartender; head waiter; laundry agent	Tenants on good farms; owners of farms who just manage to eke out a living, some by "working out," others by working in plants, etc., to supplement income from crops
6.	Less than $500 value or equity		Semiskilled factory and production workers; warehousemen; janitors; watchmen; ordinary cook	Taxi and truck drivers; baggagemen; delivery men; gas station attendants; waitresses	Sharecroppers; established farm laborers; subsistence farmers who work out at unskilled jobs, e.g., "cottagers"
7.			Laborers; unskilled miners and mill hands; section hands; migrant workers; scrub women; laundresses	Domestic servant (but not butler or housekeeper); bus boys ...... Reputed law-breakers	Migrant workers: not established and do not want to be; move with the seasons ...... Unemployed; "no occupation"

ᵃ Actors, authors, musicians, artists, etc. may be rated from 1 to 5 on the basis of reputation of their work, degree of acceptance, etc.
SOURCE: From Warner, Meeker, and Eells (31).

CHART C. Scales for Rating Factors 2, 3, and 4 Used in Determining Index of Status Characteristics

Rating	I Source of Income	II House Type	III (a) Area Lived In	III (b) Education of Father
1.	Savings and investments, inherited: 50 percent or more of income	Large houses (9 rooms) in good condition with adequate grounds	Select residential area of highest repute in community	Completed 1 or more years of graduate work at college or university
2.	Savings and investments, gained by earner (not retirement pensions)	Large houses in medium condition. Medium houses (7 rooms) in good condition. Best apartments	Better suburban and apartment house areas; homes with large grounds	Graduated from 4-year college, university, or professional school
3.	Profits and fees—including higher executives who share profits	Medium houses in medium condition. Large apartments in well-kept buildings	Preferred residential areas, adequate grounds; good apartment buildings	Attended college 2 or more years, or equivalent higher education
4.	Salary or commission, including retirement earned thereby	Large and medium houses in fair condition. Apartments in buildings in medium condition	Residential neighborhoods with no deterioration; reputed to be average	Graduated from high school, or equivalent secondary education
5.	Wages based upon hourly rates or piece-work; time-card personnel	Small houses (5 rooms) in good condition. Good apartments in remodeled houses	Area beginning to deteriorate; business or industry beginning to enter it	Attended high school; completed at least one year but did not graduate
6.	Private aid or assistance; may be supplemented by part-time work	Small houses in medium or fair condition. Apartments in fair condition	Area considerably deteriorated but not a slum area; depreciated reputation	Third to eighth grade (older persons). Shifting to eighth grade (young adults)
7.	Public relief and nonrespectable income, according to reputation	All houses and apartments in bad condition. Store fronts, etc. Dwelling not intended for homes	Slum area of the community; neighborhood in bad repute	Below third grade (older persons). Shifting to below eighth grade (young adults)

Source: From Warner, Meeker, and Eells (*31*).

328

REFERENCES

1. Allen, R. M., *Personality Assessment Procedures*, New York: Harper, 1958.
2. Brown, S. F., unpublished paper, read at the Eighth World Congress of the International Society for the Rehabilitation of the Disabled, New York, 1960.
3. Davis, H., and S. R. Silverman, *Hearing and Deafness*, rev. ed., New York: Holt, Rinehart, and Winston, 1960.
4. Davison, A. H., "The relationship betwen unimanual and bimanual handedness," *Journal of Experimental Psychology*, 1948, *38*:276-283.
5. Doll, E. A., *The Vineland Social Maturity Scale*, Philadelphia: Educational Test Bureau, 1946.
6. Goodstein, L. G., "Functional speech disorders and personality: a survey of the research," *Journal of Speech and Hearing Research*, 1958, *1*:359-376.
7. Goodstein, L. G., "Intellectual impairment in children with cleft palates," *Journal of Speech and Hearing Research*, 1961, *4*:287-294.
8. Heltman, H., "Contradictory evidence in handedness and stuttering," *Journal of Speech Disorders*, 1940, *5*:327-332.
9. Hirsh, I. J., *The Measurement of Hearing*, New York: McGraw-Hill, 1952.
10. Institute of Child Welfare, *Minnesota Scale for Paternal Occupations*, Minneapolis: University of Minnesota Institute of Child Welfare, 1950.
11. Johnson, W., "Are speech disorders 'superficial' or 'basic'?" *Asha: A Journal of the American Speech and Hearing Association*, 1961, *3*:233-236.
12. Johnson, W. (Ed., assisted by R. Leutenegger), *Stuttering in Children and Adults: Thirty Years of Research at the University of Iowa*, Minneapolis: University of Minnesota Press, 1955.
13. Johnson, W., and Velma L. Bissell, "Iowa Hand Usage Dextrality Quotients of one hundred high-school students," *Journal of Educational Psychology*, 1940, *31*:148-152.
14. Johnson, W., S. F. Brown, J. F. Curtis, C. W. Edney, and J. Keaster, *Speech Handicapped School Children*, rev. ed., New York: Harper, 1956.
15. Johnson, W., and D. Davis, "Dextrality quotients of seven-year-olds in terms of hand usage," *Journal of Educational Psychology*, 1937, *28*:346-354.
16. Johnson, W., and D. Duke, "The dextrality quotients of fifty six-year-olds with regard to hand usage," *Journal of Educational Psychology*, 1936, *27*:26-36.
17. Johnson, W., and D. Duke, "Revised Iowa hand usage dextrality quotients of six-year-olds," *Journal of Educational Psychology*, 1940, *31*:45-52.
18. Johnson, W., and A. King, "An angle board and hand usage study of

stutterers and nonstutterers," *Journal of Experimental Psychology*, 1942, *31*:293-311.

19. Johnson, W., et al., *The Onset of Stuttering: Research Findings and Implications*, Minneapolis: University of Minnesota Press, 1959.

20. Mecham, M. J., "Measurement of verbal language development in cerebral palsy," *Cerebral Palsy Review*, 1960, *21*(3):3-4.

21. Neelley, J. N., "A study of the speech behavior of stutterers and nonstutterers under normal and delayed auditory feedback," *Journal of Speech and Hearing Disorders*, 1961, Monogr. Supp. 7, 63-82.

22. Newby, H. A., *Audiology*, New York: Appleton-Century-Crofts, 1958.

23. Rosenzweig, S., *Psychodiagnosis*, New York: Grune and Stratton, 1949.

24. Shane, M. L. S., "Effect on stuttering of alteration in auditory feedback," in W. Johnson (Ed. assisted by R. Leutenegger), *Stuttering in Children and Adults*, Minneapolis: University of Minnesota Press, 1955.

25. Schuell, Hildred, "Aphasic difficulties in understanding spoken language," *Neurology*, 1953, *3*:176-184.

26. Schuell, Hildred, "Diagnosis and prognosis in aphasia," *Archives of Neurology and Psychiatry*, 1955, *74*:308-315.

27. Sheehan, J. G., "Projective studies of stuttering," *Journal of Speech and Hearing Disorders*, 1958, *23*:18-25.

28. Spadino, E. J., "Writing and Laterality Characteristics of Stuttering Children," *Contributions to Education*, No. 837, New York: Teachers College, Columbia University, 1941.

29. Spriestersbach, D. C., "Research in articulation disorders and personality," *Journal of Speech and Hearing Disorders*, 1956, *21*(3):329-335.

30. Templin, Mildred C., "Certain Language Skills in Children," *Institute of Child Welfare Monograph Series*, No. 26, Minneapolis: University of Minnesota Press, 1957.

31. Warner, W. L., M. Meeker, and K. Eells, *Social Class in America*, Chicago: Science Research Associates, 1949.

11 THE EXAMINATION REPORT

In this chapter we present an outline for the examination report, together with a number of suggestions about the preparation of the report and the uses to be made of it.

The examination report serves two major purposes: it is a record and it is a communication. As a record it serves as a baseline against which to compare future reports and to evaluate future developments; it may be used in the preparation of annual or other periodic reports of the clinical program; it may be shared, ethically and judiciously, with students in professional training courses; it may be utilized in research. As a communication, the examination report is addressed to appropriate professional persons or agencies, on request and with approval of the person being served or his parents or others responsible for him. Both as a record and as a communication it should be clear, valid, and no longer than necessary.

Here are a few suggestions that you may find useful in writing the examination report:

1. Use the fewest possible words to give a serious-minded reader the information he needs. Avoid personal comments that are beside the point and forego cleverness. Include the more important facts and

omit needless detail. Go to the point without unneeded howevers and neverthelesses. Write short and simple sentences. Use common words. If you must use a technical term put it in a context that makes its meaning clear, or else define it; your reader may not be a speech pathologist. Keep the tone of your report basically impersonal, but if you can make a statement more clear and simple by using a personal pronoun, use it.

2. Don't be critical of other professional specialists or agencies.

3. Don't reveal intimate information given to you in unmistakable confidence. Let the person, or those responsible for him, give any strictly confidential information they may have to other examiners or agencies themselves. In describing especially significant aspects of the problem, however, such as parent-child relationships, be as clear as possible, and in case of doubt ask permission to pass along specific details that you consider essential to adequate understanding of the case.

Follow the basic rule of releasing the examination report only with permission or on request of the person served. If a copy of the report, or of some part of it, is requested by someone other than the person served, obtain his permission before complying with the request. In referring a person to another specialist or agency for an examination, it is understood that the person served consents to the exchange of information between you and the other specialist or agency. In case of doubt, obtain explicit consent. Also, it is understood that when a person is referred to you for examination or consultation, you are free to report your findings to the referring practitioner or agency. Again, in case of doubt, because of the nature of your findings perhaps, obtain permission.

Some clinicians routinely ask all persons they serve to sign a general form giving them permission to make certain uses of the information obtained from them or about them. Without regard to the question of the legal status of this or any other form of release or permission employed in clinical relationships, we present an example of such a release form.

AUTHORIZATION OF USE OF CLINICAL
AND SCIENTIFIC MATERIAL

Date _____

I hereby authorize _____ (name of clinic) to make customary and constructive use, exercising due discretion, for educational, scientific, and professional purposes, and in the public interest, of information, photographs, sound recordings, films, and other records or materials pertaining to, and in consideration of, my enrollment, examination, instruction, and scientific participation, or that of my minor child(ren), _____ (name or names), or that of _____ (name or names), for whom I am legally responsible, in _____ (name of clinic).

I further consent to the release of relevant confidential material to qualified professional personnel in furtherance of clinical services in behalf of me, or any other person(s) named above, as deemed necessary by _____ (name of clinic).

Witness:

_____

Name: _____

Address: _____

_____

Relationship, if not the
person(s) in question: _____

The following is a suggested outline for the examination report. In using it you will, of course, adapt it to the particulars of each specific case.

EXAMINATION REPORT

Start the report with the name, sex, birthdate, age (years, months), and address of the examinee; and the full name(s) of the informant(s), stating the relationship of each to the person whose history is under review.

Problem

Briefly and clearly indicate the type of communication problem. Describe it in the informant's own words, if possible. Be specific. A statement such as "He does not make his *s*'s well and he does not sound his *r*'s" is more clear and specific than "He doesn't talk plainly," and more understandable to some readers than "He presents a functional articulatory disorder with lateral [s] and omission of [r]."

Referral

Give the full name and the relationship or title of the individual or agency who referred the person to your clinic.

History

If it is the policy of your clinic to include the complete case history in the examination report, write it, unless otherwise directed by your supervisor, in accordance with the case history outline presented in Chapter 2. Organize it under the major headings of History of Problem, Developmental History, Medical History, School History, Social History, Family History, and Comments on the Interview. Include a statement of the socioeconomic status of the family.

If it is your clinic policy to include a summary of the case history in the examination report, write it as an abstract without divisions and headings. Make the abstract no longer than a page to a page and a half, typed single-spaced. Include only the most important relevant findings, both positive and negative (noncontributory), from each part of the history.

Examinations

Speech, Voice, and Language Examinations: Summarize the results of each test or set of observations of speech, voice, or language. Name each test and explain it briefly so the reader may visualize what was done. State concisely the significance of the findings. Present first the general facts indicated by the General Speech Behavior Rating. Proceed then to summarize the most pertinent or significant other test findings, and finally include additional notable but less important test results.

For example, in a report of the testing of a 5-year-old child with an articulation problem, begin with the results of the General Speech Behavior Rating (Form 2, p. 78) ; then continue with the results of the articulation test (Form 3, p. 104). In reviewing the articulation test, explain how the speech responses were elicited; list the scores earned and the comparable normative values; list all omissions, substitutions, and distortions of sounds, indicating the positions in the word in which the errors were made; summarize the information about the consistency of these errors and the child's response to auditory stimulation. Clarify the meaning of phonetic symbols, which a layman or a specialist in another field may not understand, in some such way as this: "He substituted *t* for *th*, saying *t*umb for *th*umb." Also indicate the general intelligibility of the person's speech.

Abstract the more important information concerning language behavior recorded on Form 9 (p. 196), and evaluate it with reference to appropriate norms. If tests for dysphasia, or aphasia, were administered summarize and explain the pertinent findings. Include a summary and interpretation of obtained measures of rate and disfluency of oral reading and speaking, as recorded on Forms 10 and 11 (pp. 234-236).

If the series of tests for stutterers was given, name or briefly describe each procedure and summarize and explain the results. For instance, "His mean score of 2.5 on the Iowa Scale of Attitude Toward Stuttering indicates a fairly strong tendency to be intolerant of stuttering."

Examination of Oral Speech Mechanism: Extract pertinent information from Form 4 (p. 127), listing deviations noted and their possible significance in relation to the person's speech problem.

Audiological Examination: Summarize essential findings of the audiological examination. On the basis of the audiologist's report, indicate the results obtained, and the probable validity of the test. Following are typical entries:

CASE A: On a sweep-check test with a pure-tone audiometer set at 10 decibels above zero, hearing was found to be essentially normal.

CASE B: As the child's responses to the pure tones of an audiometer were judged to be unreliable, other testing methods were employed. He responded correctly (by dropping a marble into a box) to whispered commands given behind his back at a distance of 8 feet. It is believed that his hearing is essentially normal. If there is a hearing loss, it is probably of minor significance in relationship to his speech problem. Retesting in 6 months is recommended.

If a test of hearing threshold was administered with a pure-tone audiometer and some hearing loss was discovered, summarize the results in a simple table such as the one below. The figures in the top line represent the tonal frequencies tested (125 to 8000 cycles per second), *R* and *L* indicate the right and left ears, and the numbers in the columns refer to hearing loss in decibels for each ear at the various frequencies tested:

	125	250	500	1000	2000	4000	8000
R	10	10	15	15	20	25	30
L	5	5	10	15	20	20	40

Other information may be extracted from the audiogram, such as the person's "average pure-tone loss for speech" (the average of the values in decibels for the three speech frequencies, 500, 1000, and 2000 cycles per second) in the better ear. If speech audiometry was used, state the type of stimulus (phonetically balanced word lists or spondees) and report and evaluate in practical terms the speech reception threshold in decibels. Enclose all direct quotations from the audiologist's report in quotation marks and credit them to the audiological examiner.

Psychological Evaluation

On the basis of the psychologist's report, give the full name of each test administered. Report the results of intelligence testing by stating the obtained mental age (MA) and intelligence quotient (IQ). Indicate the general level of intelligence of the person tested. In addition, quote verbatim those portions of the psychologist's report that describe details of the person's behavior during the test which bear on the question of the probable validity of the results obtained. Enclose all extracts in quotation marks and credit the remarks to the psychological examiner. The findings from personality tests should be summarized largely in the psychological examiner's own words, with quotation marks.

Impression

Make a brief statement of the conclusions about the nature of the communication problem, its probable etiology, and the degree of its severity. Identify the person or persons responsible for this conclusion. Examples of such entries are the following:

Stuttering—severe

Functional articulatory problem—mild

Articulatory problem—moderately severe—whether its basis is primarily functional or organic has not yet been determined

Speech retardation—severe—referable to general mental retardation

Recommendations

Summarize the decisions reached by the clinic staff on the basis of the findings of the examination. Indicate whether there should be referral to other specialists or agencies for further examinations, referral to a speech clinician near the speaker's home, counseling of the parents, a particular program of therapy for the speaker, or some other form of help. Indicate the nature of any counseling done after the examination with the person served or his parents or other responsible individuals. Make clear the present status of the problem, and the disposition made of it following examination. State all recommendations in clear and specific terms.

NOTE: If entries for the *Impression* and *Recommendations* sections are prepared for you by one or more other members of the clinic staff copy them verbatim but without quotation marks.

INDEX

Adams, Lois Hickman, 253, 293
Adaptation of the stuttering response, *see* Stuttering
procedure for measuring, 269 ff.
Agnosia, 185
Ahlstrand, Ann, 269, 270, 295
Ainsworth, S., 245, 253, 273, 293, 294
"Air charge," 58
Aldrich, C. A., 66, 71
Allen, R. M., 316, 329
Amatruda, C. S., 72
American Cancer Society, 59
American Speech and Hearing Association, 18
Ammons, H. S., 198
Ammons, R. B., 198, 262, 293
Ammons Full-Range Picture Vocabulary Test, 177
Anderson, J. E., 17, 21, 67, 71
Anderson, Patricia W., 97, 108
Angle's classification of dental occlusion, 115 ff.
Ansberry, M., 245, 295
Anxiety, concerning expected stuttering, 255
informant's, 32
Aphasia, appraisal of language impairment in, 185 ff.
tests for, 186
Apraxia, 186

Armstrong, E. M., 66, 73
Arnold, P. R., 198
Arresting consonants, *see* Consonant, arresting
"Arthur, the Young Rat," 206
Articulation, 15
correctness of, 81
development of, 81 ff.
errors, 89–92
problems, 80
testing of, 80 ff.
Articulatory disorders and personality adjustment, 314
Articulatory errors, consistency of, 92
Ataxia, 47
Athetosis, 47
Audiological evaluation, referral for, 310
Audiology, 310–313
Audiometer, 310
Auditory feedback, 311
delayed, 311
Auditory stimulation, response to, 92 ff
Autobiographical method, 24
Avoidant speech reactions, 253

Bain, K., 71
Baker, H. K., 159
Baldwin, B. T., 64, 65, 71
Barbara, D. A., 245, 293

341

Format by Jeanne Ray
Set in Linotype Century Expanded
Composed, printed and bound by The Haddon Craftsmen, Inc.
HARPER & ROW, PUBLISHERS, INCORPORATED

71 72 73 15 14 13 12 11